Contemporary Bioethics

Mohammed Ali Al-Bar · Hassan Chamsi-Pasha

Contemporary Bioethics

Islamic Perspective

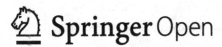

Mohammed Ali Al-Bar
Medical Ethics Center
International Medical Center
Jeddah
Saudi Arabia

Hassan Chamsi-Pasha
Department of Cardiology
King Fahd Armed Forces Hospital
Jeddah
Saudi Arabia

ISBN 978-3-319-36381-3   ISBN 978-3-319-18428-9   (eBook)
DOI 10.1007/978-3-319-18428-9

Springer Cham Heidelberg New York Dordrecht London

Printed on acid-free paper

Springer International Publishing AG Switzerland is part of Springer Science+Business Media
(www.springer.com)

Foreword

Contemporary Bioethics: Islamic Perspective, by Dr. Mohammed Ali Al-Bar and Dr. Hassan Chamsi-Pasha, is a timely contribution in the field of Islamic bioethics. The book is authored by two prominent practitioners of medicine in Saudi Arabia with an impressive knowledge of Islamic religious sciences and legal-ethical rulings on various topics of clinical significance. Rapid advancement in the innovation of medical technology has given rise to the critical need for expansion of the bioethical field to keep up with medical practice and research while relating the ethical decisions to their religious sources and reliable medical knowledge. Muslim bio-ethicists are struggling to keep pace with and produce answers to the questions posed by the medical establishment. The early phases of Islamic bioethics saw a number of medical professionals taking up to write on various issues in medical practice and research. Some of these early works were supplemented by Muslim legal scholars who teamed up with medical professionals to write responses to religious questions for clinical cases that required careful analysis of Islamic tradition and jurisprudence to provide dependable rulings. The present works are now being authored by some medical professionals who also have a good understanding of the religious sources that provide spiritual and moral guidance for complicated medical cases.

Contemporary Bioethics: Islamic Perspective is such an endeavor that provides the readers a theoretical framework and practical decisions made by leading Muslim jurists. Accordingly, the first half of the study presents the Islamic sources that are utilized by Muslim legal scholars in deducing appropriate rulings on various medical cases on which bioethicists around the world have offered solutions. In the second part of the book, the authors have compiled and discussed Islamic rulings in various controversial fields of modern medical practice and research. This combination of theory and practice in Islamic bioethics makes *Contemporary Bioethics: Islamic Perspective* an indispensable reading for those who work on bioethics from an Islamic ethical-legal point of view. In the Western world, questions range over concerns such as stem cell research, cloning, cessation of life support, and fertility treatments. Often contentious and filled with fervor, proponents and opponents of controversial medical advances struggle to prevail in the disagreement. The means of resolving the argument are usually achieved through official legislation. The predominant reason for government authority in resolving bioethical issues correlates with the plurality of ethnicities, religions, social values, and ideologies of most Western countries. While religion in particular motivates and influences at the individual level, in secular bioethics no religious figure has the authority to enact law. Religious authorities can unquestionably influence the law but do not promulgate or enforce laws.

Unlike in Western countries, there is no established apparatus that institutes, monitors, and regulates the field of bioethics in the Muslim world. The very reason for the lack of such an establishment stems from a fundamental flaw in the application of traditional rulings in the field of bioethics. Since the 1970s, the Muslim scholarly community has come together to establish a physician-jurist consultation group that meets under the auspices of the Supreme Islamic Juridical Council. The council meets regularly to undertake important investigations of pressing questions in the field of medical practice and research and provide reliable juridical decisions in accord with Islamic religious texts. Although the body has no power to enact laws, it certainly functions as an advisory body for Muslim governments in their healthcare policies.

In the West, the field of bioethics is largely based on utilitarianism, an ethical principle that places primacy of consequences of an action over the action itself. Utilitarianism is the major source of resolving ethical questions in the West. In light of the characteristic Western approach to bioethics, it is important to note that in *Contemporary Bioethics: Islamic Perspective*, Dr. Al-Bar and Dr. Chamsi-Pasha have combined medical practice and research and scrutinized these in light of Islamic religious values, laws, and ethics. It is important to underscore and evaluate the contribution made by these two medical doctors drawing from their professional knowledge of medicine and profound understanding of Islamic tradition in the cultural context of Islamic Sunni countries. In other words, their study combines the theory and practice of clinical ethics in an important part of the Arab-Muslim world. In order to address bioethical issues within Muslim society in Islamic Sunni countries, the authors focus on medical as well as cultural issues that inform Muslim attitudes toward human body in relation to family, community, religion, and science. They have attended to the sensibilities of Islamic jurisprudence and have approached Islam from both legal and ethical perspectives.

Let us see the context of this important contribution in comparison to other recently published works on Islamic bioethics. In the past decade the literature on Islamic bioethics has come to its own. Several monographs written by both secular and confessional students of religious ethics, medical anthropology as well as historians of medicine, and medical law have appeared in English and other major European languages. In particular, ethnographic studies working on specific Muslim societies have enriched our understanding of the way ethical dilemmas at critical moments of patients' illness have been handled by healthcare providers, in consultation with close family members and communal religious leaders. More pertinently, some medical anthropologists have acted as sensitive conveyers of this culture of pain, suffering, and relief to those living in the affluent Western societies where the entire worldview is founded on the human ability to defeat the evil of illnesses through costly medical intervention. In contrast, in many parts of the Muslim world where unspeakable poverty levels have denied any medical care to suffering patients and financial relief to their families, these ethnographers have worked as advocates of mercy and compassion. After all, bioethics has to engage in negotiating proper recognition of human suffering. Human affliction goes beyond the technicalities of who can afford to pay for expensive treatment or which state has better policies to alleviate everyday suffering in the healthcare institutions. In the developing world, in most cases, healthcare institutions are professionally geared toward maintaining a culture of treatment for those who can afford it.

In the midst of this growing literature one can feel the void of authoritative religious-moral guidance on various topics that arise in the departments of critical care in hospitals regarding the bioethical aspects of the problematized clinical cases that require satisfactory resolution for the wellbeing of the patient as well as his/her family. In the recent anthropological study, Sherine Hamdy's sustained fieldwork in Egypt entitled: *Our Bodies Belong to God* explores the ethics of organ transplant. The author demonstrates the confusion that exists in the area of authoritative religious-ethical opinions that could provide critical guidance to both public health officials as well as healthcare providers to resolve some of the urgent moral dilemmas that face patients and their families. In fact, Hamdy takes the reader through the maze of ethical minefields confronting Egyptian doctors, torn between their own religious-cultural sensibilities and the professional obligations to do everything possible to relieve their patients from long-term affliction caused by hard to cure diseases. However, to address bioethics within Egypt, Hamdy narrows the expansive field of Islamic ethics by focusing narrowly on organ transplantation, particularly kidney and cornea, as a method of assessing Egyptian attitudes toward the human body in relation to religion and society. Hamdy's fieldwork in the area of transplant is highlighted by the fact that she had to consult the written literature produced by Egyptian religious scholars to understand the ethical-legal implications of organ transplant based on organ donation or organ acquisition through the legal or illegal thriving black market managed by every possible agent engaged in money-making schemes.

Compared to this and other similar studies on Muslim bioethics, the present volume, *Contemporary Bioethics: Islamic Perspective*, advances a meticulously documented necessity of engaging bioethics as a discipline. The authors combine Islamic textual analysis with juridical methodology to engage dominant secular bioethics in Muslim healthcare institutions. *Contemporary Bioethics* integrates Islamic textual resources with medical information in order to provide careful analyses of the political, economic, and cultural terrains that are necessary for bioethicists to effectively promote social justice. In many Arab countries, national media attention is directed at the views of Islamic legal scholars, whose answers to religious questions on various issues in bioethics are part of the larger political project. This political project has to direct ethical queries to medical and Islamic authorities who are challenged to solve problems of allocation and managing of meager resources to address social inequalities in corruption-ridden governance. Islamic revivalism since the 1970s has prompted medical practitioners and educated people in the Arab world to actively engage in learning about Islamic views independently, bypassing the religious scholars connected with the state bureaucracy whose views are distrusted as being politically motivated. In a country where ethics is still dominated by legal rulings (fatawa) of Islamic jurisprudence and where bioethics still awaits definition within healthcare institutions that could determine the outcome of morally problematic procedures, the contribution made by *Contemporary Bioethics* is both timely and critical for medical professionals and the larger educated public that is thirsty of biomedical information at the level of everyday resolutions of moral dilemmas touching life and death decisions in Muslim societies. Naturally, culture plays a leading role in seeking realistic solutions. The authors of *Contemporary Bioethics* have admirably interwoven medicine and religion to provide a sense of legalistic-ethical discourse on subjects dealing with biomedical issues. What is understood in Muslim societies as right or wrong still abides with legally formulated technical terms such as *halal* (permissible) and *haram* (forbidden). It is to Dr. Al-Bar and Dr. Chamsi-Pasha's credit that they have been able to translate for their readers the medical culture in Sunni Islamic countries in a comprehensible language that can benefit any educated reader of the subject.

January 2014/Rabi I, 1435   Abdulaziz Sachedina
                                                    Professor and Endowed IIIT Chair
                                                                 in Islamic Studies
                                                    George Mason University, USA

Acknowledgments

We have to forward our deepest thanks to the Chair of Medical Ethics, headed by Prof. Adnan Albar, who supported this work and took charge of publishing it under the Chair of Medical Ethics, King Abdulaziz University, which is supported by a generous grant from Sheikh Mohammed Hussein AlAmoudy, who supported many chairs in Saudi universities.

Our thanks and gratitude to Prof. Abdulaziz Sachedina, Professor and Endowed IIIT Chair in Islamic Studies George Mason University, for his elegant Foreword.

Our deepest thanks and gratitude to sister Ms. Cumiya Johnson, the Office Manager of CEO Dr. Walid Ahmad Fitaihi of the International Medical Center for typing the whole manuscript despite scribbling and poor handwriting.

We extend our thanks to Dr. Shihab Ghanem and his son Dr. Wadhah Shihab Ghanem for reading the first three chapters diligently and commenting on them and to Dr. Abdullah Srour Aljoudi for reading through the book and giving his important comments.

Mohammed Ali Al-Bar
Hassan Chamsi-Pasha

Acknowledgments

Contents

Part III Selected Topics

Part I
Introductory Chapters

Chapter 1
Introduction

بسم الله الرحمن الرحيم

The present study undertakes to examine biomedical issues as they have emerged in the last three decades. In the Muslim world, as in any part of the globe, advancements in biomedical technology has meant a number of new issues in the medical treatment and procedures that impinge upon Islamic values as taught by the Qur'an and the Sunna (the Tradition of Prophet Muhammad). Our investigations in bioethical issues require Muslim ethicists to examine a number of judicial decisions made by Muslim scholars in response to the growing number of cases in the clinical settings as well as national health policies adopted by various Muslim governments in the last two decades. The field of bioethics is new even in the Western countries where its principles and rules are being worked out in a standard approach to secularly mediated resolutions of morally problematic issues regarding, for instance, embryonic inviolability or end of life decisions in connection with terminally ill patients.

For several centuries, the world, and particularly Europe, has benefited from the great contributions made by Muslim physicians in the field of medicine. These contributions were not only based on technical skills but also on the role of eminent Muslim physicians in establishing medical ethics. Many prominent physicians of the Islamic civilization involved themselves with professional ethics; among them were al-Ruhawi, and al-Razi (Rhazes). Both wrote the earliest and most thorough books on medical ethics over a 1000 years ago [1].

In this study we hope to bring these and other ethical issues on which Islamic scholars have provided religious-moral guidance by investigating the foundational sources of Islam like the Qur'an and the Sunna.

Ethics in this Study

It is important to begin our study by elucidating some key concepts with which we will be concerned in this research. The most important term that we need to formulate in view of its central role in Islamic legal-ethical decision-making is ethics. Although the term ethics is clearly a heritage of all humanity experiencing

© The Author(s) 2015
M.A. Al-Bar and H. Chamsi-Pasha, *Contemporary Bioethics*,
DOI 10.1007/978-3-319-18428-9_1

moral dilemmas in their everyday relations with other persons, in this study we have taken ethics to mean that inquiry which examines the rightness and the wrongness in human conduct. Human conduct is informed by moral principles which determine the outcome of particular acts or activities. Furthermore, according to Beauchamp and Childress, ethics is a "generic term for various ways of understanding and examining moral life [2]." In this latter usage, then, it is appropriate to speak about normative and non-normative ethics, depending upon the sources of this understanding. Normative ethics based on the source of these norms, attempts to understand which general moral norms should we accept and why. In contrast, ethical theories attempt to identify and justify these norms revealing justificatory reasoning that provide resolution to moral dilemmas. However, ethics is concerned with examining human conduct and, therefore, it seeks to find ways of predicting practical aspects of human activity by investigating moral problems, practices and policies in professions, situations, and public policy. In other words, ethics is concerned with applications and in this sense bioethics is a branch of applied ethics concerned with resolving problems in the area of living sciences, including research and practice in the field of medicine.

In contrast to normative ethics, non-normative ethics which takes human experience, culture, and history as important sources of moral decision-making takes the form of descriptive ethics which studies how people reason and act. Thus, for instance, anthropologists, sociologists, psychologists and historians study the norms and attitudes of societies towards moral issues in different societies and epochs and the factors that are used to justify their actions in different professions and in matters connected with larger public. The other branch of non-normative ethics is meta-ethics. Meta-ethics involves the analysis of conceptual language and methods of reasoning in ethics. It addresses the meaning of right and wrong, virtue and vice, the good and the bad, and so forth in the larger global context. In short, it addresses the ethical epistemology and forms of justificatory reasoning.

In this study, we use ethics and morality interchangeably to refer to norms about right or wrong in human conduct that are so widely shared in a certain society. These norms differ, at least in details, from one society to another, and from one era to another in the same society. However, many principles, rules and virtues remain constant across different cultures and different times. For instance, almost all persons know that lying, stealing and killing an innocent person is immoral; and veracity, fidelity and saving a human life is a great virtue and a highly commended moral act. Our interest in this book is to discuss the sources of common principles of morality and ethics to show that commonalty unites all human beings in understanding the difference between moral and immoral. This is the scope of our first chapter, where we explain and elaborate:

1. **Intuitive nature (al-fitr' a)**: This is a fundamental Qur'anic idea, which speaks about the basic nature of all human beings by which human beings can discern certain things to be morally right (honesty, truth telling, doing good, benevolence, etc.) and certain things to be wrong (lying, cheating, stealing, killing an innocent person or being unjust).

2. **Reason** (*intellect, mind, al-'aql*): God endowed humanity with the ability to use reason to differentiate between right and wrong, and to discern the proper course of action. Those who refuse to use their minds and follow their egotistic desires, and blind themselves with self-importance follow their instincts and hedonistic desires and deviate from the true path, becoming unable to minimally distinguish right from wrong. To be sure, even if they know the truth of the matter, they are inclined to follow their carnal desires and lust for material ends and tramp over whatever remains of their conscience.
   The Qur'an extols humanity to strive to control egotistic and hedonistic desires, and it deplores those who are arrogant, mischievous and having insatiated desire for wealth and power, which they use to crush the poor and weak. Muslim theologian, Abu Hamid al-Ghazali, has admonished people correctly when he says: "If you cannot reach the level of Angels, then do not fall into the level of beasts, scorpions and snakes [3]." We will have more opportunity to cite the Qur'an and the Sunna, in addition to theological and philosophical heritage of Islam, when we undertake to elaborate this point further.
3. **Revelation** (*wahy, Tanzil*): Muslims believe that all communities had received Allah's (God's) guidance through revelation given to the Prophets and Messengers of God. In Islam, Adam is not only first human being; he is also the first Prophet who delivered God's message of monotheism to his descendants.

It is important to state from the outset that Muslims do not believe in original sin. Adam committed an act of disobedience by eating from the fruit of the tree which God had ordered him not to eat. According to the Qur'an, he and his wife, Eve, repented and God accepted their repentance and they became pure. God bestowed on Adam and Eve and their children His Grace and Blessing "We honored the progeny of Adam, provided them with transport on land and sea; given them for sustenance things good and pure; and conferred on them special favors above a great part of Our creation" (Qur'an/17:70). Furthermore, Muslims believe that God sent to every nation and people, prophets and messengers to guide them to worship one God and follow the path of righteousness. In other words, Muslims believe in all these prophets and that they brought the same religion in its essence, and worshipped only one God. This belief is the source of unity among human beings under the unity of God's religion, which is essentially the same. However the followers of these religions distort God's religion and bring back polytheism in different forms and shapes, by changing the pristine clear messages of the prophets altering the good teachings with adulterated misconceptions both in theology and morality. It is significant to note that, as the youngest of the monotheistic traditions, Islam addresses the whole humanity and respects all the prophets from Adam to the last Prophet Muhammad and considers all nations to have witnessed God's uncompromising unity confirmed in all the messages and teaching of God's true envoys on earth. Belief in God's unity (*Tawhid*) is the basis not only for Muslim theology; but it is also the basis of morality and ethics in Islam. We will return to this subject in greater detail in the first two chapters: "The Sources of Common Principles of Morality and Ethics" and "The Origins of Islamic Morality and

Ethics." There we shall explain how Islamic theology and Islamic religious law—the Shari'ah are integral and based on morality and ethics.

Karen Armstrong in her book, *A History of God* explicates this point about the relationship between ethics and belief in one God. According to her, "the assertion of unity of God (*Tawhid*, monotheism) is not only a denial that deities were worthy of worship. To say that God is one is not just a mere numerical definition; it is a call to make that unity the driving factor of one's life and society" [4]. In another place she observes: "In practical terms, Islam meant that Muslims had a duty to create a just, equitable society where the poor and vulnerable are treated decently. The early moral message of the Qur'an is simple: It is wrong to stockpile wealth and build a private fortune, and it is good to share the wealth of society fairly by giving a regular portion of one's wealth to the poor" (Holy Qur'an Surah 92/18, Surah 9/103, Surah 63/9, Surah 102/1) [5].

Some Important Concepts Related to Islamic Legal-Ethical Tradition in this Study

The Shari'a: (lit. "a way or well-trodden path to a source of water") refers to the normative religious law of Islam with the Qur'an and the Sunna (The Tradition of Prophet Muhammad including his sayings, acts and approvals) as its sources. The norms of the Shari'a are immutable, since they have supernatural source in God's revelation for humankind. Islamic jurisprudence (*al-fiqh*) engages in understanding (lit. sense of the word *fiqh*) of these revealed texts and formulating rules and rulings to cover all human activity in the area of human-God relations (*'iba da t*) and human-human relationships (*mu'a malat*). In Islamic rulings acts are classified as obligatory, recommended, permissible, reprehensible, and forbidden.

1. **Obligatory Acts**: The research in and understanding of the revealed texts makes it possible to declare certain acts as required (*fardh*, *wajib*) and certain other acts as recommended or even forbidden. The rule of thumb is that where there is a clear command in the Qur'an or the Sunna (for instance performing the five daily prayers) then performance of that action becomes obligatory. Obligatory acts include paying the annual alms (*zakat*) to the poor, fasting during the month of Ramadan between dawn and dusk for a month; performance of the annual pilgrimage—the Hajj, once in a lifetime, if he/she has got the means to perform it.
2. **Recommended Acts**: These are the acts that are performed as supererogatory acts (*mustahab*, *mandub*). It includes all those acts that are good to perform, but they are not required. For instance, it is recommended to fast on Mondays and Thursday every week. Likewise, on certain important days of the Muslim calendar, it is highly recommended to perform extra prayers and fasting. Those who perform these acts are rewarded for their piety by God. But if they cannot, for any reason, perform them, they do not become blameworthy.

3. **Permissible Acts**: These acts are neutral and permissible (*mubah*) in the sense that whether one performs them or not, it does not matter since they constitute neither blame nor recrimination. It includes all daily life activities. Everything is allowed unless there is a clear text prohibiting it. This is also equivalent to the legal presumption of innocence until the proof of guilt is established. Things are presumed allowed in the absence of prohibition.

4. **Reprehensible Acts**: These acts, although better to avoid (*makrooh*), do not constitute blame or sin. It simply requires a person to think before performing it since there is no clear order of avoiding it. Certainly, being reprehensible, if avoided then God would reward the person for abstaining from it, but will not punish the person who did it.

5. **Forbidden Acts**: These are forbidden explicitly in the Qur'an or the Sunna (*haram*). If a person performs such an act, then he/she will be punished either in this world or in the hereafter, unless he/she repents. Repentance is direct between God and human, and He (God) accepts repentance at any time except at the time of death when it is too late.

Islamic jurisprudence (*al-fiqh*) consists of two sets of inquiry: one set of inquiry deals with case studies (*furu'*), and the other relates the cases to the legal principles and precedents derived from the foundational sources of Islamic tradition (Usoo' l). These include:

(a) **The Qur'an**: Muslims believe that the Qur'an contains the revelation that the Prophet Muhammad received directly from God. Accordingly, it is regarded as the most authentic source of religious and moral directives that can be extrapolated to formulate judicial decisions touching all practical matters in everyday life of the community.

(b) **The Sunna**: This source consists of all the sayings, deeds and silently approved directives and prescriptions provided by the Prophet Muhammad. This is collectively known as the "Tradition" in the forms of *hadith* -reports that describe the context in which certain rulings were made by the Prophet and reported by his contemporaries including his close associates. After the Qur'an, the Sunna serves as the most important source for deriving legal-ethical rulings in Islamic jurisprudence.

(c) **The Ijma'**: This is the consensus of the companions of the Prophet after his death on certain issues not found in the Qur'an and the Sunna. In the later period this consensus included the agreement of the learned scholars, the ulema, who are regarded as the most learned and most pious to render their opinions in the form of their collective agreement. However, as the Islamic world spread all over the different regions, it became difficult to garner the agreement of all Muslim scholars.

(d) **The Qiya's**: This is analogical reasoning that allows the jurists to extrapolate fresh decisions from a case already known through the Qur'an or the Sunna which shared similarity with the new case for which the solution had to be found.

Besides the four well-recognized foundational sources for legal-ethical decision-making which were accepted by legal scholars belonging to different Sunni legal schools (Hanafi, Maliki, Shafi and Hanbali), the jurists belonging to specific schools had recognized subsidiary rules and principles based on the Qur'an and the Sunna to resolve practical questions. Among these well-known rules and principles are:

1. **al-Mas' a lih' al-Mursala** (unrestricted public interest and benefit): This was formulated by the Maliki (1) jurists who justified this principle on the basis of the public and personal interests of the people. The principle was also accepted by the Hanbali jurists as legitimate since it was based on the Qur'an, the Sunna, scholarly consensus and analogical reasoning.
2. **al-Istih' sa' n** (bases of juridical preference): This was formulated by the Hanafi jurists. It simply means that under a given research one can prefer one ruling over the other through analogical deduction, by comparing its final solution and its practicality. It is important to keep in mind that Muslim jurists accepted these two principles as long as they did not contravene the foundational sources like the Qur'an and the Sunna.
3. **al-Istih' h' a' b** (presumption of continuity): This rule was developed to provide the assumption of continuity of a ruling if nothing to nullify it had occurred. Hence, if one were ritually clean to undertake any religious obligation that required such a state, and if a person knew that he/she were in such a state then he/she can continue to assume the state of purity, unless the contrary were proven. This rule also applies to the presumption of innocence until proven guilty.
4. The principle of **'Urf** or **'A' da**: This is a major source of problem resolution that embodies considerations based on custom, tradition or local habits. This category includes all the professional codes and practices pursued by specialists in the field. Nevertheless, 'urf is accepted as a source of judicial decision making so long as there is no provision of the matter in the revealed texts (the Qur'an or the Sunna).
5. **Sadd al- Dhara'i'** (blocking the means): is another reasoning procedure that some jurists considered to be a source of legislation, especially in the Maliki school. Most jurists do not mention blocking the means as separate rule, but included its denotation in *al-mas' lah' a*, that is, public good.

The basic primary sources of Islamic jurisprudence have been elaborated sufficiently in the context of this study. To be sure, these principles are expounded to discover and promote the objectives of the sacred law of the Shari'a. It is important to proceed to discuss the major objectives and aims of the Shari'a. These are:

(1) Preservation of Faith (*di' n*)
(2) Preservation of Life (*al-nafs*)
(3) Preservation of Mind (*al-'aql*)
(4) Preservation of Progeny (*al-nasl*)
(5) Preservation of Honor (*al-irdh*)
(6) Preservation of Property (*al-ma' l*)

It is important to underline the fact that these aims of Islamic teachings are related to medical practice and research. They were studied to guide both the physicians and the community in matters that were open to ethical and legal evaluation in the modern times.

Chronology of Bioethical Issues that were Resolved Through Legal-Ethical Juridical Methodology

A number of issues in the field of bioethics which include questions regarding abortion, organ transplantation, in vitro fertilization, end of life issues, advanced directives, stem cell research, brain death, genetic engineering, genetic finger printing and so forth. These are all new questions that faced the Islamic scholars in the second half of the 20th century and the beginning of the 21st century (C.E.). As the growing literature shows Muslim jurists have been active in studying these contentious subjects and providing religious and ethical guidance in the form of fatwas (religious decisions) that are followed by healthcare providers in the Muslim world. As far back as 1959 fatwas appeared from Grand Mufti of Egypt on corneal transplantation and blood transfusion. A similar fatwa was issued by the Grand Mufti of Tunisia in 1959. At the same time a number of rulings were issued on organ transplantation that continued until 1990. Leading juridical authorities in different centers of Islamic learning participated in formulating religious responses to the growing problems created by phenomenal advancement in biotechnology and medical practice. Following this early interest in bioethical issues the governments of the region formed an advisory body that functioned under the Organization of Islamic Countries (OIC). The *Majma'al-Fiqh al-Islami* (the Islamic Juridical Council of the Muslim World League in Mecca) discussed many critical issues in medical ethics, published fatwas and studies on these subjects in its quarterly journal, which was published from the beginning of the third session 1980 CE/1400 AH on the subject of contraception. The following year in 1981 the Council issued rulings regarding the use of alcohol, porcine material and blood in medicine. In 1982, the Council reviewed in vitro fertilization which took almost 3 years to investigate different aspects of the subject.

In 1985 organ transplantation was studied and different aspects of this subject and brain death continued to be studied until 1987. In 1987 post mortem and anatomy were given a thorough review. The subject of inter-sex and trans-sex was discussed in 1989. In 1990, the Juridical Council studied the subject of abortion with specific reference to congenital anomalies. In the same year they studied the interference of the husband in preventing his wife from taking certain medications or accepting certain surgical procedures. Many judicial decisions and regulations from the Ministry of Health in Saudi Arabia reiterated that an adult competent lady is the one who should give consent to therapy. The husband, father, brothers or sons cannot give consent in her name so long as she is a competent adult. However, in matters of reproduction a mutual decision and consent from both the spouses was necessary.

In 1992, the Council discussed the use of umbilical cord blood and placenta for medical purposes and research, making it permissible for the larger good of the society. In 1995, the regulations for exposure of private parts 'awra) especially of females, in hospitals, operating room (OR) and so forth were studied to provide the ethical guidance in that situation. In 1998, the DNA fingerprinting, the paternity disputes, the genetic engineering were carefully discussed to allow for pre-natal genetic testing and related issues. The Council also studied the use of animal gelatin investigating its sources to determine its permissibility in pharmaceutical production. In 1999 medicaments containing alcohol, narcotics and anxiolytics, were discussed to understand the need to permit their content in some of the life-saving medications, and when definite need is apparent.

As the biotechnology was moving toward understanding the pluripotent stem cells and their use in replicating organs and tissues, it was in 2003 that the Council discussed the legality of stem cell research, hereditary blood diseases and porcine heparin. The gender selection was studied in 2006 and 2007. In 2010, the jurists studied the separation of conjoined twins and its complications. The meeting in December 2012, 21st session, studied the end of life issues and postponed issuing the rulings on the matter until further clarifications were provided by the medical professionals. In the same year issues related to the early marriage of girls and its medical complications, the minimum and the maximum period of pregnancy to deliver a viable fetus were scrutinized. It postponed the decision on early marriage (before 18 years old) until further discussions and studies are forwarded. The minimum period of viable pregnancy is settled in Islamic jurisprudence, as 6 lunar months from consummation of marriage, since the time of the Sahaba (companions of the Prophet Muhammad PBUH), but the question of maximum period of pregnancy was always a bone of contention. The Majma agreed that the maximum period of pregnancy is 1 year from the last cohabitation between married couple. However the judge should decide on the case. The Majma (21st session), December 2012 also discussed the power of the guardian when he is not acting in the best interest of the person under his custody, and decided that the custody (guardianship) should be given to another person. In case of emergency, the health provider should act immediately to save the life or organs of the minor or incompetent.

The guardian should not expose any person under his custody to any danger or research which is going to harm the minor or the incompetent. If he insists on this act, he should be replaced by another guardian through the court.

The decision for medical or surgical treatment in all these contentious cases should be decided by a trustworthy medical committee.

The second important corpus is the International Islamic Juridical Council under the OIC = Organization of Islamic Countries which represents all Islamic countries. The organization has studied medical issues and ethical problems since its inception in 1985 when they studied assisted reproduction, in vitro fertilization, milk-banks for babies, and instruments for resuscitative measures in situations like brain death. In the latter case, the discussion went on for two sessions when rulings were issued on these matters. The 1986 ruling on brain death was a landmark decision since it equated brain death with cardiac and respiratory death. It opened the way for cadaver transplants. The ruling was passed in October 1986 and by November of that year the first case of cadaver (brain death) transplant occurred in Saudi Arabia for kidney transplantation.

In 1988, a detailed ruling on organ transplantation was issued, which clearly rejected any trading or trafficking of organs and stressed the principle of altruism. However, the Council allowed governments to encourage organ donation by awarding medals, services or even a certain fixed amount of money to compensate for loss of earning and suffering during the preparation and donation of organs. In 1990, the Council discussed transplantation of nerve tissues, transplantation from anencephalics and transplantation from aborted fetuses and left over pre-embryos from IVF projects. Stem cell research was discussed by the Council in 2003. It also studied transplantation of internal and external sexual organs. Whereas the Council allowed transplantation of uterus (womb), it refused transplantation of gonads (ovaries and testes) as they carry all the genetic materials from the donor. In addition, it also rejected the permission for external sex organs transplantation. In Jeddah, a surgeon transplanted a womb from one woman to another in April 2000, but the operation failed and ended in a disaster, as there was no prior experimentation on animals.

The Council also discussed contraception and sterilization in 1988. In 1992, it studied the consent in medical and surgical cases, and the futile cases when there was no hope for cure. In 1993, it discussed the traffic accidents (the highest world figures are from Saudi Arabia and Gulf Countries). It also discussed confidentiality in health services, the liability of the medical and healthcare professionals, the opposite sex health professionals, and the HIV cases which were discussed more elaborately in 1995. In 1997, it discussed problems of fasting during illness and the drugs that may affect fasting and its route of administration. Cloning was also discussed in 1997, along with slaughtering of animals for food. In 2007, lengthy discussions took place on plastic and cosmetic surgery and a number of rulings were issued on these subjects. In 2009, the emergency medicine was discussed with its problems of consent of minors and adults, and in pregnant women, and the emergency of doing caesarian operations to save the baby. In September 2012, the Council discussed genetic engineering and genetic fingerprinting and genetic diseases, but did not issue any rulings on these matters.

The International Islamic Juridical Council OIC re-discussed the issues on genetic in its 21st session held in Riyadh 18–22 November 2013, and studied the recommendations of the seminar held in Jeddah in 23–25 February 2013 regarding the human genome, genetic engineering, genetic counseling, genetic surveys, premarital genetic testing during pregnancy and after delivery. It passed a detailed Fatwa on all these issues after lengthy discussions, with the physicians and genetics'.

The International Islamic Juridical Council also discussed in this session (21st) 18–22 November 2013 the following issues and passed Fatwas on them:

1. The use of prohibited substances e.g. alcohol, porcine material or any other prohibited "Najas" substance after changing its composition, which ends in a new substance differing from the original one e.g. change of alcohol (acetyl alcohol) into acetic acid (vinegar).
   The Majma made Fatwas, recommendations and asked for further studies in dubious substances and issues.
2. The slaughtered animals after being electrocuted with non fatal electric shock. The Majma reiterated a previous Fatwa No 3/10 of 1995, and recommended detailed procedures that certify an Islamic slaughter of a living animal, which was not already dead by electrocution.
3. The huge responsibility of those causing traffic accidents both under the Shari'a law and in the Day of Judgment (Hereafter).

The Council policy is to consult physicians, scientists and religious scholars by writing to them on the specified subject long before the meeting. The research work is distributed to all attendants, usually prior to the time of discussion, then a physician or scientist makes a resume of the scientific papers and a religious scholar makes a resume of the religious papers. The discussions are recorded. All the data along with the rulings are published in their quarterly journal (actually many volumes for each session have already been published). It includes all the subjects discussed during the sessions of that year and is printed (usually a few years after the session). CDs were introduced in the late nineties and continued into the new millennium. The subjects are varied on economics, financial matters, social problems, family problems and public domain including medical and health problems. They get involved in astronomy to decide the beginnings of lunar months, and so forth. The literature produced covers issues of wide scope and scholars have asked separate publications according to the subjects and domains discussed. Because of the legal language of these articles physicians and scientists have not made any use of these voluminous books. There have been recommendations to publish CD-ROMs with necessary glossary to explain technical language of the publications so that more specialists can use this valuable literature on medical ethics. To elaborate on the substance of this important publication the articles treat the subject from different angles: scientific, ethical, religious (theology) and jurisprudence, discussing both the objectives of the Shari'a, the juridical methodology providing juristic arguments in support of one or the other ruling.

The third important corpus in studying medical and ethical perspective is the Islamic Organization for Medical Sciences of Kuwait. It held its first conference in January 1981, under the rubric of Islamic Medicine. Subsequently, it held five conferences of wide participation from many Islamic and Western countries. It searched medical jurisprudence, history of Islamic medicine, the Hippocratic and Oath of a Muslim physician, and so forth. In addition, the organization held numerous symposia on selected topics related to the medical advancement and the moral dilemma that this phenomenal progression had caused in clinical setting. The attendants included Islamic scholars (Ulama), physicians and scientists. Among the topics that were discussed in these symposia, include: the legality of milk-banks, gender selection, technically assisted reproduction, surrogacy, sterilization, abortion, and so on. With the advancement in biotechnology, topics like brain death, "do not resuscitate order", trans-sex and inter-sex found interest among Muslim religious scholars and medical professionals. The organization published the proceedings of these conferences and symposia, a book on Islamic Code of Ethics, a large volume on alternative medicine, a volume on ethics of research and a number of studies on history of Islamic medicine. The work of the Organization was also recognized by the international health organizations like WHO, ISSCO, UNESCO and the International Islamic Juridical Council OIC and the Islamic Jurisprudence Council of Mecca (Islamic World League) and the World Medical Association, with whom the organizers collaborated in holding several joint sessions and meetings.

The fourth significant source for medical jurisprudence and Islamic bioethics are the rulings of the Grand Muftis of Egypt which have been collected and published in many volumes along with subjects including medical and health issues. Some authors have collected the rulings on medical and health issues and published them. For instance, Abdulaziz Abdulmohsin published the rulings of Saudi scholars on medical issues. There are numerous books and booklets authored by different medical and legal scholars on specific issues dealing with, for instance, organ transplantation, methods of assisted reproduction (in vitro fertilization), plastic and cosmetic surgery, stem cell research, cloning, abortion, sterilization, liability, the medical codes, blood transfusion, allowed and prohibited medicine, the fasting of the ill, the pregnant and lactating woman and so on. The topics also include ritual matters such as the performance of ritual prayers during illness and so forth. There are many Masters and Ph.D. thesis in many Universities about these subjects which may be important in these fields This extensive literature is mainly in Arabic, some in Persian, Urdu and Turkish languages; very few in English and other languages.

Today there is an increasing interest in medical ethics from Islamic perspective in the West. Both Muslims and non-Muslim healthcare providers have shown sustained interest in Islamic viewpoints in medical practice and research to cater to the health care needs of the Muslim population in Western countries. Moreover, Islam is growing in numbers and has surpassed other minority religions in North America. There were many conferences and symposia held mainly in USA (and Europe) on Islam and Bioethics. Many publications have been published in English. Some of the earliest works include, for instance, Dr. Hassan Hathout's, "Islamic Basis for Biomedical Ethics" and his co-authored book with Andrew Lustig: "Bioethical Developments in Islam". Gamal Serour is another prominent physician whose article on "Islam and Four Principles of Healthcare Ethics" is an early work that lays down the boundaries of Islamic bioethics. Daar and Al-khitamy's article "Bioethics for Clinicians: Islamic bioethics" and a number of articles about medical, ethical and philosophical topics in academic journals indicate the growing interest in Islamic biomedical ethics. Prof. Abdulaziz Sachedina in his excellent book, "Islamic Biomedical Ethics" has poignantly criticized the literature (in English), where many Muslim physicians writing on the subject have tried to emulate and mimic the Western secular bioethics, which does not fully resonate with the local and regional Muslim values. According to him, "Translation and grafting of the secular bioethics to the Muslim medical and healthcare institutions is unproductive without first investigating native epistemic and cultural resources to teach and disseminate bioethics in Muslim societies" [6]. He goes on to criticize the adoption of Western understanding of autonomy and human rights. "Western notion of universal human rights rests in a secularized public sphere…the modern idea of the autonomous self, envisions social actors as self-contained matrixes of desires who direct their own interest. In Islamic communitarian ethics autonomy is far from being recognized as one of the major bioethical principles…Islamic communal discourse sought to define itself by legitimizing individual autonomy within its religiously based collective order by leaving an individual free to negotiate his/her spiritual destiny, while requiring him/her to abide by a command order that involved the play of reciprocity and autonomy upon which a regime of rights and responsibilities are based in the Shari'a [6]." In his elucidation of the role of Shari'a and theology in formulating the new field of bioethics Sachedina clarifies: "Islamic biomedical ethics cannot ignore judicial opinions and the sources that provide their legitimization as being Islamic… the Fatwa literature needs to be investigated for the purpose of exploring and understanding the legal reasoning behind the rulings [6]."

Among other studies that deserve mentioning include: *Muslim Medical Ethics from Theory to Practice*" [7] edited by Brockopp and Eich. This is an important work published through a collaborative effort beginning with the First International Conference on Medical Law and Ethics in Islam held at The University of Haifa, Israel (occupied Palastine) in March 2001, and continuing through the publication of a sequel entitled: *Islamic Ethics of Life: Abortion, War and Euthanasia* (both published by the University of South Carolina Press). A number of scholars contributed to this scholarly work which recognized the importance of going deep into aims of Islamic teachings, the principles of Islamic jurisprudence, and the Islamic jurisprudence itself with its axioms. It also paid attention to theology and the Muslim creed in formulating the ethical background. Some of the articles added a new dimension which is medical anthropology in Muslim world. Their studies focus on the application of legal, moral or ethical norms in medical practice. The anthropologists have focused on categories such as class and gender as well as the comparison of cases from the whole Muslim world. The fundamental importance of these studies lies in their actor-oriented approach showing that the acts of Muslim patients are influenced by a wide variety of factors; religious norms expounded by the Ulema form one of the factors, but perhaps not the most important one. Another important book in this field is "Islamic Bioethics; Problems and Perspective" by Dariusch Atighehetchi. These studies are, therefore, instrumental in forcing researchers to abandon mono-casual and monolithic explanations of Muslim behavior [7]."

The field work undertaken by the anthropologists expanded the scope of research in Iran, Tajikistan, Pakistan, and among Muslim migrants in Western countries. The work of Sherine Hamdy, "Our Bodies Belong to God" [8] is an illuminating example of how the anthropological approach sheds new light on medical problems faced by ordinary people in Egypt. Her field work exposed the societal problems in organ transplantation in Egypt. She also examined the fatwa literature and made it clear that collecting of these rulings given by the Ulama are only a part of solving the problem of patients suffering from poverty and disease without any net of social security or medical services provided by the government or medical insurance. She was kind enough to present me (MAA) her superb work during a symposium on Islamic medical ethics held in Qatar in 2012 with collaboration of Georgetown University, Qatar and Qatari Government.

The Present Study

The present volume builds on a number of books that both authors wrote or co-authored with colleagues on different issues in Islamic medical jurisprudence. Dr. Albar has closely worked with both the International Islamic Juridical Council OIC and the Islamic Juridical Council of Islamic World League for almost 30 years. He also participated in the activities of the Islamic Organization of Medical Sciences for a similar period. All these works were in Arabic except a book in English titled "Contemporary Topics in Islamic Medicine" which included topics on organ transplantation, the problem of alcohol and its solution in Islamic religious law, Islamic approach to AIDS prevention, Islamic medical jurisprudence and so on. This study starts off by elaborating, "The Origins of Islamic Morality and Ethics". It discusses the common principles of morality and ethics derived from divinely endowed intuitive reason through the creation of *al-fit' ra* (nature); and endowment of human intellect (*al-'aql*). Whereas, these natural sources are God's special gifts to human beings, God's revelation given to the prophets is the supernatural source of divine guidance through which human communities are guided at all times through history. Hence, according to Islam, Adam, Noah, Abraham down to Muhammad, are all God's envoys to humanity to lead them to live a pious and moral life.

We have stressed the importance of each one of these three sources in formulating the creed, moral and ethical issues and religious practices. The Ten Commandments of the Torah (Bible-Old Testement) are explicitly pronounced by every prophet and messenger of God.

Furthermore, we explained the effect of Islamic creed which has six pillars as follows:

1. *Shaha' da* is the statement of faith which declares that there is no god except God (Allah) and Muhammad is the Messenger of God (Allah) (Subhanaho wa Tala).
2. Prophethood (*nubuwwa*) is the belief in all the prophets and that they brought essentially the same message regarding the Unity of God (*Tawhid*) and the necessity to worship Him and none other than Him.
3. Revelation (*tanzi' l, Wahy*) is the belief in the scriptures that were revealed to Abraham, Moses, Jesus and Muha'mmad. Muslims also hold the Psalms of David as divinely revealed.
4. Resurrection (*qiya' ma* or *ma'a'd*) is the belief in the Day of Judgment and the hereafter when the good people will enter the Paradise, and the wretched wrongdoers will dwell in the Hell forever.

5. Angels (*mala' 'ka*) are God's special creation (created from Light), and Muslims believe that God has appointed angels as protectors of human beings and the divine agents who bring revelation to the Prophets.
6. Destiny (*qada'* and *qadar*) is the belief that God determines the blue print for each human being while on earth and guides humanity to fulfill their responsibilities to God and to one another.

We have expounded what Muslims believe in and their different schools of thought. Certainly, the creed forms the basis of understanding the human responsibility for the volitionary performances. We have taken care to probe this matter since it entails the core of morality-the understanding of good (*h'usn*) and evil (*qubh*). These topics are part of the Muslim theology, known as *'ilm al kala' m*.

In the second part of the book we have concentrated on the objectives of the Islamic religious practice—the maqasid -which include: Preservation of Faith, Preservation of Life, Preservation of Mind (intellect, reason), Preservation of Progeny (al-nasl), Preservation of Honor (*al-irdh*) and Preservation of property.

We have utilized numerous studies dealing with Islamic legal methodology and jurisprudence to formulate the second part of this study [9–12] e.g. "Maqasid alShari'ah as Philosophy of Islamic Law" by Prof. Auda [9], who was kind enough to present me (MAA) with his elegant book, Prof. Tariq directed me to his wonderful book "Radical Reform: Islamic Ethics and Liberation" [10]. The rich and deep discussions of Maqasid and Usul (principles) of Islamic Jurisprudence in these books and the valuable book of the late Dr. Ghanem (Ph.D. Law) "Outlines of Islamic Jurisprudence" [11]: Islamic Law in a Nutshell, were great help to us. We cannot miss mentioning the book of Dr. Yacoub, Fiqh of Medicine [12]. This section ends with the subsidiary sources of Islamic legal-ethical methodology and applied jurisprudence.

In the third part of the book we discussed selected hot and controversial topics such as abortion, Assisted Reproduction devices, genetics, organ transplantation, brain death and end of life issues. We reviewed the current medical evidence in each subject followed by detailed discussion of the ethical issues.

Notes and References

1. Chamsi-Pasha H, Albar MA (2013) Islamic medical ethics a thousand years ago. Saudi Med J 34(7):673–675
2. Beauchamp T, Childress J (2001) Principles of biomedical ethics, 5th edn. Oxford University Press, New York, pp 1–3
3. Al Ghazali, A Ihya 'Uluom al-Din. Kitab 'Aja'ib al-Qalb, vol 3/9, Beirut Dar al-Ma'rifah(nd)
4. Armstrong K (1993) A history of god. Baltimore Books, New York, p 151
5. vide supra, pp 142–143

6. Sachedina A (2009) Islamic biomedical ethics: principles and application. Oxford University Press, New York, pp 10–14
7. Brockopp J, Eich T (2008) Muslim medical ethics from theory to practice. University of South Carolina Press, Preface IX, X and Introduction 1–7
8. Hamdy S (2012) Our bodies belong to god: organ transplants, Islam, and the struggle for human dignity in Egypt. University of California Press, Los Angeles
9. Auda J (2008) Maqasid al-Shari'ah, as philosophy of Islamic Law. The International Institute of Islamic Thought, London-Washington
10. Ramadan T (2009) Radical reform, Islamic ethics and liberation. Oxford University Press, New York
11. Ghanem I (1983) Outline of Islamic jurisprudence Islamic Law in a Nutshell, 3rd edn. Saudi Publishing House, Jeddah
12. Yacoub AA (2001) The Fiqh of medicine: responses in Islamic jurisprudence to developments in medical sciences. Ta-Ha Publication, London

Chapter 2
The Sources of Common Principles of Morality and Ethics in Islam

Introductory Remarks

All nations have common principles in morality and ethics. The source of these moral and ethical attitudes can be traced back to three main sources:

1. Intuitive Reasoning (al-fitra) or the basic innate constitution of all human beings. In every person there is an innate intuition that can guide him/her to right or wrong in, at least, the basic morals. Killing an innocent person is repudiated and considered as an abominable, detestable crime, by all normal human beings whose innate constitution has not been distorted by wrong beliefs, practices, and attitudes. The Qur'an extolled the unblemished innate nature in many verses, including, for example, the following:

    Our Sibghah (religion) is the Sibghah (Religion) of Allah (Islam) and which Sibghah (religion) can be better than Allah's? And we are His worshippers. (Q. 2:138)

    So direct your face toward the religion, inclining to truth. [Adhere to] the fitrah of Allah (i.e. Allah's Islamic Monotheism) upon which He has created [all] people. No change should there be in the creation of Allah. That is the correct religion, but most of the people do not know (Q. 30:30)

    In a tradition, the Prophet said: "Everyone is born with the basic innate nature which is inclined to submit to God; then his parents bring him up as a Jew or as a Christian or Magian. (Narrated by Bukhari and Muslim) [1].
    The untainted nature can discern that lying, breaking promises, stealing and so forth are bad and wrong and that veracity, keeping promises, fidelity and honesty are good and right. The basic principles of ethics lie deep in every soul. The intuition and innate constitution guide those with normal unblemished nature to the right conduct and keep them away from malevolent behavior.

2. Faculty of Reason (al-'Aql): The ability to reason and derive a decision by using one's mind. The Qur'an extolled those who are wise, thoughtful and ponder

© The Author(s) 2015
M.A. Al-Bar and H. Chamsi-Pasha, *Contemporary Bioethics*,
DOI 10.1007/978-3-319-18428-9_2

over matters as a result of their accepting the call of the prophets of God. Thus, the Qur'an says:

You who believe. If you heed Allah, He will give you criteria (by which you will judge right from wrong), and will cleanse you of your sins and forgive you. (Q. 8:29)

However, the Qur'an also speaks about those who refused to use their faculty of reason and willfully transgress the boundaries set by God's commands. Such people will find their abode in Hell:

They will say: If only we had really listened and used our reason (minds), we would not have been companions of the Blaze. (Q. 67:10)

The reason should be used to reflect on creatures of the Lord and his signs spread all over:

And in Your creation and all the creatures He has spread about, there are signs for people who use their reason (Q. 45:4)

There are signs for people who use their reason. (Q. 16:1)

There are those people who are blind to the truth because they refuse to see it despite the fact that they have normal eyesight, and refuse to hear despite the fact they have normal hearing:

And surely, We have created many of the jinns and mankind for Hell. They have hearts wherewith they understand not, they have eyes wherewith they see not, and they have ears wherewith they hear not (the truth). They are like cattle, nay even more astray; those! They are the heedless ones. (Q. 7:179)

And Allah guides not the people who disbelieve. They are those upon whose hearts, hearing (ears) and sight (eyes) Allah has set a seal. And they are the heedless! (Q. 16:108).

The blind and the seeing are not the same. Nor are those who believe and do right, the same as evildoers. (Q. 40:58)

It is only people of understanding who heed. (Q.13:19)

Truly it is not their eyes that are blind, but their hearts which are in their breast. (Q. 22:46)

Similar themes can be gauged in the biblical literature. Hence, for instance, one reads in the Gospel of Matthew about what Jesus (PBUH) said: "The reason I use parables in talking to them is that they look, but do not see, and they listen, but do not hear or understand. Isaiah said: This people will listen and listen but not understand; they will look and look, but not see because there minds are dull, and they have stopped up their ears and have closed their eyes." (Matthew 13/13–16).

It is logical to derive that people of wisdom acquire morality. They are honest, just, sincere, benevolent, modest, never inflicting harm (non-maleficence) except with very good reason to thwart greater harm. They are usually tolerant and forgive the misdeeds of others. The one who possess sagacity and discernment has the ability to analyze an event, or behavior in the best possible way. He can draw the best conclusions and make the right decisions.

Human beings are endowed with the faculty of reasoning by which one can discern right from wrong. However this pure faculty could be enmeshed and lured by instincts and carnal desires, egotism, search for pleasure, selfishness and hedonism. All the vices will ensue if the carnal desires, egotism, arrogance, pride, hegemony, unsatiated desire for wealth and power, are not controlled by reason and revelation. Both are needed to control the beast in each one of us hidden deep in the egotistic arrogant selfish desires. Man should strive hard to control his desires and aspire to those exalted who always do good and refrain from harming others: "And those who strive in Our (cause), We will certainly guide them to Our paths; for verily God is with those who do right" (Q. 29:69).

The first and foremost requirement in the development of moral-spiritual is to work on the control of the lower self from "doing harm" to any creature (humans, animals or ecosystem), except in self-defense and in order to thwart aggression. This striving is followed, or may go hand in hand, by doing good to others (beneficence). The Prophet Muhammad (PBUH) told one of his companions that if you are not capable of doing good to others, at least do no harm to them [2]. According to the famous Muslim theologian, al-Ghazali: "If you cannot reach the level of angels, then do not fall into the level of beasts, scorpions and snakes. If your soul is content to come down from the highest heights, at least, do not let it be content into the lowest depths (to the rank of beasts, snakes and scorpions). Perhaps you will be saved by the middle way where you have neither more nor less than what suffices" [3]. The Qur'an says:

> We have indeed created man in the best of stature, then We abase him to the lowest of the low. (Q. 95:4,5).

Certainly belief in Oneness of God guides the believers to noble virtues and righteous deeds, and admonishes them to refrain from vices and heinous deeds. The Prophet said: "I solemnly declare that a person who inflicts harm to his neighbor is not a believer of God" [4]. In another tradition he said, "A woman entered Hellfire, because she incarcerated a cat until it died of hunger and thirst" [5]. Still in another tradition, a prostitute of Bani Israel was thirsty so she came to a well, and got water for herself to drink. When she finished she found a dog very thirsty, so she went back to the well and got him water in her shoe and quenched its thirst. God was pleased with her deed and let her enter Paradise [6].

Muslim Philosophers like Ibn Tufail believe that any normal human being can recognize God, with his divinely endowed nature and his reason. He wrote the Story of Hayy bin Yaqzan whose mother delivered him on a remote island, and died in post partum. A gazelle felt sympathy for this newly born, and reared him like a mother. When he grew up, she died, and he was stunned, and dissected her body to know what happened. He went on pondering and by using his intuitive reason he reached the conclusion that indeed there was a Creator for this world, and he worshipped Him silently until a learned sage came to his island. They became friends and Hayy learned a language from him. Both were amazed when they found that Hayy reached to the conviction of a Supreme Being, the Creator of this world, without any guidance from anybody or revelation except his own intuition and reason.

Ibn Sina, Ibn Tufail, Al Kindi, Al Farabi, Al Razi, among many other Muslim philosophers believed that human being can recognize God and most of His attributes, without revelation if he uses his intuition and reason properly, and if it is not masked by carnal instincts, and false beliefs. They thought that the multitude of common people needed revelation, but the intellectuals and the philosophers can reach to the same conclusion without the guidance of a Prophet or his representative. Ibn Sina believed that revelation is also needed for men of intellect, not to reach the recognition of God, but to describe for them the proper code of life. Ibn Sina came to this conclusion in his later days, when he almost became a mystic Sufi.

Ibn Sina defied the other philosophers (or at least some of them) who saw that the revealed religion suits only the common people, while men of intellect are suited for philosophy. Ibn Sina held that a Prophet like Muhammad (PBUH) is superior to any philosopher, as the Prophet is not dependent on human reason, which can err, but is wholly dependent on revelation from God, which will never err. In his "book al-Isharat" signs (Admonitions) he became a mystic Sufi and became critical of the rational approach to God. Ibn Sina worked out a rational demonstration for the existence of God, based on Aristotle's proofs, which became standard among later medieval philosophers in both Judaism and Islam [7]. However, neither he nor the Islamic philosophers ever doubted the existence of God, and that unaided normal human reason can arrive at knowledge of the existence of Supreme Being. Reason was man's most exalted activity and it has an important role in the religious quest. Ibn Sina thought it was a religious duty for those who had the intellectual ability to discover God for themselves by using reason and to free the conception of God from superstitions (added to true religion) and anthropomorphism. Ibn Sina and others like him, wanted to use reason to discover as much as they could about the nature of God.

This attitude seems strange in modern philosophy. Reason is used in Western modern philosophy in a more mundane and pragmatic way as in a utilitarian consequentiality school, or to stress the importance of deontology, the categorical philosophy of Kant and his followers to establish the basis of ethics and morality on secular grounds. It is ironic that post modernist philosophers of the West in the twentieth century attacked "Reason" and all the philosophies built on Reason [8].

3. Divine Revelation (al-wahy, Tanzil): Muslims believe that God guides humanity by sending a number of prophets and apostles, who are the bearers of the revelation. Muslim believe that since the beginning of history there have been a hundred and 24,000 minor and major prophets who came to guide humanity about their origin and final return to God. These prophets receive the revelations from God. However, the major Prophets are sent with a universal message from God, and a Shari'ah (Code of Life) to organize the community of faithful—the Umma, into a universal body of the believers. These prophets brought monotheistic faith in One God, but as time passed by their followers distorted the pure monotheism and brought back their old deities to be worshipped along with God. The first such prophet of God was Adam and the last is Muhammad (PBUH). A Muslim should believe in all of them, whether he knows their names, origins or not. The Qur'an

mentions a number of them. Thus, it mentions, for instance Noah (Nuh), Abraham (Ibrahim), Ishmael (Ismail), Isaac (Ishaq), Jacob (Ya'qub/Israel), Joseph (Yusuf), Moses (Musa), Zacaria (Zakariyah), Jesus (Isa), John the Baptist (Yahya), Jonah (Yunus), Lot and so on. All these are mentioned in the Hebrew Bible (with difference in their stories). Others who were not mentioned in the Hebrew Bible, like Hud, Salih, Shu'yib are considered of Arab origin. Nevertheless, all of them stressed belief in one God, the Supreme Lord of all the worlds and creatures. The Qur'an is replete with the admonition of the messengers of God to their nations from the time of Noah, Hud, Salih, Shu'ayb, Lot, and every Prophet and Messenger of God who proclaimed the unity of God by declaring:

Invoke your Lord with humility and in secret. He likes not the aggressors. And do not do mischief on the earth, after it has been set in order, and invoke Him with fear and hope; Surely, Allah's Mercy is (ever) near unto the good-doers. (Q. 7:56–57)

Muslims believe in all these prophets and the divine messages they brought with them. The Qur'an says:

Say we believe in God, and His revelation given to us, and to Abraham, Ishmael, Isaac, Jacob, and the Tribes; and that given to Moses and Jesus, and that given to all prophets from their Lord. We make no difference between one and another of them; and we bow to God in submission (islam). (Q. 2:136–138)

The Apostle believes in what has been revealed to him from His Lord; as do the men of faith. Each one of them believes in God, His Angels, His books and His Apostles. We make no distinction between one and another of His Apostles. And they say we hear, we obey; we seek your forgiveness. (Q. 2:285).

In the tradition reported on the authority of the Prophet, he said: My example and the example of the preceding Prophets is similar to a man who enters a wonderful building, which he admires, but for a cleft in the wall, which needs to be sealed by a slab (or a slate). The building represents the past prophets and I am only the slab which fills the gap" (narrated by Muslim in his authentic collection of traditions) [9]. The Prophet Muhammad is the culmination of a long history of prophethood and messengers of God. This is captured by the Qur'an when it declares:

This day I have perfected your religion for you, completed My favor upon, and have chosen for you Islam, as your religion. (Q. 5:3).

Islam is the religion that unites the entire humanity from Adam till doomsday and considers all nations to have witnessed One God through the messages and teachings of their respective prophets:

There is no nation that was not given an admonisher. (Q. 35:24).

All peoples are the progeny of Adam who was elevated to be the vicegerent of God on earth:

Behold thy Lord said to the angels: I will create on earth a vicegerent. (Q. 2:30).

And He (Allah) taught Adam the nature (names) of all things. (Q. 2/31).

Adam was endowed with the knowledge which the angels did not know, and for that reason God ordered them to bow to Adam in respect and veneration. (Q. 2:30–34). And not only Adam was honored by Allah, but also his progeny:

We honored the progeny of Adam, provided them with transport on land and sea, given them for sustenance things good and pure, and conferred on them special favors above a great part of our creation. (Q. 17:70).

It is in this sense that Islam teaches respect for the human body. In a tradition the Prophet rebuked a man who broke a bone from the cemetery without any good reason and told him, "The guilt of breaking the bones of the dead is equal to the guilt of breaking the bones of the living" (narrated by Abu Dawud *Sunan Abi Dawud, Kitabal-jana'iz*), [10].

In other words, due respect and reverence should be given to the funeral as exemplified by the Prophet who stood up in veneration for the passing by of a funeral of a Jew, at a time when Jews were waging war against him (and tried to assassinate him and then poison him but failed). One of his companions exclaimed: "It is only the funeral of a Jew". The Prophet (PBUH) retorted: "Is it not a human being?" [11] (*Sahih al-Bukhari, Kitab al-jana'iz*).

The unity of human beings is established in many verses of the Qur'an and the traditions of the Prophet. The value of a human being depends on his good deeds, and not on his wealth or position:

Oh mankind, We created you from a single (pair) of a male and female, and made you into nations and tribes that you may know each other. Verily the most honored of you in the sight of Allah (God) is he who is the most righteous of you. (Q. 49:13).

Karen Armstrong in her book "*A History of God*" [12] says: "In practical terms, Islam meant that Muslims had a duty to create a just equitable society where the poor and vulnerable are treated decently. The early moral message of the Qur'an is simple: It is wrong to stockpile wealth and build a private fortune, and good to share the wealth of society fairly by giving a regular proportion of one's wealth to the poor". (Holy Qur'an 92/18, 9/103, 63/9, 102/1).

The zakat (alms giving) and salat (prayers) are two of the five Pillars of Islam. These five are (1) *Shahada* (i.e. witnessing that there is no God but Allah and that Muhammad is His Messenger), (2) *Salat* (Regular five prayers each day) (3) *Zakat*: Compulsory alms giving which is a definite share of the wealth to be distributed every year to the needy and poor. (4) Fasting during the month of Ramadan (the 9th lunar month in the Islamic calendar) from dawn to sunset (5) *Hajj* (pilgrimage) to Makkah, at least, once in a lifetime, if a person has the amenities and means to go there.

Each of these has a great moral value, for example, prayers are done five times a day in congregation. There are no priests or clergy to lead the congregation. Any Muslim who knows the prayer and the rules of this ritual can lead them. The imam stands in the front while the rest stand behind him close to each other (shoulder to shoulder) with no difference between race, color, wealth or even age. Women usually stand in the back rows inconspicuously. However, it is recommended for them to pray in the privacy of their home.

The aim of Salat is multiple: Adoration of Allah, speaking to Him directly by reciting His word, the Qur'an, sense of equality and legality. The Salat should prevent those who pray from shameful and unjust deeds.

Establish regular prayers for prayers restrain from shameful and unjust deeds. (Q. 29/45).

The Zakat (literally purification and growth) frees Muslims from worship of wealth and teaches them to share their wealth with the needy and poor:

Take (O Muhammad) from their wealth a charity by which you purify them (Q. 9:103).

Zakah expenditures are only for the poor and for the needy, and for those employed to collect it, and for bringing hearts together (for Islam, usually the new reverts), and for freeing slaves, and for those in debt (for a good cause), and for the cause of Allah, and the wayfarer. (Q. 9:60).

Have you seen the one who denies the Day of Judgment, for that is the one who repulses the orphan, and does not encourage the feeding of the indigent. So woe to those who pray, (but) who are heedless of their prayers. Those who only make show (of their deeds), and refuse (even) neighborly needs (*Surah Al-Ma'un – Almsgiving* Q. 107: 1–7).

Similarly fasting a whole month from dawn to sunset, abstaining from food, drink and sex with a spouse, teaches each Muslim to develop a disciplined life and to forebear and remember the poor and needy who do not even get their meals. The month of Ramadan is celebrated with communal meals, congregational prayers and giving a lot to the needy and indigent.

Every Muslim has to make hajj, at least once in a lifetime, if he can afford the journey and expense. All those who go to Hajj, put off their clothes, garments and get into the simple traditional pilgrim's white dress that eradicates all distinction of race or class. Furthermore, the person who adorns the required attire get liberated from the egotistic preoccupations of their daily lives. They all cry out in unison, "Here I am at your service O Allah"; and then start to circumambulate around the Ka'aba (the holiest shrine in Islam) seven times, along with multitudes (almost tens of thousands at a time, the total being more than 3 million).

Ali Shariati, the late Iranian sociologist of religion described his experience succinctly. "As you circumambulate and move closer to Ka'aba, you feel like a small stream merging with a big river. Carried by a wave you lose touch with the ground. As you approach the center, the pressure of the crowd squeezes you so hard that you are given a new life. You are now part of the people, you are now a man, alive and eternal... You have become part of this universal system. Circumambulating around Allah's house, you soon forget yourself...you have been transformed into a particle that is gradually melting and disappearing. This is absolute love at its peak." [13].

This is the true significance of the affirmation of *islam*, which literally means "surrender/peace." Every Muslim has to surrender himself/herself in obeisance to Allah, The Creator, The Sovereign, The Merciful, The Exalted who has ninety-nine beautiful names or attributes:

He is Allah, other than whom there is no deity (no other God) Who knows (all things), both the unseen and the witnessed. He is the Most Gracious, Most Merciful. He is Allah other than whom there is no deity, the Sovereign, the Pure, the Perfection, the Bestower of Faith, the Overseer, the Exalted in Might, the Compeller, and the Superior. Exalted is Allah above whatever they associate with Him. He is Allah, the Creator, the Inventor, the Fashioner; to Him belong the best names (attributes). Whatever is in the heavens and earth is exalting Him and He is the Exalted in Might, the Wise (Q.59:22–24).

According to Karen Armstrong [14]: "There was no obligatory doctrines about God; indeed the Qur'an is highly suspicious of theological speculation, dismissing it as Zanna/Self-indulgent guesswork about things that nobody can possibly know or prove. The Christian doctrine of the Incarnation and the Trinity seemed prime examples of Zanna, and not surprisingly, the Muslims found these notions blasphemous. Instead…God was experienced as a moral imperative. Having practically no contact with either Jews or Christians and their scriptures, Muhammad had cut straight into the essence of historical monotheism."

Further down she writes: "In the Qur'an, however Allah is more impersonal than Yahweh…" We can only glimpse something of God in the signs of nature, and so transcendent is He that we can only talk about Him in parables. Constantly, therefore the Qur'an urges Muslims to see the world as epiphany:

Verily in the creation of the heavens and of the earth and the succession of night and day in the ships that speed through the sea with what is useful to man; and in the waters which God sends down from the sky, giving life thereby to the earth after it had been lifeless, and causing all manner of living creatures to multiply there on; and in the change of the winds, and the clouds that run their appointed courses between sky and earth. (In all this) there are signs, indeed for people who use their reason. (Q. 2/158, 159).

"The Qur'an constantly stresses the need for intelligence in deciphering the "signs" or "messages" of God. Muslims are not to abdicate their reason, but to look at the world attentively and with curiosity. It was with this attitude that later enabled Muslims to build a fine tradition of natural science, which has never been seen as such a danger to religion as in Christianity. A study of the workings of the natural world showed that it had a transcendent dimension and source, whom we can talk about only in signs and symbols; even the stories of the Prophets, the accounts of the Last Judgment, and the joys of Paradise would not be interpreted literally, but as parables of higher ineffable reality." The Prophet said that Jannah i.e. Paradise is something that no eye has seen or heard of or evencrosses the imagination of any human being) [15].

The Qur'an emphatically denied any association with God, neither as wife or son:

Say: He is the One God, the Eternal Refuge (the uncaused cause of all beings). He begets not, and neither is He begotten, and there is nothing that could be compared to Him (Q. 112:1–3).

"But they have attributed to Allah partners- the jinn, while He has created them. And they falsely, having no knowledge attribute to Him sons and daughters. Praise and glory be to Him (for He is) above what they attribute to Him. He is the originator of the heavens and earth. How can He have a son when He has no consort? He created all things and He has full knowledge of all things".

That is God (Allah), your Lord, the Creator of all things, so worship Him, and He is the Disposer of all things. Vision perceives Him not, but He perceives all vision, and He is the Subtle (above all comprehension) yet acquainted with all things (Q. 6:100–103).

According to the explanation provided by Karen Armstrong [16], The perception of God's uniqueness is the basis of the morality of the Qur'an. To give allegiance to material goods, or to put trust in lesser beings was Shirk (idolatry), the greatest sin of Islam...Muslims must realize that Allah is the ultimate and unique reality... There is no deity but Allah the Creator of the heaven and earth, who alone can save man and send him the spiritual and physical sustenance that he needs. Only by acknowledging Him as as-Samad (The uncause cause of all being) would Muslims address a dimension of reality beyond times and history... She continues: "There is no simplistic notion of God, however, this single deity is not a being like ourselves which we can know and understand. The phrase "Allahu Akbar" (God is Greater) that summons Muslims to Salat (prayers 5 times a day) distinguishes between God and the rest of the reality, as well as between God as He is in Himself (al-Dhat) and anything that we can say about Him; yet this incomprehensible and inaccessible God wanted to make Himself known. An early tradition (hadith of the Prophet) says: "I was a hidden treasure; I wanted to be known. Hence, I created the world so that I might be known" [17].

By contemplating the signs (ayat) of nature and the verses of the Qur'an, Muslim could glimpse that aspect of divinity...we only see God through His activities, which adapt His Ineffable being to our limited understanding. The Qur'an urges Muslims to cultivate perpetual consciousness (taqwa) of the Face or the Self of God that surrounds them on all sides "Wheresoever you turn, there is the Face of Allah" (Q. 2:115)...Qur'an sees God as the Absolute, "Who alone Has True Existence".

The Qur'an stressed the continuity of the religious experience of humankind, and teaches that God sent Messengers to every people on the face of earth. The Qur'an orders Muslims to argue other faiths with respect and friendly attitude, "Do not argue with the Peoples of the Scriptures except in the most kindly manner- unless it be such of them as are set on evil doing- and say: We believe in that which has been bestowed upon us, as well as that which was bestowed upon you; for our God and your God is one and the same, and unto Him that we surrender ourselves". (Q. 29:46). Indeed, the religion of God introduced the compassionate ethos which was the hallmark of the more advanced religion: brotherhood and social justice were its crucial virtues. A strong egalitarianism would continue to characterize the Islamic ideal [18].

Gender Equality, the Hallmark of Islam

During pre-Islamic period, known as the Age of Ignorance (*jahiliya*), the majority of women were on par with slaves; they were disdained and the birth of a female child was considered as a calamity. Some would hide in disgrace, others would kill the newly born female child immediately after birth; still worse he might keep her and then he would take her and bury her alive.

The Qur'an condemned this callous disgraceful behavior:

And when the female (infant) buried alive (as the pagan Arabs used to do) shall be questioned. For what sin she was killed? (Q. 81:8–9)

If one of them receive the tidings of a female, his face darkens, and he is in wrath inwardly. He hides himself from his folk because of the bad news. He contemplates: Shall he keep the child in contempt or bury it (her) in the dust? Verily evil is their judgment. (Q.16:58,59)

They despised women because they could not fight. Moreover, since feuds and fights were almost a daily phenomenon between different tribes, there was deep-seated fear that if they get conquered, the enemy would enslave children and women. The men, when they felt the defeat, they fled the battlefield. Consequently, disgrace would befall the whole tribe for ages.

The Qur'an not only forbade the killing of female children (infanticide), it also gave women legal rights of inheritance (which they were deprived from when there was a male inheritor) and divorce. The Prophet encouraged women to play an active role in the affairs of Ummah. The first person on earth to believe in the prophethood of Muhammad (PBUH) was his beloved wife Khadija, who supported him all through his life. In fact, when the Prophet had the first encounter with revelation in the Cave of Hira in Makkah, he came back trembling from the harsh new experience with the Archangel Gabriel. Khadija supported him and he was afraid of being attacked by bad spirits turning him into insanity. It was Khadija who reassured him saying: "Nay...never will Allah let you down. You are kind and considerate towards kin. You help the poor and forlorn, and bear their burdens. You are striving to restore the high moral qualities that your people have lost. You honor the guest and go to the assistance of those in distress. This cannot be that you are attacked by an evil spirit" [19].

She took him to her cousin Waraqa bin Nawfal, an old learned sage, who had adopted Christianity, and after hearing from Muhammad (PBUH), he reassured him that he had received a revelation from God, similar to that revealed to Moses and the Prophets, and that his tribe (Quraysh) will drive him out of Makkah. He wished to be alive then, to support him.

The first batch of Muslims included slaves, Sumayyah, her husband Yasir and her son Ammar, who were exposed to torture by Quraish. Sumayyah was the first martyr in Islam. She was followed by her husband Yasir, but Ammar was saved.

Khadija herself suffered greatly when Quraysh prevented Muslims to have any dealings with people of Makkah and its traders. This was a total boycott of the

Hashimites, the Prophet's clan. No food was allowed for them, and all of them suffered greatly. After 3 years of full siege it was lifted when the Prophet informed Quraysh that their written oath (to deprive Muslims from their necessities and push them into hunger) which was hanged in Ka'ba was eaten by moth except the name of Allah. Both Khadija and the Prophet's uncle, Abu Talib, who also supported him, died in that same year.

A number of women of Medina supported the Prophet and even fought battles with him. The Qur'an stressed the equality of men and women in the sight of Allah, and the women continued to play a pivotal role in the community. The Qur'an says:

> Indeed the Muslim men and Muslim women, the believing men and the believing women, the obedient men and women, the truthful men and women, the humble men and women, the charitable men and women, the fasting men and women, the men who guard their private parts and the women who do so, and the men who remember Allah often and women who do so, for them Allah has prepared forgiveness and great reward. (Q. 33:35).

It is remarkable to note that the supervisor of the markets of Medina, at the time of 'Umar (the Second Caliph) was al-Shaffa bint Abdulla of Quraysh, and that of Makkah was another woman by the name of al-Samra bint Nuhaik al-Asadiyah [20]. The Qur'an addressed women explicitly, and sections were named for women The Women Chap. 4) which discussed a number of the marital problems and the role of women. Another chapter entitled Divorce (Chap. 65) discussed the divorce and completed what has been alluded to earlier in Chap. 2. The chapter entitled: Maryam (Mary, Chap. 19) narrated the story of Mary and the birth of Jesus (PBUH). Chapter 3, entitled The Family of Imran relates the circumstances connected with the mother of Mary (PBUH) who wished to have a boy to serve in the temple, but instead she delivered Mary and she gave her to the sanctuary. The wife of Zakariyah delivered Yahya after being barren, and her story is told in Chaps. 3 and 19. The story of the woman who argued with the Prophet (PBUH) was given in Chap. 58.

It is instructive to note that when God mentions an example of the best believers, He only mentions Mary and the wife of the aggressor tyrant Pharaoh who brought up Moses. According to Arabic tradition, Asia the daughter of Muzahim reared Moses, and believed in him as the Messenger of God. (See the Qur'an, Chap. 66).

Similarly, when God mentions the example of the unbelievers, He only mentioned two women who transgressed and refused the prophethood of their husbands; they were the wife of Noah and the wife of Lot, who perished with her people. (Q. Chap. 66). The sister of Abu Sufyan, the leader of Quraish, (Abu Lahab's wife) who threw stones and placed thorns on the route of the Prophet Muhammad (PBUH) was mentioned in the Chap. III).

The Qur'an is replete with stories of believers and non-believer transgressors from both sexes. Accoridng to Karen Armstrong, the Qur'an quite frequently addressed women explicitly; something that rarely happens in either the Jewish or Christian Scriptures [21].

Qur'an abhorred fornication and adultery which was banned. Both the male and female who practiced this heinous act were to be punished by 100 lashes, if they confess, without any duress, or, if the actual act is witnessed by four adult persons of integrity (which is almost impossible), as required by the Qur'an (Q. 24:2–5).

Likewise, prostitution is banned, and those who had slave girls and forced them into prostitution were required to stop the evil practice. In such cases the oppressed slave girls were to be exonerated from any blame as they were actually forced into the evil act while they had wanted to get out of it. God is all Merciful but harsh punishments await the doers of evil deeds unless they desist and stop forcing the poor slave girls into the dirty trade (Q. 34:33).

The Prophet restored the humanity of women and emancipated them at every level of social life. Emancipation of both male and female slaves was declared as a commendable act of piety and love of God, which He would reward in the Hereafter. The Qur'an encouraged freeing of the slave as acts of expiation when wrongs were committed unintentionally. Such acts included unintentional manslaughter or having sex with one's wife during the fasting.

Succession to the Prophet Muhammad (PBUH) and Appearance of Different Schools of Thought Among Muslims:

After the sudden death of the Prophet Muhammad (PBUH) in 632 C.E., majority of Muslims in Medina chose Abu Bakr, Muhammad's close friend and his father-in-law, to be their leader; but some of the companions believed Ali, the cousin and son-in-law of the Prophet should be his successor. However, Ali himself recognized Abu Bakr as the caliph. Similarly after the death of Abu Bakr (CE 634), 'Umar was nominated as the successor by Abu Bakr and the muslims approved and gave him allegiance. Ali also gave allegiance to 'Umar. When 'Umar was assassinated by Abu Lu'lua the Magian Persian slave in CE 644, he appointed a committee of six companions, including 'Uthman and Ali (both of whom had married the Prophet's daughters) among whom the next caliph was to be chosen. The majority chose 'Uthman, as he was of more lenient nature than Ali. 'Uthman was old when he became caliph, and after 6 years in power, he delegated many of his responsibilities to Marwan ibn al-Hakam (a young Umayyad), and appointed many of his relatives as rulers in different parts of the empire. Unfortunately, many of them were not as good as he wished. Uthman was slaughtered in a revolt, and Ali was chosen as caliph by the companions of the Prophet in Medina, but Mu'awia, the Umayyad governor of Syria refused to give allegiance on the pretext, that the mutineers who killed 'Uthman should first be brought to justice. He knew that Ali could not put a thorough investigation of the case, as the mutineers were multitudes from Iraq, Egypt and even some from around Medina. He had to establish his rule first. Mu'awia, who governed Syria from the time of 'Umar and under 'Uthman was powerful and used his resources to appease the soldiers and men of influence.

Imam Ali was assassinated by Abd al-Rahman ibn Muljam, an ultra fundamentalist (Kharijee) who refused any truce between the fighting parties.

Following 'Ali's assassination, his son Al Hasan was selected by the people as the successor of Ali, but his men were divided, and finally he agreed to relinquish the caliphate to Mu'awiya, on condition he should be openly acclaimed as the successor after Mu'awia. Mu'awia was a shrewd political leader who could rule a vast empire, with good administration. Mu' awia was accused of poisoning Al Hassan through his wife Ja' da bint Al Asha' th Al Kindy [22–24].

Following the death of Al Hasan the way was cleared for Mu'awiya to appoint his son Yazid as the heir to the throne. Yazid was known for his love for good wine, concubines and music. When he came to power, the people of Iraq sent for Husayn ibn Ali, to offer their allegiance as the proper caliph [25].

Many of the companions e.g. Abdullah ibn Omar, Abdullah ibn Abbas warned him not to leave Makkah to Iraq as those who gave their allegiance in Iraq will betray him as they had betrayed his Father (Imam Ali) and his brother (Imam Hasan). Husayn thought his duty was to rise against the corrupt Yazid, especially that more than 100,000 gave him their allegiance.

By the time he went to Iraq, the mutiny was suppressed by U'bayd Allah ibn Ziyad, the new governor of Iraq, in the name of Yazid.

The hundreds of thousands who paid their allegiance to Husayn backed out. Husayn had already left Madina for Iraq. He and his small band of followers, including his family, were besieged and killed in Karbala, Iraq by the huge Umayyad army. Members of the family of the Prophet who survived the tragedy were taken as prisoners back to Damascus where Yazid was on the throne. The head of Husayn was taken to Yazid, where he poked the mouth, lips, eyes and nostrils with a rod in front of Zainab, Husayn's sister. And had it not been for Zainab, Yazid would have slaughtered the only remaining son of Husayn, Ali Zayn al-Abdin, who was ill at the time of the battle of Karbala.

This catastrophic blow to Muslims all over was manifested by the revolution of the people of Medina and Makkah against this brutal rule of Yazid. Yazid sent a strong army which included many mercenaries to crush the revolution. They did with the strongest possible force.

The brutal army finished the carnage and went to Makkah which was saved by the news of the sudden death of Yazid [25].

All the pious Muslims were against the rule of Yazid. Even the son of Yazid, Mu'awiya the second, who was appointed as the new caliph, refused the throne and declared that he could not condone the massacres or behavior of his father He was poisoned by the Umayyad house soon after this incident [26].

The followers of Ali in Iraq, who betrayed his son Al Hasan and his other son al-Husayn, felt remorse up to this day and considered themselves, in a way the cause of the catastrophe of Karbala. They chain themselves and cut their bodies with knives and swords annually, on 10th of Muharam, the day on which al-Husayn was massacred.

Zaid, the grandson of al-Husayn was instigated by those Shi'ah of Iraq, in an exactly similar way to what happened to his grandfather. He was warned by Imam Jaffer al Sadiq (his nephew) not to be lured by them. He even told him that he himself refused their call for him to revolt against the Umiyad ruler (Hisham ibn AbdelMalik) as they are cowards and hypocrites who will fail him. More than 100,000 paid their allegiance, but before the battle started, they asked him about his opinion on Abu Bakr and U'mar. He praised them, and they took this opportunity to recline from fighting, as he refused to curse Abu Bakr and U'mar. He declared them rafidah i.e. those who refused the true path. Only some three hundred remained with him and he was massacred with all his family and followers. His body was taken from the grave, crucified on a post in Basra, and then the body was thrown in the trash of al-Basra [26].

His followers are known as Zaydiyah, and one of his descendants al-Hasan al-Utrush established a government and dynasty in Daylam, in Northern Iran near the Caspian Sea. Later another branch established long lasting Imamates in Yemen which remained for almost a thousand years (sometimes ruling only a small mountainous part of Yemen in Saada), and at times ruling the whole of Yemen up to Dofar, (now in Oman).

The Zaydi School, the first Shi'ah Sect, were moderate and never cursed the Sahaba (the companions of the Prophet [PBUH]) and accepted the traditions (hadiths) of the Prophet narrated by Al-Bukhari, Muslim, etc. i.e. Sunnah people. In Fiqh (jurisprudence) they are similar to Sunni schools.

They were strictly Mu'tazilah who claimed to be Ahl al 'Adl waal-Tawhid i.e. the people of justice and monotheism. They defended the free will of men, so that God will judge them by their deeds. God is also very rational, and they refused predestination to emphasize God's essential Justice. They extolled Reason and were considered free thinkers. At the time of the Abbasid caliph alMa'mun, who encouraged philosophy, medicine, astrology and science by translating books from different languages (Greek, Latin, Syriac, etc.), the Mu'tazila became the doctrine of the caliphal state, and they tried to impose it on other Muslims.

The champion of the Sunnah, Ahmad ibn Hanbal refuted their <u>doctrines</u> about:

(1) The Creation of the Qur'an: According to this doctrine, the Mu'tazilites claimed that there was no eternal word of God (Logos), and that all the revealed books were created by God in time and place, as the need arose. Hence, they were not eternal.

(2) Predestination: According to this doctrine, the Mu'tazilites refused any hint to predestination. Ahmad ibn Hanbal, though not a strict believer of predestination (Jabriyah), claimed that Allah preordained things and nothing can happen without His permission or order.

(3) Anthropomorphic Description of God: According to this doctrine, Ahmad ibn Hanbal accepted all the attributes of God that were mentioned in the Qur'an or Hadith, as they are without any explanation. If God in the Qur'an is described as having a face, then God has a face, hands and feet and He sits on the throne. He "sees", "hears", "speaks" and we shall see Him in Paradise. There is no way except to take these descriptions literally, though he acknowledges fully that nothing is similar or comparable to Him. " There is nothing whatever like unto Him and He is the One that hears and sees (all things)" (Qur'an 42:11). The perception of God's uniqueness is beyond doubt, but what the Mu'tazila maintained is tantamount to saying that the concept of the transcendent God could never be seen in this world or the Hereafter.

Ibn Hanbal's followers maintained that reason was not an appropriate tool for exploring the unfathomable nature of God. They accused the Mu'tazilites of draining God of all mystery, and making Him an abstract formula that has no deep religious value. Ibn Hanbal was stressing the essential ineffable God, which lay beyond reach of all logic and conceptual analysis.

(4) Rationalistic Conception of God: According to the Mu'tazilite doctrine God became rational being not very different from a rational man, thus emptying God of His transcendence. The Mutazilis replied that such an attitude is almost blasphemous as God is depicted as a dictator, whose actions cannot be explained, and that He can be unjust. Their opponents retorted that if everything is His own and in His domain, whatever He does is wise and just though we may not be able to discern the wisdom behind such an act.

They cite misfortunes that befalls human beings, natural disasters, the evil and mischief that is abundant and all around. The innocent children could suffer from painful diseases, or put into hardships by becoming orphans, maimed by wars and explosive mines as happens in modern world. The evil and mischief is evident all through human history, and if that has been ordained by God, or at least by his permission, the Mu'tazili will say then that God is a tyrant despot and dictator. To them God cannot ordain or allow any evil. He gave human beings free will and reason to do whatever they want; accordingly, they will be judged by God in the hereafter.

The polemical arguments between the rationalists and traditionalist continue; to include accusation by the traditionalists that the Mu'tazilites were dualist (*Mathanawiya*) who believed in two Gods: one is the God of goodness and the other is the God of evil. Of course, the Mu'tazilis rejected these allegations. Perforce, the good and the bad, the Mu'tazilis say, are inherent in humans, but they have the divinely endowed reason and revelation to choose between the two, and be accordingly judged by God. Unfortunately, the Mu'tazilis in power used the caliphal authority to torture the imam of the Sunna (traditionalists), Ahmad ibnHanbal to accommodate their views, and that horrified the people by this unjust behavior. Since then the Mu'tazilis fell into disrepute. Later Ahmad ibn Hanbal was absolved by al-Mutawakkil, who apologized of what his predecessors had done to him, and took his side openly. Ahmad ibn Hanbal, however, refused the royal patronage and any monetary rewards from the caliph Nevertheless, he kept his allegiance to the caliph since he believed that rebellion would bring more harm to Islam and to the people.

The Ithna 'Ashariyya—Twelvers—of Iraq

The Shi'ites believed that the post of Imam (Khalifa) was too important to be left to the people to decide. As a matter of fact, they believed that God Himself appointed the Imam by commanding the Prophet to declare Ali to be his appointed heir. The process of designation was continued by Ali, who did the same and appointed al Hasan, his son, by the order of God. Similarly, al-Hasan appointed his brother al-Husayn and al-Husayn appointed his son, Ali Zayn al-Abdin, who was followed by Muhammed al-Baqir, and then Imam Ja'far al-Sadiq. According to them, Imam Ja'far established their *madhhab* and that is the reason they are called Ja'fariah or Imamiyah. Ja'far appointed his son Musa al-Kazim, followed by his son Ali al-Rida till the line reached the 12th Imam Muhammad al-Mahdi, who disappeared in a "tunnel" in Samarra in Iraq for over 1,100 years and will appear at the End of Time (like the Messiah of Jews, Christian's Jesus and Sunni Muslim's Mahdi and Jesus).

The Ja'fari (Imami or Twelver) Shi'ites use reason in their jurisprudence only, which is similar in a way to Sunni Schools (Qiyas: analogy).

The essential doctrine in their creed is the belief that God Himself has designated those purified twelve (Ali and his descendants from Fatima, the daughter of the Prophet). The Sunni Muslims believe that the Muslim Community should choose their leaders.

The Ja'fari (Imami or Twelver) believe that the Qur'an has both exoteric and esoteric dimensions which require allegorical or metaphorical interpretation of the (Qur'an) which is far from using reason. However,they agree and adopt part of the Mu'tazli theology, but they are not Mu'tazili. In fact, a number of their doctrines is far removed from Mu'tazili theology.

The Kharijites: This is the fraction that disagreed with Imam Ali during the battle of Siffin in 36 AH and rebelled against him and later assassinated him. The Kharijites constitute of the Arab tribes who rebelled against the caliphal authority. They fought the Umayyad dynasty with unprecedented bravery and caused, at least partly, its demise. As zealots, they did not hesitate to fight those who disagreed with them even for trivial things, and called their adversaries non-believers. They were divided among themselves under different leaders and were wiped out by the rulers who were threatened by their ferocious battles against corrupt rulers. Today, there remains only one moderate faction who are known as Ibadiyya and this faction which is indeed a minority can be found till this day in Oman, Tanzania, Algiers, and some in Tunis and Libya.

The Ibadiya are Mu'tazili in their creed. They maintain that the Imam is to be chosen by the highest group of their learned scholars, and then the public. This leader should be one of the best scholars, of perfect character, bravery and able to lead the congregations in prayers and to fight in the battles. From early times, they refused what the Sunni claimed that he should be of Quraish or even an Arab. Of course, they refuted bluntly the idea of the Imams designated by God as the Shi'ites believed. In their doctrine of leadership—they resemble the Zaydi school, except that the Zaydis believe that the Imam should be chosen from the descendants of al-Hasan or the descendants of al-Husayn. Few among the Zaydi School accept any qualified Muslim as their leader and Imam. They can dispose their ruler (Imam) if the council of Ulema (learned people) decided to topple him at anytime.

The Isma'ili Shi'ite believe like the Twelver faction that the Imams are appointed by God and that there are only seven instead of the twelve of the Imamiya faction. They put Isma'il instead of Musa al-Kazim, who they accuse of being corrupt, and that was the reason his father, Ja'far al-Sadiq replaced him with his brother Isma'il.

Isma'ili's are an esoteric group, with secret associations. The assassins of Syria and Iran were one of their blood thirsty, well-organized secretive societies. They differed greatly among themselves and had many factions, the most important of these are the Fatimids which founded a dynasty that started its rule from Maghreb-Tunis and settled in Egypt where it expanded to rule the whole of Syria, Hejaz (including Makkah and Medina) and Yemen. In Yemen, the Sulaiyhal-Yemeni dynasty ruled in the name of Fatimids. One of its rulers was Queen Arwa (Sayyida bint Ahmed) who was beautiful, very clever and wise. She ruled Yemen for 50 years (20 years during the period in which her husband al-Mukarram Ahmad, the ruler, was paralyzed and 30 years after his death). She established the Bohra Ismailis of India, and that is why they pay her allegiance, and come to Yemen annually to visit her tomb, and her palace in Gibla in Yemen.

There are other offshoots of Ismali faith e.g. Druze, Nuseriah (Alawiyin). They are mainly found in the mountainous areas of Palestine, Syria, Lebanon and Turkey. They themselves claim they are not Muslims and certainly they are far from Islam.

Another Isma'ili sect which completely vanished were the Qarmatians, because of their extremism, vandalism and obscenity. They were courageous and caused havoc in Iraq and even invaded Makkah, killed the Pilgrims, and took the Black Stone from the most sacred mosque in Makkah to their home in al-Ahsa (the Eastern Province of Saudi Arabia of today) for 23 years. They allowed incest and shared among themselves the bounties, money, women, drinking alcohol, and allowed every type of vice that could be imagined. Fortunately, they were wiped out and annihilated by the Fatimids, and in Yemen by many factions.

The assassins were exterminated by Salahuddin two centuries later, and finally the Mongols who invaded Persia and Iraq in the thirteenth century under the leadership of Hulaku, exterminated many in Alamut Castle in North Iran near the Caspian Sea.

The Ismailis of today are the AghaKhani's of India, the Bohra of India (both are found in many other places), the Ismailis of Nejran (Saudi Arabia) and Northern Yemen. The Ismailis believe in the esoteric dimension of religion, and claim to possess a different esoteric explanation of the Qur'an. The Imami Shia also believe in the esoteric dimension of the Qur'an; but the Ismailis have surpassed any imagined limit in the interpretation of Islamic revelation. Isma'ili thinkers use Greek philosophy, ancient Zoroastrian myths of Iran and neo-platonism to formulate their religious myth. Thus for instance, they speculated about the Prophet and the Imams based on Al-Farabi's theory of emanation and regarded them as the "souls" of this celestial scheme. In the highest Prophetic sphere of the first heaven was the Prophet. In the second heaven was Ali, and each of the seven Imams presided over the succeeding spheres in due order. The last sphere is for Fatima, the daughter of the Prophet who was married to Ali, and who was the mother of Hasan and Husayn. She was, according to this scheme of emanation, therefore, the Mother of Islam and corresponds with Sophia, the divine wisdom. There were a number of Ismali thinkers including Abu Ya'qub al Sijistani (from Afghanistan), Hamid al-Din Kirmani (Iran) and Ikhwan al-Safa, the Brethren of Purity. The latter was a group of an esoteric society that rose in Basra, and had authored a number of epistles which included mathematics, science, philosophy and Isma'ili esoteric faith. However, the sect, unlike the Twelver Shi'ites of Iran has little influence in politics of our world of today,

Ahl al-Sunna wa al-Jama'ah, (the People of Tradition and Community) the Sunni Muslims:

They are the largest sect of Muslims and compose at least 80 % of all world Muslim population. They maintain the Five Pillars of Islam as follows:

(1) *Shahada*: This is the foundation of the Muslim faith. It is bearing testimony that "There is no diety except God, and Muhammad is the Messenger of God.
(2) *Salat:* Five religiously prescribed daily prayers.
(3) *Zakat*: Alms-levy to support the poor and needy.
(4) Sawm fasting from dawn to dusk during the month of Ramadan, the 9th lunar month of the (Hijra Calender).
(5) (*Hajj*/pilgrimage to Makkah) at least once in a life-time if one can afford.

The Sunni Muslims also believe in the six fundamental beliefs of the creed:

(1) Belief in One God, as the only God and Creator of all creatures, and believing in the ninety-nine attributes of God.
(2) Belief in all the prophets (124,000), as mentioned in Hadith of the Prophet, and apostles of God (more than 300), though we may not know their names and locations.
(3) Belief in all the Scriptures—(the scriptures revealed to the prophets of God). Muslims believe that the scrolls were given to Ibrahim (Abraham), the Torah to Moses, the Gospel to Jesus, the Psalms to David and the Qur'an revealed to Muhammad. Muslim believe these scriptures to be the word of God (before distortions).
(4) Belief in the Angels of God who were created from light (nur). They always obey God by their nature and hence always do good. Muslims know about the high ranking angels who have been mentioned in the Islamic tradition. Hence, Gabriel is the angel who brought revelation to Muhammad, Mikhael is the Angel of Mercy (Rain), Israfil blows the horn the Angel of Death (Izrail) and Munkar and Nakir, the two angels who are responsible for questioning people when they are lowered in their graves at the burial.
(5) Belief in the Day of Judgment and the Hereafter. Muslims believe that God will resurrect every dead body with new properties suitable for eternal life, who will be judged for their deeds while living on earth. The good people among them will be rewarded with life in Paradise; and those who did evil on earth shall be punished in the Hellfire. However, Muslim wrong doers will not be forever in Hell. Once they are purified they are taken to paradise.
(6) Belief in Destiny ordained by God. Everything that befalls us or any creature of God, is predestined and ordained by God, long before He created all creatures. The question of preordained destiny will be taken up again in this study as it is one of the divine mysteries that has divided opinions among Muslim sects. The Sunni also believe in the Pillar of Ihsan (Doing the best).

This pillar teaches that you worship God as if you see Him all the time. If you cannot see Him, then you are certain that He watches you all the time. This stage is only reached by few who constantly seek God, and feel God's presence in their life. They almost do no sin or evil, and if they do so they immediately repent and reach out to God.

This high stage is alluded to in a sacred tradition which is inspired by God but it is not verbatim from God as is the Qur'an): "*My servant draws near to me by means of nothing dearer to me than that which I have established as a duty to him. And my servant continues drawing nearer to me through supererogatory acts until I love him: and when I love him, I become his ear through which he hears, his eye with which he sees, his hand with which he grasps and his foot whereon he walks*" (narrated by al-Bukhari and others).

The transcendent God also has an immanent presence in a way. The aforementioned tradition indicates that a purified person becomes a saint whose actions and desires are in conformity with what God has prescribed in the Qur'an and the tradition. Hence, it is accurate to say that there is no belief in immanentism in Islam which maintains that God exists in and extends into all parts of the created universe, including the individual. Those who believed thus were considered heretics.

The Qur'an, the word of God, represents the presence of God in the midst of all Muslims, and each one of them has access to the Qur'an and can recite, this eternal word of God. By doing so, each Muslim can connect with God directly, especially during prayers (salat).

Majority of the Muslims, which includes Kharijites, Za'hirites and Zaydis believe what the Sunnis believe, with differences in interpretation. The Imami Shi'ites believe in some pillars of Islam, Iman and Ihsan, with differences in their interpretation, naming, and additional conditions such as witnessing Ali ibn Abi Talib as Walii (true adherent to Allah) and the true heir of the Prophet Muhammad.

All the Muslims agree that caliphate (Imamate) is not a political affair; rather, it is part of religion. The Shi'iite, as we mentioned earlier, believe that the Imams are appointed by God through the Prophet, who declared Ali, as the Imam. In contrast, the Sunnis believe that the matter of caliphate was left to the community leaders to choose the proper caliph through the process of "shura" consultation. They also maintain that he should be from Quraysh, the tribe to which the Prophet belonged, and that he should be a man of integrity and rectitude. Once he is recognized as a caliph he cannot be overthrown unless he is accused of blasphemy, apostasy, of being completely incapacitated by illness, blindness or mental disease. In other words, the Sunnis are against revolutions, since it leads to more bloodshed and worse tyranny. They yielded to the tyrant rulers, and avoided more harm, and bloodshed. However, if a revolutionary movement could succeed in overthrowing the ruling power, then they supported it by giving their allegiance.

The Origins of the Belief in Predestination (*al-qadar*) Among Muslims

To be sure, the Qur'an and the the Sunna provide a complex doctrine of God's omnipotence and omniscience, which led to support the notion of predestination.

There are a number of the verses in the Qur'an which appear to support such a belief:

The command of God is a destiny decreed. (Q. 33:38).

Indeed all things We created with predestination. (Q. 54:49).

In a tradition quoted on the authority of the Prophet he said, "You should believe in predestination, its good or bad, as ordained by God" (Sahihal-Bukhari, Kitab al-Iman; Sahih Muslim, Kitab al-Iman).

But there are other verses that emphasize the human responsibility:

Consider the human self, and how it is formed, and how it is imbued with its wickedness and its righteousness. He has succeeded who purifies it, and he has failed who buries it in corruption and darkness (Q. 91:7-10).

Verily God does not change men's condition unless they change their inner selves (Q. 13:11).

Every soul will be held responsible for what it had done (Q. 74:38).

The first people who used predestination as an excuse for their sins of blasphemy and worshipping idols with God were the unbelievers in Makkah who made excuses for their disbelief by saying:

If God had willed, we would not have associated with him any deity, we or our fathers. So did those before them until they tasted Our punishment. Say: Do you have any knowledge that you can produce (that supports your allegation)? You follow but conjectures and you only guess and lie. (Q. 6:148).

God condemned their attitude of arguing and making excuses for themselves to worship deities other than God. The hypocrites of Medina also argued with the Prophet about predestination, and found excuses for their behavior by saying that they should not try to do the good, since God had already willed for them to be wretched. On one occasion during the caliphate of Ali, he was asked about pre-destination by an old man. To this he responded: "God gave His orders to do the good and shun evil, but never enforced us to do it. We have a choice. However, God certainly knows what we are going to choose". This is the doctrine of divine omniscience.

Historically, the Umayyad dynasty encouraged the doctrine of predestination, and justified their rule by claiming that God had already given them the power to rule, even if they were transgressors. Moreover, they taught that resisting the authority of the ruler was like resisting the authority of God. This sect was known as al-Jabriyah, who claimed that man has no choice, and God has already forced him to do whatever he is doing. Even if they commit crimes, it is not their fault, since they are simply performing what God has preordained. This group almost disappeared after the overthrow of the Umayyad dynasty.

Another group known as al-Murji'ah, claimed that once you declare the belief in God and the prophethood of Muhammad then whatever bad deeds you do will not affect you. They were also supported by the majority of Umayyads rulers who indulged in sins and tyranny, but continued to testify their faith by tongue. This group also didn't persist for long after the collapse of Umayyad rule. The critics of the Umayyad establishment stressed free will and moral responsibility.

Truth of the Matter Regarding the Doctrine of Predestination: It is clear from reading the Qur'an that there are a number of verses that could be interpreted as supporting predestination and others that could be cited in support of free choice. Thus, for instance, the following passage:

> If good comes to them, they say: "This is from God"; and if evil befalls them they say: "This is from you." Say: "All (things) are from God." So what is (the matter) with these people that they can hardly understand any statement? What comes to you of good is from God, but what comes to you of evil is from yourself. (Q. 5:7879)

This verse has been explained in the commentary by Ibn Kathir [27]: "The hypocrites of Medina say when they get good things it is from God, but when bad things or mishaps befall them, they say: it is because of you, O Muhammad, as we have left our old religion and followed you. This is similar to what Pharoah and his people said to Moses. God denied their false allegations and said "Everything that befalls you from mishaps and natural disasters is from God, as it is ordained to be a test for you in this life. Hardships, misfortunes and natural disasters befall all humans, good and bad, believers and non believers; and it is only a test for their patience and faith. Then God explained that what befalls you of good fortune is by the Grace of God, but whatever befalls you of hardships is because of your misdeeds and corruption on earth. But God forgives a lot".

Imam Ali ibn Abi Talib explained the doctrine to the old man that predestination signifies the full knowledge of God of whatever we are going to do. But it does not mean that God forced us to do good or bad.

According to Ibn Qayyim al-Jawziya, [28] and a number of other Muslim thinkers destiny of God could be divided into two main parts: (1) Cosmic part which is related to the laws of nature in the whole cosmos including of course the earth and human beings. This constitutes the laws of nature, earthquakes, floods, tsunamis, storms, dry seasons, etc. For human beings, it constitutes all those matters related to our parents, nation, language, the era we are born or our genetic make-up, our ailments or the society we were brought up in.

It is the old recurrent question of nature and nurture and philosophy of determinism appears in different guises e.g. the determinism of Marx which is dependent on the tools of production, economic issues, or the determinism of the genetics, that we are fashioned according to our genes, and our choices and character depend wholly on hidden influences of the genetic make up. Some even claim "we are what we eat" and find excuses that determine our behavior or inclinations on this genetic make-up, or "the effect of that type of food". Ibn al-Qayyim agrees that we cannot control natural causes which, he says are ordained by God in His omnipotence and omniscience and His sublime wisdom. (2) The injunctions of Shari'ah, which God has ordained through the prophets and the scriptures. For that He gave human beings the choice of obeying or disobeying, believing or refusing to believe; doing good or spreading evil and mischief on earth. God says in the Qur'an:

And say: The truth (has now come) from your Lord. Let then, him who wills, believe in it, and let him who wills reject it. (Q.18:29).

There shall be no compulsion in (acceptance of) religion. The right course has become clear from the wrong. (Q. 2:256).

Are you going to compel people to be believers. (Q.10:99)

It is evident that the people have free will to accept Islamic faith and revelation or refuse it. There is no compulsion in acceptance of religion. In other words, all the commands of God regarding faith and Shari'ah are not to be enforced on human being, as they have free will. But God will judge them for what they do whether bad or good on the Day of Judgment. Accordingly, there is no compulsion or predestination as regards choosing the right or wrong, the true religion or the false deities, doing good or doing evil. Human being is entrusted with reason that can guide him to the true path.

Though there is a wide range of things that has been predetermined for man e.g. his color, his faculties, his misfortunes, ailments, natural disasters, his genes, the era or the nation that he is born, or the society in which he lives, or the language he has grown up with (mother tongue); nevertheless there is still free choice of man to hold him responsible for his deeds. If that free will is abolished or curtailed for any reason, then that responsibility is lifted, even by law and definitely in the Day of Judgment, for God is oft forgiving and just.

Imam Nawawi, a famous Muslim traditionist, in his commentary on the tradition reported in Sahih Muslim [21, 29] explains: "The predestination (al-'qada' wa al-qadar) does not mean that God forces man to do good or bad, and takes away his ability to choose. It simply means that God with His omniscience and previous knowledge knows exactly what he (a man) will do; and whether he will believe or not, or, will do good or evil, and what will be their choices and preferences. He exactly knows what is going to happen. But that does not mean that He compels him to take such a path. Moreover, and He never ordained that he will go astray and pay no heed to the revelation, and do all the evil deeds. Certainly Allah ordered them through His Apostle to believe, do good and spread peace, and give charity and help the needy and so forth, but He gave him the choice to accept or reject the true path, to do the good or enmesh himself in carnal egotistic desires and actions and spread evil and mischief on earth. The Day of Judgment will come when he will pay for all his arrogance and mischief".

Predestination and Science

We suggest a new approach to the question of predestination, using the findings of physiology of the nervous system (NS), which illustrates the integration of the autonomic NS with the central NS The autonomous nervous system [30] is a system that controls the involuntary part of our bodies. It is a part of the peripheral NS and runs along with these nerves, but relays signals in different ganglia (stations). It is divided into Sympathetic System thoracolumbar division which originates from thoracic and lumbar spinal cord, travels along with different nerves and relays the signals in separate ganglia. The medulla of the suprarenal gland is an important part of the Sympathetic NS. It affects the circulatory system (heart and blood vessels) whereby it can raise the blood pressure or increase the heart beats according to any situation that requires more pumping of the heart as in fight-flight situations. If there is a need for fight-flight, then all the blood in the reservoirs (liver, spleen, muscles) is pumped to the circulation, the blood pressure increases and the heart rate quickens, and becomes very fast. The muscles get more nourishment; the stored sugar (glycogen) is immediately released from the muscles and the liver. The suprarenal gland increases its output of epinephrine (adrenaline) and nor epineph-rine (nor adrenaline), which also increase the blood pressure, and cause tachycardia (fast heart beats) and the pupils widen, the muscles stiffen (contracts) thereby ready for the fight-flight. These muscles are voluntary striated muscles nourished by different nerves to do their job, but they are affected by the sympathetic NS.

The non-voluntary muscles of the gastrointestinal tract and urinary tract get less blood and nourishment in such a situation. The profuse secretion of epinephrine-nor epinephrine also affects the emotional state of the person and affect a separate system in the brain called the limbic system and certain nuclei in the brain which play a role in the psychological and emotional state of the person.

All the internal organs and viscera are not controlled by the volition. The heart and circulatory system are controlled by multitudes of hormones, nerves (sympathetic and Para sympathetic), a lot of reflexes, and by an innate system in the heart muscle itself with a special conductive system with pacemaker tissue starting from a node in the atrium (SA node) down to the node at the junction of the atria and ventricles (A-V node), and then a system of fibers through both ventricles. The heart will continue to beat even if all the nerves to it are sectioned. Even if the heart is cut into pieces, the pieces will continue to beat (idioventricular rhythm) [31].

The work of the heart is outside the domain of volition. Similarly the respiratory system is not affected by volition except for moments when a person holds his breath intentionally, but is forced by the rise of CO_2 in his blood sensed by centers in the brain (medulla), to go on breathing.

The gastrointestinal system is out of control except at the beginning when a person starts to drink or eat, but once the bolus of food or drink pass in the gullet (esophagus), then everything goes under the control of the involuntary autonomic nervous system. At the end when the person wants to excrete the refuse i.e. defecate, the voluntary system is called upon and the sphincters will not allow defecation unless the place is appropriate for this act. Similarly the urinary tract is completely involuntary except at the time of voiding urine, when the sphincters in the neck of the bladder control this act. However, if the pressure is increased in the urinary bladder, the person will urinate anywhere. In short, almost all the systems of the body are controlled by involuntary mechanisms. Volition only comes in a small percentage of the body activities.

The nervous and the skeletal muscular systems are partly under control of volition. The decision to raise my hand or write a paragraph or run, comes from the higher centers of the brain in the frontal lobe. The order is relayed to a motor area of the brain (precentral gyrus) down to the specified nerve centers in the spinal cord, through specific tracts, and from thence to the appropriate muscles to contract, and the antagonistic muscles to relax. At the same time, the basal ganglia (in the brain) and the cerebellum make these movements smooth and not overshooting. There is a synergy between many systems just to raise one finger or pronounce one word, in which the voluntary and involuntary systems of the body cooperate.

This knowledge offered, by the Science of Physiology, gives an idea of how things are complicated even in simple tasks of volition. The involuntary or pre-destined part of our bodies and life is huge, and we will not be held responsible for things which are outside the domain of our volition and control. God will judge us only on the part over which we have control and volition. The responsibilities among persons also differ, according to their abilities, intelligence, wealth, power, health and so forth. Those endowed with higher abilities, power, wealth and so on, will definitely be held more responsible, than the poor, ignorant powerless person. All, however, will have their just share of responsibility on the Day of Judgment.

The Attributes of God

Muslim theology takes up the question about God's attributes (sifat and names). These are God's beautiful names that describe God's essence and His actions. Hence, the doctrine that states God's uniqueness simply asserts that there is nothing that could be compared to Him is His essential uniqueness (tawhid). God is the ultimate unique reality:

> Say: He is the One God; God, the Eternal Refuge; He beget not, and neither is begotten;
> And there is nothing that can be compared to him (Q.112:1-3)

There is no deity but God, the Creator of heaven and earth, who alone can save man and send him spiritual and physical sustenance that he needs. Allahu Akbar (God is Supreme) is the call of the minaret, which is repeated five times daily, distinguishes between God and anything else. He is the Real Existence, while all the other creatures are ephemeral even if they last for thousands and thousands of years, as they will vanish one day. Their existence depends on His will, and they are always in need of Him, the *Samad* (the Eternal Refuge).

The name Allah is the essence of all the names and attributes:

> All that lives on earth or heaven is bound to pass away; but forever will abide your
> Sustainer's self, full of majesty and glory (Q. 55:26-27)

The world only exists because He is al-Ghani (rich and infinite); He is the giver of life (al-Muhyi), the Knower of all things (al-'Alim), the Producer of Speech (al-Mutakallim). Without these attributes there would not be life, knowledge or speech.

It is an affirmation that only God has true existence and positive value...The God worshipped by Muslims cannot be contained by human categories and refuses simplistic definition. Allah is the only true reality, beauty or perfection [32].

The assertion of the unity of God was not simply a denial that other deities were not worthy of worship. To say that God is One, is not just a mere numerical definition: it is a call to make that unity the driving factor of one's life and society [33].

One of names of God in the Qur'an is al-Nur (The Light). In the famous Light verse of the Qur'an (Q. 24:35), God is described as the source of all knowledge as well as the means whereby humans catch a simple glimpse of transcendence:

> God is the light of the heavens and earth. The parable of His light, as it were, that of a niche containing a lamp; the lamp is enclosed in glass, the glass shining like a radiant star; a lamp lit from a blessed tree-an olive tree that is neither of the East nor of the West-the oil whereof (is so bright that it) would well-nigh give light (of itself), even though fire had not touched it; light upon light. (Q. 24:35).

The participle "as it were (*ka* in Arabic)" is a reminder of the essentially symbolic nature of the Qur'anic discourse about God. Therefore, the Light is not God himself, but refers to the enlightenment which He bestows on a particular revelation (the Lamp) which shines in the heart of an individual (the Niche). The light itself cannot be identified wholly with any one of its bearers, but is common to them all. As Muslim commentators (especially al-Ghazali) pointed out, light is a particularly good symbol for the divine Reality, which transcends time and space. The image of the olive tree in this verse was interpreted as allusion to the continuity of revelation, which springs from the "root" and branches into multifarious variety of religious experience that cannot be identified with or confused by any one particular tradition or locality; it is neither of the East nor the West [34].

Some of the attributes describe the essence of God (*al-dhat*). For instance, Power, Knowledge, Will, Hearing, Sight and Speech were attributed to God in the Qur'an. However, they were distinct from God's unknowable essence, which always would elude simplistic understanding [35]. The Qur'an is the eternal word of God. The Mu'tazilite theologians alleged that Qur'an is not eternal but was created by God, like any of His creatures. This is one of the items where Mu'tazali differed greatly from other Sunni theologians. For example, al Karabasi [36] a later Mu'tazili declared that the written and spoken Arabic of the Qur'an was uncreated in so far as it partook of God's eternal speech, but once it is written or recited by humans, their action and doing so is definitely created, as humans are but the creatures of God. This notion is agreed upon by a number of Sunni theologians like Abu al-Hasan al-Ash'ari (260–330) and Abu Mansur Al Maturidi (d 337), and even Ahmed ibn Hanbal said it at one stage, but later refused to say anything except that the Qur'an is the actual word of God [37]. Some of his followers, later on, claimed that even the recitation or the written Qur'an is the eternal word of God. It seems more of a bickering, for all the Sunni, and most of other sects apart from Mu'tazilis, agree that the Qur'an is the pristine eternal word of God. The actual writing or reciting by humans is an act done by mortals and creatures of God and hence, their act is perforce created. God said in the Qur'an:

But there comes not to them a newly revealed message from (God) Most Gracious, but they turn away therefrom (Q. 26:5).

The word "anew" (muhdath in Arabic) denotes to some that it is not the everlasting old eternal word of God. In fact, the Mu'tazilis were responding to polemics of Christians (Youhanna Al Dimshqi/Jonathan of Damascus) who argued that the Qur'an said that Jesus is the Word of God, and the Muslims say that the Qur'an is the eternal word of God and is an attribute of His essence. Similarly, Jesus is the word of God and is an attribute of His essence. That type of argument led the Mu'tazilis to claim that the Qur'an is a creation of God, and not an attribute of His essence.

The Mu'tazila also refused the separation of the 99 attributes (names) of God into attributes of essence, and attributes of property or character (al-Sifat). They claim this paves the way to claiming many forms for God, that will end to what the Christians or other idol worshippers say. According to Abdulaiz Sachedina's extrapolation [38], the Mu'tazili doctrine of the "created Qur'an" signified the historical Qur'an which only reflects the historical circumstances of the original divine command, and should be, therefore, interpreted in lieu of the cultural and historical environment at the time of revelation. "Quantitive and Qualitative changes in the modern Muslim world have raised questions about the relevance of traditional readings of the revelation to contemporary ethical and social exigencies".

He is not alone in this assertion. Some of the liberal modern secular Muslim thinkers like Muhammad Abid Al Jabri of Morocco, who wrote a book expounding this theory, also maintains a similar interpretation. "Fahm Al-Qur'an Al-Hakim". Another scholar who is a Syrian architect by profession, Muhammad Shahrur in his book, "The Book and the Qur'an…A Contemporary Reading" written in Arabic: "Al Kitab wal Qur'an…Kira'a Mu'asera".* Both of them tried to put the Qur'an in historical perspective and hence tried to remove the sanctity of the Qur'an, despite their effort not to expose these new allegations about the Qur'an and cover them with some praise, here and there. There are others like Mohammed Arkoon, Nasr Abu Zaid, Garoudi, Hassan Hanafi, and others who maintain similar doctrine, have played minimal role in influencing a small minority of Arab intellectuals [39].

Most Sunni, Zaidi, and the Imami Twelver Shia scholars bluntly refuse such allegations, and consider such ideas, as being instilled by Western secularism, who want to put the Qur'an in par with their altered adulterated scripture, which, according to their historians and even some theologians, were written by a multitude of writers in difficult times [40–43].

Objective Good and Evil

The Mu'tazilis and and other Sunni scholars, with the exception of al-Ash'ari, believe that there is rational good and rational evil, discerned by divinely endowed intuition and reason. Ibn Taymiya and his disciple Ibn al-Qayyim also upheld rational good and evil. Lying, breaking promises, stealing, arrogance, injustice are all evils or bad things that every normal person can discern. Similarly doing well, saving an innocent life, charity, justice, veracity, keeping promises and truthfulness are all good things commended by intuition and reason. Al-Asha'ri, however, claims that what some people consider good, others will consider bad or evil, under the influence of one's culture, education, tribe, or nation and the time. Human beings change their attitudes towards things from time to time and from one place to another. Sexual relations outside wedlock, were considered bad and evil. Nowadays they are the norm. Homosexuality, lesbianism, same sex marriage are nowadays normal behavior in many cultures, whereas they are still taboo in other cultures. Usury was considered a dreadful thing in all revealed religions but in modern times, it became the bedrock of modern economics and banking and so forth. Al-Asha'ri claims that it is only through revelation that we can discern the bad from the good, the wrong from the right; otherwise humans will differ.

Al-Maturidi (another Sunni leader) said that things are divided into three categories: (1) Things that the human intellect (reason) can discern that they are good: (2) things that human reason can know they are wrong; and, (3) things which are not clear or things about which people will change their opinion, sometimes accepting them as good and at times refusing them as bad. In other words, divine revelation guides humanity about such matters. However, we surely need clarification for the doubtful things, or things about which humans differ among themselves. In the final analysis, it is only the revelation that can guide humanity with correct answer.

The Position of a Sinner

Muslims are advised to repent for the sins they commit, as soon as possible. Indeed, in Islam humans should avoid committing sins because intention to do so is considered another sin. It is God alone who forgives, and expiates sins and misdeeds. If repentance is sincere God may show how some sins lead to positive impact of maturing spiritually. But what if a Muslim continues to sin without repentance until he dies? Muslim scholars differ among themselves, depending on the school of thought they represent. For example, the Kharjites maintain that a sinner will go to Hell and will never get into Paradise, even if the sin is not a major sin The Sunni-Mu'tazilis maintain that if a person has committed a major sin, then his abode will be Hellfire for ever. On the other hand, other Sunni thinkers maintain that if the sinner is a believer of Islam and God, then his condition will be judged by God. He may pardon him or punish him, but he will not be in Helfire forever. He will after sometime of chastisement, be brought out of Hell, and will be sent to paradise. The Prophet Muhammad or other good people of the sinner's family or friends may intercede and God will accept this intercession.

The Position of Philosophy in Islam

Although Mu'tazilite thinkers emphasized rationality and intellectualism in knowing religious teachings and developing strong belief through rational argument, overall, Muslim scholars looked upon the field of philosophy as outside the orbit of Islamic teachings. They were critical of philosophical speculation about God's existence and other metaphysical issues. Nevertheless, Muslim jurists endorsed natural and mathematical sciences, more particularly, medicine, mathematics, astronomy, which were all branches of philosophical studies. Muslim traditionalists were suspicious of the philosophical claims of superiority in reaching the metaphysical and moral truth. They did not accept those philosophers who declared that matter was eternal, and will not be destroyed, and that God does not know the details of things that happen on earth as He is transcendental and above all creatures. Some philosophers did not believe in body resurrection, and maintained that all the rewards and punishments are spiritual only. However, a number of Muslim philosophers rejected such ideas and theories, and, hence, were accepted by the traditionalist scholars. Al-Ghazali was well known for his criticism of philosophers and he wrote a critical work demolishing philosophers' metaphysical claims in his book entitled: "The Incoherence of Philosophers".

Ibn Rushd of Cordova who came almost a century after Ghazali responded to Ghazali's "incoherence" by composing a refutation entitled: "The Incoherence of the Incoherence" Ibn Rushd was a grand jurist, a physician and a philosopher. He supported the philosophy of Aristotle and wrote a book to explain it and make it more acceptable to religious people. The book was translated into Hebrew and Latin and was adopted by the Church. Thomas Acquinas supported the explanation of Ibn Rushed (Averros) and Aristotle's ideas became part of the Christian dogma about the world. However the Muslim religious scholars didn't accept Aristotle's philosophy even after being Islamiciezed by Ibn Rushed.

Mysticism (Tasawwuf)

When luxury invaded the Muslim communities, many devout Muslims became ascetics, refused to indulge in these indulgences and love for Dunya (this life). They preferred the Hereafter and strived hardly to curb the lust for fortune, property and profanity. They were respected most of the time, and tried hard to purify themselves first, and then spread their teachings to others, using the Qur'an, the Hadtih of the Prophet, and his exemplary character and Sahaba (companions of the Prophet [PBUH]). They had a great success in the masses, and sometimes a wonderful success with the elite and even some of the despotic rulers, cried in repentance. There were stories of some who gave all their wealth to the poor and needy and became themselves ascetics. The Philosophical part of the Mysticism appeared later and was limited to few, but they were definitely antagonized by the religious scholars. However, many of the Sufis were religious scholars themselves and that explains their acceptance all over the Islamic world.

Notes and References

1. Narrated by Abu Huraira in Sahih AlBukhari and Sahih Muslim in AlAjlooni (Ismail) (1983) Kashf AlKhafa wa Muzeel AlIlbas, 3rd edn, vol 2/165 AlRissalah Publication, Beirut
2. AlBukhari: Sahih AlBukhari Kitab AlAdab, Kitab AlZakah narrated by Abu Moosa AlShari Sunan AlNesa'yi, Kitab AlZakah
3. AlGhazali M Ihya Oloom AlDeen, Kitab Aajayib AlQalb, vol 3/9. DarAlMarifah, Beirut. (no date mentioned)
4. Narrated by Abu Suriaih in Sahih AlBukhari and Musnad Ahmed in AlAjlooni (Ismail): Kashf AlKhafa (reference no. 1) vol 2/450
5. Narrated by Abdulla ibn Omar in Sahih AlBukhari, Sahih Muslim, Musnad Ahmed. In: AlAjlooni (Ismail): Kashf AlKhafa (Vide Supra) (vol 1/484)
6. Sahih Muslim narrated by Abu Huraira Hadith No. 2245, Musnad Ahmed ibn Hanbal 2/507
7. Armstrong K (1993) "A History of God", Baltimore Books, New York, p 181
8. Taylor (editor) Encyclopedia of Postmodernism, p 101, quoted in Gaser Oudah, Magasid AlShari'ah, The International Institute of Islamic Thought, Herndon, Virginia, 2012, pp 303–304
9. Sahih Muslim, vol 4/190, Sahih AlBukhari, vol 4/162, quoted in AlAhdal (Abdulla): AlImam Ho'wa AlAsas, Dar AlAndulus AlKhadra, Jeddah, Saudi Arabia, 2nd print 2009, p 285
10. Abu Da'ood: Sunan Abi Da'ood, Beirut, Dar AlFiker: Kitab AlGanayiz, vol 3, Hadith No. 3207 and Musnad Ahmed ibn Hanbal, Dar AlMaarif, Cairo (n.d.), Vol. 6/58
11. Sahih AlBukhari, Kitab AlGanayiz, Matabi Asshab, Cairo 1958, vol 2/107
12. Armstrong K "A History of God" (Vide Supra), pp 142–143
13. Ali Shariati: AlHaj translated into Arabic and English, quoted by Karen Armstrong "A History of God" (Vide Supra), pp 156–157
14. Armstrong K "A History of God" (Vide Supra), pp 143–144
15. Narrated by Abu Huraira: Sahih AlBukhari, Sahih Muslim Musnad Ahmed
16. Armstrong K "A History of God" (Vide Supra), pp 149–150
17. AlAjlooni (Ismail): Kashf AlKhafa wa Muzeel AlIlbas, vol 2/173, not true Hadith, but correct meaning, mentioned by Ibn Abbas in Tafsir
18. Armstrong K "A History of Religion", p 157
19. Sahih AlBukhari, Kitab Bedu'o AlWahiy (vol. 1/pp 1–3) Matabi Asshab Cairo, 1958
20. AlMawardi: Adab Aldeen wa AlDawlah quoted in Dr. Samurayik: Madkhal li Marodoo AlHosbah, Nadwa (Symposium) of Hosba and Mohtasib end AlArab, University of Baghdad, 1987, Baghdad
21. Armstrong, K "A History of God", p 158
22. AlMasoodi, Ali ibn AlHussein: Morooj AlThahab wa Marden AlJawhar, vol 2/349, Dar AlMaarifa, Beirut (n.d.)
23. Ibn Abi Usaibi'a: Eyoom AlAnba'a fi Tabagat AlAttiba, Beirut, pp 171–175
24. AlMasoodi, Ali ibn AlHussein: Morooj AlThahab wa Maaden AlJawhar (Vide Supra), vol 3/5, and AlZahabi: Se'yar Ma AnNubala, vol 2/274 with many details and Ibn AlAtheer: OSD AlGhabah, vol 2/15
25. AlZahabi, Mohammed ibn Ahmed: Se'yar A'lam AnNubala, Musasat AlRisalah, Beirut, 7th edn, vol 4/37, 1990
26. Ibn Katheer: AlBidayah wa AlNihayah, Muktobat AlMaarif, Beirut (n.d.), vol 8/337–338
27. Ibn Katheer: Tafseer AlQur'an AlAzeem, Issa AlBabi AlHalabi, Cairo (n.d.) Surah AlAnaam (Cattle) 6/148, vol 1/526–528

28. Ibn AlQayim: Shifa AlAleel fi Masa'el AlQada wa AlQadar, Dar AlTurath, Cairo (n.d.), pp 585–591
29. Imam Nawawi: Sahih Muslim Bishareh AlNawawi, Dar AlFiker, Beirut (n.d.) vol 1/155, Kitab AlIman, Hadith Gabriel
30. Ganong W (1999) Review of medical physiology, 19th edn. Appleton & Lang, London, Sydney, Toronto, pp 214–220
31. Vide Supra (pp 76 and pp 522–524)
32. Armstrong, K "A History of God", p 150
33. Vide Supra, p 151
34. Vide Supra, p 151
35. Vide Supra, pp 164–166
36. Vide Supra, p 165
37. Abu Zuhra: Tareekh AlMazahib AlIslamiyah (n.d. and no mention of publisher) pp 150–186
38. Sachedina Abdulaziz (2009) Islamic Biomedical Ethics. Oxford University Press, Oxford, p 28
39. Ou'dah, Jabir: Magasid AlShari'ah in Arabic by Abdulatif AlKhiyat, The International Institute of Islamic Thought, Herndon, 2012, pp 292–293
40. Encyclopedia Britannica, 15th edn, 1982, vol 2/891
41. Hick J (ed) (1985) The Myth of God Incarnate, SCM Press, London (7th Impression)
42. Hyam M (1987) The Myth Maker Paul & The invention of Christianity. Harper, San Francisco
43. AlKitab AlMuqudas: AlAhd AlJadeed, Dar AlMashreq, Beirut, 19th edn. 2000: Introduction (Universal edition agreed by Vatican & International World Council of Churches [Arabic])

Chapter 3
The Origins of Islamic Morality and Ethics

The Objectives of the Religious Law (The Shari'ah)

The Value of Man

Islam differs from many other religions in providing a complete code of life. It encompasses the secular with the spiritual, the mundane with the celestial. Man is the vicegerent of God on earth "Behold thy Lord said to the Angels: I will create a vicegerent (khalifa) on earth" (Q. 2:30). He endowed Adam with knowledge of all things, as the Qur'an relates: "And He taught Adam the names-all of them" (Q. 2:31). The Angels had no knowledge of those things. Accordingly, Adam was on a higher level than the angels. It was for this reason that God commanded the angels to bow in obeisance for Adam: We said to the Angels prostrate before Adam; so they prostrated except for Iblies (Satan, the Devil) who is from the Jinn. "He refused and was arrogant and became a disbeliever" (2:34). Allah said: What prevented you from prostrating (to Adam) when I commanded you? (Iblies) said: "I am better than him. You created me from fire and created him from clay" (Q. 17:12).

The satanic claim to superiority is the source of arrogance. Islam considers it the worst sin since through arrogance all other sins are committed. Adam and his progeny were honored by God, as the Qur'an says: "We honored the progeny of Adam ... and preferred them over many of what We have created with (definite) preference" (Q. 12:70). According to the Qur'an there is no original sin. Adam repented from his mistake of eating from the fruit of the forbidden tree, by the deceit and trick of Satan. (Q. 7:19–23). Adam and Eve both repented and God accepted their repentance, and were forgiven. The Qur'an has recorded what Adam and Eve said to God:

> Our Lord, we have wronged ourselves; and if You do not forgive us and have mercy upon us, we will be surely among the losers (Q. 7:23).

© The Author(s) 2015
M.A. Al-Bar and H. Chamsi-Pasha, *Contemporary Bioethics*,
DOI 10.1007/978-3-319-18428-9_3

God warned the children of Adam not to repeat the mistake of their father and obey the luring of Satan:

O children of Adam, let not Satan tempt you as He removed your parents from Paradise. We have made the devils allies to those who do not believe (Q. 7:27).

In another passage, God warns the children of Adam not to follow Satan (Iblies) as he is their enemy:

Will you take him (Satan) and his descendents as allies other than Me, while they are enemies to you? Wretched it is for the wrongdoers as exchange (Q. 18:50).

Freeing humanity from the original sin, empowering human beings, and giving them full responsibility of their actions is the message of the Qur'an: "Every soul will be held responsible for what it had done" (Q. 74:38)—is the essence of morality and ethics in Islam.

In the previous chapter, the subject of predestination and free will was fully discussed. We now need to turn our attention to the philosophy of Islamic religious law by closely exploring the Purposes of the Shari'ah (maqasid).

The Aims of Islamic Religious Law

The five cardinal essentials of Islamic teachings are:

(1) Preservation of Faith (din)
(2) Preservation of Life (al-nafs)
(3) Preservation of Mind (al-'aql)
(4) Preservation of Progeny (al-nasl)
(5) Preservation of Honor (al-'irdh)
(6) Preservation of Property (al-mal)

Anything that is deleterious to the above should be avoided, and anything that will preserve the above is meritorious and should be done.

Ibn Qayyim [1] said: "Al-Shari'ah fundamentals are built on keeping the interests (masalih) of the people during this life and hereafter. These objectives are built on justice, mercy, wisdom and interest of the creatures. Therefore, any situation which perverts from justice to injustice, from mercy to cruelty, from wisdom and utility to chaos and futility is outside the scope of Shari'ah."

The aims of Shari'ah were discussed fully by Muslim scholars 1,000 years ago. For instance, Imam al-Juwayni (d 478/1185) said: "The aims of Shari'ah are nothing but the interests of the entire humanity [2]." Imam alGhazali (d 505/1111) discussed al-maqasid under the principle of the public interest [3]. Imam al-Tufi (d 716/1316) defined public good as the way that fulfills the objectives of the teachings of God and His Prophet, and that public interest may be taken as even more important than what we might understand from textual proof based on Islamic revelatory sources like the Qur'an or the Sunna [4].

The objectives of the Shari'ah could be divided into three parts [4]:

(1) **Necessities (daruriyat)**: These include preservation of faith, life, mind, progeny, property. They are essential for life, religion, and community.
(2) **Needed Things (hajiyat)**: These are needed for the community, or for persons. They can live without procuring them, but they are recognized needs for the welfare of society and individuals.
(3) **Recommended (tahsiniyat)**: They are also needed by the society or individuals to make life more comfortable and, more beautiful, and try to reach the level of satisfaction and happiness for both the individual and society.

Contemporary Muslim scholars discuss three levels for objectives of Islamic teachings [5]:

(1) **Common aims** which involve the necessities and the needs of individuals and public, and justice, universality, and making things easy when obstacles arise.
(2) **Partial aims** which search for the telos or rationale of certain texts of the Qur'an or Hadith. An example is the prohibition of wine, the rationale is intoxication, and henceforth any intoxicant substance, e.g., spirits, beer, or even drugs that can cause intoxication are all considered prohibited.
(3) **Special aims** which seek the interests of children, or wives or family as a whole; or means that will deter criminals from inflicting their crimes; or means that will prevent mismanagement of contracts; or prerogatives of persons or companies that will end in harming the whole community.

Contemporary Muslim scholars stress the interest of the communities rather than the interests of individuals or certain groups. Many would expand their view to humanity anywhere. Instead of the Islamic emancipation of slaves, which is no more relevant nowadays, they stress liberty (freedom), as a wider scope which involves all human beings [6, 7]. Sheikh Mohammed AlGhazali (d 1996) called for making justice and liberty in the forefront of aims of Islamic teachings [8]. Sheikh Yusuf al-Qardawi (born 1926) called for the dignity of humans, purifying the human soul from its vices, the equality of women, building human cooperation for a just non-belligerent new world as the most salient topics of aims of the Shari'ah [9].

It is important to emphasize that intention (niyya) is very important in any deed in Islam. The Prophet said: "Deeds are judged by intention [10]." An action though maybe good apparently, but done with bad intention will be judged by God on the Day of Judgement, and will be punished. On the contrary, if someone intends to do a good deed, but when performing it, he unintentionally produced some harm, then he will be pardoned. The prayer in the Qur'an touches upon this theme: "Our Lord do not impose blame upon us if we have forgotten or erred" (Q. 2/286). The Muslim community should not accept injustice or tyranny. The Qur'an states clearly: "Let there be a community among you who call to the good, enjoin the right and forbid the wrong. They are the ones who have success" (Q. 3:104). In a tradition reported on the authority of the Prophet he said: "The highest form of striving (in God's path, the jihad) is to speak up for truth in the face of a ruler who deviates from the right path [11]." He also said: "If any of you sees something evil, he should set it right by his hand; if he is unable to do so then by his tongue, and if he is unable to do even that, then within his heart-but this is the weakest form of faith [12]." In addition, he said: "If people see a wrongdoer, but do not try to stop him, it is most likely that God will punish them all [13]."

The point to be stressed is that justice should be the norm in Muslim communities, and if injustice and aberration occur it should be corrected. However, during Islamic history, the despots ruled over with injustice and tyranny. Many revolutions were crushed, as we have alluded to in the previous chapter (revolution of al-Husayn, and his grandson Zaid ibn Ali Zain Abdeen ibn al-Husayn, the revolts of the Kharijites, and so on). The Sunni school discouraged revolutions, since they led to more bloodshed, tyranny, and despotism. However, they legitimized the revolution that was successful.

The Importance of the Preservation of the Five Objectives

(I) Religion: Islam is the religion of all the Prophets and Messengers of God. Islam means submission to God. Since monotheism is the religion of God from primordial times, then it should be defended, expounded and proclaimed. However, there is no compulsion in religion, as the Qur'an declares: "There shall be no compulsion in (acceptance of) the religion. The right course has become clear from the wrong" (Q. 2:256). In another passage the Qur'an says:

> And say: The truth is from your Lord, so whoever wills let him believe; and whoever wills let him disbelieve (Q. 18:29). Are you going (O Muhammad) to compel the people to believe? (Q. 10:99). You are not in control of them (Q. 88:22). And do not argue with the People of the Book (Scripture) except in a way that is best... and say: We believe in that which has been revealed to us and revealed to you. And our God and your God is one, and we are Muslim (in submission) to Him (Q. 29:46).

The Qur'an is replete with such verses, which promote freedom of religion. Jews, Christians, Zoroastrians, and Sabians were all given the Freedom of Faith. Similarly Magians, Hindus, and Buddhists and all idol worshipers outside Arabia, were never forced to adopt Islam. The Muslim conquerors of Persia, India, Afghanistan, and Central Asia found different religions, but they were all given freedom of religion and faith. Similarly Muslims conquering Egypt, North Africa, and Sudan gave all these different populations freedom of faith, and even freedom to have their own laws. The head of Jews (Ga'on) was ruling over the Jews in Baghdad and every Muslim capital. Similarly the Patriarch of Alexandria ruled over Copts of Egypt, and Patriarch of Antioch ruled over the Christians of Syria. Not only that they ruled in religious matters, but they also ruled on family affairs, litigations, and over all their mundane affairs if they wished to present their cases to their leaders.

The Qur'an says: When the Jews came to the Prophet to adjudicate in a case of a Jewish woman who committed adultery, the Qur'an responded in these words: "But how is that they come to you for judgment while they have the Torah, in which is the judgment of God (which was stoning for adultery). Then they turn away, (even) after that; but those are not in fact believers (in Torah)" (Q. 5:43). The Jews said to themselves let us go to Muhammad in this case of adultery. If he gave a judgment other than stoning (which is the rule of Torah) accept it, but if he insists on Torah rule, then abandon it.

And God told the Prophet: "Judge between them or turn away from them. And if you turn away from them-never will they harm you at all. If you judge, judge between them with justice. Indeed God loves those who act justly" (Q. 5/42).

They were given the choice to have their own judges; but if they came to you O Muhammad (PBUH) (or any Muslim judge) then judge with justice. The Jews in Medina had a peaceful pact with the Prophet Muhammad (PBUH), but they didn't keep their pact. Some of them tried to assassinate him, while others tried to bewitch him and even poison him, but many remained peaceful. A hypocrite stole a shield, and when he was accused of stealing, he threw the shield into his Jewish neighbor's house, and accused the Jew of stealing the shield. His family supported him, and the Prophet was swayed to believe him when they found the shield in the house of the Jew.

But the revelation came and exposed the whole truth in Chap. 4: 105–113:

> We have revealed to you the Book in truth so you may judge between the people by that which God has shown you. And do not be for the deceitful an advocate. And do not argue on behalf of those who deceive themselves. God loves not that who is a sinful deceiver. They conceal their evil from the people, but not from God. He is with them (in His knowledge) when they spend the night conspiring and preparing their unacceptable speech. Here you are arguing on their behalf in this worldly life but who will argue for them on the Day of Resurrection, or who will (then) be their advocate? Whoever does a wrong or wrongs himself but then seeks forgiveness of Allah will find Allah Forgiving and Merciful. And whoever earns (commits) a sin only earns against himself...But whoever earns an offense or a sin then blames it on an innocent (person) he has taken upon himself a slander and manifest sin. Was it not for the favor of Allah upon you (O Muhammad) and His Mercy, a group of them would have misled you. But they do no mislead except themselves and they will not harm you at all.

The innocent Jew was exonerated, and the hypocrite of Medina was incriminated, and the true balance of justice was administered. The Qur'an teaches that even with one's enemies that one hates. Justice should not be violated.

> Do not let the hatred of a people prevent you from being just. Be just that is near to righteousness and fear Allah, for Allah knows well whatever you do (Q. 5:8).

The Qur'an allowed Muslim males to marry females from the people of the Book (Jews and Christians) and allowed their food with the exception of pork and wine. (Q. 5:5). The Prophet himself married Safiya, the daughter of Huyai bin Akhtab, the Chief of the Jews, who was killed fighting the Prophet in the Battle of Khaybar. The Prophet gave her the choice of accepting Islam so that he could marry her, or remaining in Judaism and he could free her and send her to her relatives. She chose Islam and marriage with the Prophet after she saw his kindness and charity.

She became one of the wives of the Prophet and a mother of all the believers through out the ages.

The ruler of Egypt sent Prophet Muhammad (PBUH) Mariya, the Copt as a concubine. She adopted Islam and joined his house and became the mother of his son Ibrahim who died in early childhood. The court physicians from the time of the Umayyad dynasty in 680 until Muhammad Rashad, the last Caliph of the Ottoman Empire, were mostly Christians, Sabians, or Jews. Very few Muslims became court physicians. These non-Muslim court physicians amassed great wealth and influence. Bacht Yushu, the court physician of Harun al-Rashid (the Abbasid Caliph) had great influence on the caliph, and many ministers and leaders sought his intercession with the caliph. The vizier in the Umayyad dynasty and other rulers in Spain, was on many occasions a Jew or a Christian. Similarly, in Abbasid caliphate many Sabians, Christians, and Jews held important posts in the government. The Fatimids of Egypt (also ruled Syria, Hijaz, and Yemen) were fond of Jews, Christians, and many of their administrators were non-Muslims. Some of these ministers became Isma'lite Shi'ites and became leaders in this sect. Such was Ya'qub (Jacob) ibn Killis who was also the prime minster of the Fatimid caliph al-Mu'iz and his son al-'Aziz (Nizar). Saladdin had in his court many physicians (six Jews, six Christians and six Muslims) their Chief being Musa ibn Maymun (Miamonides).

(II) **Life (al-nafs)**: Preservation of the life of human beings is sacrosanct. "Do not kill the soul which God prevented except in the righteous situation" (Q. 6:32). The Qur'an declares in no uncertain terms:

> Because of that We ordained for the Children of Israel that if anyone killed a person not in retaliation of murder, or (and) to spread mischief in the land—it would be as if he killed all mankind, and if anyone saved a life, it would be as if he saved the life of all mankind (Q. 5:32).

Murder is one of the heinous crimes in Islam. Killing an innocent person is tantamount to killing the whole of humanity. Unintentional killing (manslaughter) should be redressed by:

(a) Diya (literally means compensation for loss) blood fine: which is the value of 100 camels of different ages (or 200 cows or 2000 sheep) to be paid to the the the family of the deceased. 'Umar ibn al-Khattab, the caliph, decided it would be 1,000 gold dinars in areas where camels are not available [14]. The compensation should be paid by the adult male members of the tribe (clan) of the killer (aqila), as they should bear with him this heavy burden. If a killer does not have that support then the caliph Omar made the administration to provide that. Muslim scholars today, allow insurance policy, since the tribal support and the caliphal administration are not available nowadays. This applies also to unintentional death or injury in medical practice [15];

(b) Manumission, i.e., emancipation of a slave. If not available, as is the case today, then;

(c) Fasting for two consecutive months to show his repentance for causing the death of an innocent person, though unintentionally. Murder, i.e., intentional killing, is punished by capital punishment unless the family or any one of them agrees to pardon the criminal. "O you who have believed, prescribed for you, is legal retribution for those murdered-the free for the free, the slave for the slave, and the female for the female. But if any remission is made by the brother of the slain, then grant any reasonable demand; and compensate him with handsome gratitude... In law of retribution (qisas) there is saving of life to you, O you men of understanding" (Q. 2:178–179)

Preservation of life entails seeking remedy, and that requires knowledge of medicine. Imam Shafi'i (d 204H/820 CE) said that knowledge (science) has two main branches: One of religion and the second of human body (al ilm ilman ilm al adyan and ilm alabdan). It is incumbent of the Muslim community to produce health professionals, and it is considered a sin for the whole community if they do not produce the required number of healthcare professionals. Ibn Sina (d 428H/1037 CE) in his poem "Al-'arjuza fi al-tib" defined medicine aim as "preservation of health and restoring it when it is lost [16]." He defined medicine in his textbook "Al-Qanun" as "the science, which studied the body of man in health and disease, its aim being to preserve health, ward off disease, and restore health when it is lost [17]. Abubaker Al Rhazi (d 932 CE) defined medicine as the science, which keeps and promotes the health when it is there, and restore it when it is lost [18]." It is noteworthy that they emphasized the preservation and promotion of health, which was unfortunately neglected to a great extent in modern medicine. Only recently have health authorities started to implement some measures in health preservation and promotion. Curative medicine brings more money, while health preservation and promotion gives the companies and health professionals little money, if any.

Al Izz ibn Abdul Salam, a renowned Islamic jurist (d 660H/1243 CE) in his book "Qawa'id al Ahkam (Basics of Rulings) [19]," said: "The aim of medicine, like the aim of Shari'ah (Islamic law), is to procure the maslaha (utility or benefit) of human beings, bringing safety and health to them and warding off the harm of injuries and ailments, as much as possible." He also said: "The aim of medicine is to preserve health; restore it when it is lost; remove ailment or reduce its effects. To reach that goal it may be essential to accept the lesser harm, in order to ward off a greater one; or lose a certain benefit to procure a greater one [20]." This is a very pragmatic attitude, which is widely accepted, in Islamic jurisprudence, and it is frequently applied in daily practice in all fields including medicine.

Seeking Remedy [21]

Islam considers disease as a natural phenomenon, and a type of tribulation that expiates sin. However, man should seek remedy. The Qur'an puts it succinctly: "And when I fall ill it is He who cures me" (Q. 26:80). Prophet Muhammad (PBUH) ordered Muslims to seek remedy when they fall ill. He said, "Never Allah sent a disease without sending its cure" (AlBukhari) [22]. He also said, "O servants of Allah, seek remedy for Allah in His glory did not put a disease without putting for it its cure [23]," "Some will know that cure while others will not [24]." He himself sought remedy and described medicaments of his time to his family and followers.

The jurists declared that seeking remedy may be obligatory in life-saving situations, or when there is an infectious disease that will affect the whole community. The person infected cannot abstain from treating his ailment, if it is available. In non-lifesaving situations and when there is no harm of communicable disease, seeking remedy is commendable and encouraged. However, in futile cases, it may be reprehensible (makrooh). It may be haram, i.e., prohibited if it involves sorcery, divination, or talismans as it encroaches on Islamic faith (creed).

It is also prohibited if it involves killing animals, using pork, blood, or alcohol. Only when no alternative medicament is available should these substances be allowed, and it should be prescribed by a trusted Muslim physician [25]. Not only should human life be respected and preserved, but also animals (not used for food) should be treated well and preserved. The Prophet (PBUH) said: "A man went into Paradise because he gave water to a thirsty dog" [26]. Similarly: "A prostitute of Bani Israel was forgiven and entered Paradise, as she gave water to a thirsty dog" [27]. On the other hand, a woman was thrown into the Hellfire because she incarcerated a cat until it died of thirst and hunger [28]. He also said: In every animal with a liver, there is recompense if you do good to them [27].

(III) Preservation of A'ql (Mind, Intellect, Reason, Sanity)

The preservation of A'ql (mind, intellect, sanity, reason) is of paramount importance, as with our minds (a'ql) we recognize God (Allah) and recognize the fidelity and sincerity of the Messengers of Allah. We use our minds (intellect, thinking faculty) to comprehend what Allah has sent, and to know the right from wrong. With our thinking faculty endowed by God, we recognized Him, and the world around us and discovered not only our earth, the universe, but above all our Creator.

> And in your creation and all the creatures He has spread about, there are signs for people who use their minds (reason) (Surah AlJa'athiya 45/4).

> There are signs for people who use their minds (reason) (Surah AnNahl 16/10–12).

The Qur'an has many verses (ayas), which extol using our minds (reason). But alas those who refuse their faculties of reason (intellect, mind, thinking) will be transgressors and abode Hell. "They say: if only we had really listened and used our minds (reason), we would not have been companions of the Blaze" (Surah AlMulk 67/10).

The mind (reason, a'ql, intellect, thinking faculty) should be used to reflect on creatures of the Lord and His signs all over. We are endowed with this great faculty, with which we can acquire knowledge, make inventions and build civilizations, and above all live harmonious life with justice, equity, and fraternity. However, man misuses this great faculty and spreads mischief and does evil. Preservation of a'ql (mind, intellect, reason) is the third most important aim of Islamic teachings. Masking these faculties by liquor or drugs is prohibited and is reprehensible.

Unfortunately, our great faculty of mind could be perturbed and swayed by egotistic, devilish desires, which will end in corruption on land and sea. Anything that will corrupt our minds should be prevented and that will help engender a non-belligerent peaceful just world.

(IV) **Preservation of Property or Wealth**: Wealth should not be squandered. The wealth of the person is in fact the wealth of the community and hence should be spent in the appropriate accepted way by Islamic Shari'ah (law)

The squanderers are the brothers of devils (Surah AlIsra 17/27)

Do not spend wastefully (Surah AlIsra 17/26)

Those who waste or squander their wealth should be prevented from squandering, as the wealth is not for them alone. It is the wealth of the nation: "To those weak of understanding (squandering their fortune), do not give them your property (in fact their property, but the community has to supervise how it is spent), which God made you to supervise; but feed them and clothe them, and speak to them words of kindness and justice" (Surah AlNisa 4/5).

Usually two of the relatives or acquaintances of the squanderer complain to the court and provide evidence of his mismanagement of wealth. The court will study the case, and if the plaintiff is proved right, then the court will take custody of the property (fortune, wealth) and appoint controllers. If such a thing happened to the debacle of 2008, where mismanagement was rife, the world would have been saved from the economic plight and depression. Islam prevents all devious transactions, usury, selling of imagined virtual values, and what is called derivatives. In fact, most financial transactions of the world banks and bourses are considered illegitimate and invalid if controlled by Islamic Shar'iah. Many of the industries will be banned, e.g., wine and spirit industry, breweries, tobacco industry, sex industry, gambling, etc., to name a few of the harmful deleterious industries. The world would be saved economically, financially, health wise, and global peace and justice will be forthcoming.

(V) **Preservation of Progeny**: Anything that is going to harm the progeny or lineage is prohibited. The structure of the family is a cornerstone of society, and marriage is the only recognized institution for procreation. Procreation outside wedlock is not allowed. Fornication, adultery, sodomy, and all sexual perversions are not allowed. Same-sex marriage, incest, child, and wife abuse are all condemned, and appropriate measures taken to prevent such heinous actions and transgressors and perpetrators should be deterred by appropriate punishment. If sexual relations outside wedlock become widespread, then sexually transmitted diseases will increase and new plagues will appear, e.g., AIDS pandemic. Most cases of abortion are done for girls and ladies outside wedlock. Abortion by itself is harmful to the pregnant woman.

Islam allows abortion for certain medical reasons, e.g., serious disease of the expectant mother that makes continuation of pregnancy hazardous to her health or even to her life. Similarly, if there is a severe congenital anomaly, then abortion will be allowed if agreed upon by a committee of gynecologists. This subject will be discussed in a separate chapter, later on. Anything that affects the progeny, e.g., smoking by parents, especially during pregnancy or lactation is considered prohibited (haram). In fact, smoking tobacco was considered "haram" prohibited, since its appearance in Islamic countries (about 500 years ago) and I (MA) compiled a book on most of these Fatwas until the end of the twentieth century [29]. There is nowadays a consensus among Islamic scholars to consider smoking as "haram" prohibited, as it is deleterious to health and kills 5 million persons annually as claimed by WHO.

Fundamentals of Islamic Jurisprudence (Usul al Fiqh)

All the laws (ahkam = plural of hokom) of Islam are built on the sources of Qur'an, Sunnah. The scholars of Islam if they reach a consensus on a certain point, then it is called ijma and becomes an important source. However, ijma is built on a text of the Qur'an or Sunnah, which may be evident or implied. There are many other sources of different Islamic Schools that we will discuss here after a quick explanation about the Qur'an and Sunnah.

1. **The Glorious Qur'an:** The literal word of God, revealed to Muhammad (PBUH) by the Archangel Gabriel which continued for 23 years (lunar) intermittently from the month of Ramadhan (July 609 CE) when Muhammad (PBUH) reached the age of 40 when he was meditating in the Cave of Hira in a mountain of Makkah (now called Jabel al Noor) until a few months before his death.

The first verse (aya) and Surah was Iqra (Recite/Read) "Read! In the Name of your Lord, Who has created (all that exists). Has created man from Alaqah (morsel that clings to the womb) and your Lord is the Most Generous, Who has taught (the writing) by the pen [the first person to write was Prophet Idrees (Enoch)], Has taught man that which he knew not." (Q. 96:1–5)

When the Qur'an was collected and compounded this Surah AlAlaq is Chapter (Surah) 96 in the Qur'an. It is not put in chronological order; the arrangement of the verses (ayas) and chapters (Surahs) were done according to the orders of Prophet Muhammad (PBUH) himself, which were directed by the Archangel Gabriel.

The last verse is Surah Al-Ma'ida 5:3: "Today I have perfected your religion for you, and I have completed my blessings upon you, and I have approved Islam for your religion." Some Scholars of Islam quote Surah 2 Al-Baqarah/Aya 281, as the last aya (verse) of the Holy Qur'an, "And fear a day wherein you shall be returned to Allah, and every soul shall be paid in full what it has earned, and they shall not be treated unjustly." More than half of the Qur'an (19/30) was revealed in Makkah during the first 13 years. The rest (11/30) was revealed in Medina in the last 10 years of the life of Prophet Muhammad (PBUH). The Qur'an revealed in Makkah were usually short Surahs (chapters) that stressed the dogma of monotheism, the life after death, the Day of Judgment, the salient fundamentals of Islam, while the Qur'an revealed in Medina came in long chapters (Surahs), e.g., AlBaqarah, AlImran, AlNisa, AlMa'ida, and so forth. It has lengthy ayas, regulations of life during war, prohibition of usury, details of how to write and witness contracts, laws of inheritance, prohibition of Alkhamir (intoxicants), certain foods (pork, carrion, blood, and whatever is slaughtered for idols). It gives more detail for a settled community with a formation of government, jurisdiction, and law.

Prophet Muhammad (PBUH) himself did not write or read, but he ordered a group of companions both in Makkah and Medina to write whatever ayas (verses) or Surahs (chapters) of Qur'an were revealed. Around 40 of the companions (Sahaba) wrote the Qur'an on leather, parchments, tables of stones, ribs of palm branches, and broad big bones (scapulae) especially of camels.

Many of the Sahaba (companions) by the end of the life of the Prophet (PBUH) compounded their own book of Qur'an in leather and pieces of parchment, the most notorious being Ali ibn Abi Talib the cousin of the Prophet and his son in law who married Fatima the daughter of the Prophet (PBUH). He was the first male to adopt Islam, which he did when he was a child of about 10 years, as he was reared in the house of Muhammad (PBUH). Abdulla ibn Ma'soud, an early Muslim from the Mekkan period has also his own collection "Masahaf ibn Ma'sood." From Medina, Zaid ibn Thabit and many others were well-known scribes (writers of the Qur'an). Hundreds of Muslims learn the Qur'an by heart.

When Abubakr al Siddiq became Khalifa, after the death of the Prophet Muhammad (PBUH), he waged wars against the Apostates of Arabia, and many of those pious who know Qur'an by heart, were killed in the battles. Omar was afraid that Qur'an would be lost if more of these Sahaba (companions) were killed and suggested the collection of Qur'an, which Abubakr agreed to and did. The whole collection of parchments, leather, bones, etc., were kept with Hafsa bint Omar, one of the wives of the Prophet Muhammad (PBUH). At the time of the third Khalifa Othman ibn Affan, some Muslims read the Qur'an and pronounced it in their own dialect (Arab tribes have as many dialects as their number). Othman collected the Sahaba (companions) and all agreed to write the Qur'an on the pronunciation of Quraish, the tribe of Prophet Muhammad (PBUH) himself.

Uthman commissioned seven copies, and each copy was sent to a certain locality, e.g., Egypt, Iraq Basra & Kofah, Yemen, Makkah, and of course Medina. This final compilation of Qur'an was made in 30H/650 CE. The ayas (verses) of the whole Qur'an are 6,232 and the words 77,934 with 90 Surahs (chapters) classified as Mekkan and 24 (lengthy) as of Medina. The verses dealing with religious ordinances of jurisprudence are around 500 verses only. Any translation of the Glorious Qur'an, in any language, is not considered Qur'an. It is a translation of the meaning of the Qur'an according to the knowledge and acumen of the translator. It never has the sanctity of the Qur'an, and cannot be used for recitation in prayers. Only Arabic language is the language of the Qur'an. All Muslims all over the world recite the Qur'an in Arabic in their prayers, and try to understand the meaning in a translation in their language.

Many Muslims, who even do not know Arabic, learn the whole Qur'an by heart and recite it in beautiful correct recitation!! This is one of the wonders of the Holy Qur'an. God, Exalted be His Name, said: "And We have certainly made the Qur'an easy for remembrance; so is there any who will remember?". (Q. 54:17)

The beauty of the language of the Qur'an is immutable, and its rhythm is suitable for remarkably beautiful recitations, admired by those who even do not know Arabic. The art of calligraphy was created by Qur'an's writers.

The Qur'an is the soul of the Muslim, and the center of his artistic attitudes. At the same time, it is the text from which all the ahkam (rulings) of Islamic jurisprudence are derived from. Only the knowledgeable scholar who is a master of Arabic language, who knows the meaning of every aya (verse), derived from the explanation of the Prophet Muhammad (PBUH), and his companions, and who knows when and where these ayas (verses) were revealed. Knowing the circumstances makes his understanding deep and henceforth his derivation of ahkam (rulings of jurisdiction) proper. He should know the historical appearance of these verses (ayas), so that he will know Naskh (abrogation of certain rules). The prohibition of Khamr (wine) took 3 years in Medina [30]. Alcohol was indispensable in the life of pre-Islamic Arabs. Tensions were high, tribal feuds, and fights were the norm, and for trivial causes, cousin tribes would fight each other to near annihilation. Family was disrupted. The Arabs considered liquor as a source of joy, benevolence, good food, and indispensable tool for keeping good health. A'isha, the youngest wife of Prophet Muhammad (PBUH), was quoted in Al-Bukhari [31] to have said: "If the Qur'an first told the Arabs not to drink wine and not to gamble or perform fornication or adultery, they would have said: "No, we cannot comply." The Qur'an kept putting in their hearts the fear and love of God, the description of the life hereafter with its paradise and Garden of Eden for those who obey, and Hell and its fire for those who rebel, until their hearts softened. Then they were commanded to stop drinking wine, adultery and gambling and they complied with."

Even then wine was not abruptly prohibited. The first verse was in Surah Al-Nahl 16/67, "And the fruits of the palms and the vines, you take therefrom an intoxicant, and provision fair. Surely in that there is a sign for a people who understand." This verse merely contrasted, "A provision fair (Rizqan Hasanan) with an intoxicant, thus indicating the difference [32]... The next verse to be revealed on the subject of wine was Surah AlBaqarah 2/219: "They question you concerning wine and gambling. Say: In both is heinous sin and uses for men, but the sin in them is more heinous than the usefulness." The third verse to be revealed on the subject was when one of the companions (Abdul Rehman ibn Owf) led the congregation in prayers, while he was inebriated. He made hideous mistakes in reciting the Holy Qur'an in his prayers [33]. Surah Al-Nisa 4/43 says: "Oh who believe do not pray when you are drunken until you know what you are saying." As Muslim prayers are all over the day from dawn to night prayers (Isha'), there is little time to drink except after Isha' (night) prayers. That was called by Arabs "Al Ghabuq." Certainly it reduced the consumption of alcohol in Medina. The final blow to wine drinking was delivered when a feast was held between Ansar of Medina and Muhajereen of Makkah was celebrated and Khamr was served. Once intoxicated they started boasting, followed by fighting with the bones of the feast. Later when they were restored to their senses, they were depressed and felt sinful and ashamed. At this point, the Qur'an appeared and announced that gambling and intoxicant liquors were henceforth prohibited for all Muslims through all ages. Surah AlMa'ida 5/90–91: "Satan wants only to cast among you enmity and hatred by means of AlKhamr (intoxicating liquor) and games of chance (gambling) to turn you away from prayer. Will you not then desist?" They cried: "O Allah we have desisted."

Anas ibn Malik (the servant of the Prophet said: "When wine was banned, the Arabs were still loving wine, and nothing was more difficult for them than to conform to prohibition. However, they conformed well. Every one of us who had wine at his home brought it out in the street and threw it away. For many days the lanes of Medina swelled of the intoxicant liquor [34]." Ever since that fateful day, Muslims—in general—all over the world have abided by the prohibition, and accordingly they are the least affected by alcoholism problems. Though Muslims constituted different nations and cultures, the majority of them kept their abstinence through the ages. This is due to the gradual prohibition of wine, step-by-step, which in 3 years succeeded to convert the Muslim Arabs who loved wine as a source of joy, magnanimity, courage, and indispensable tool of keeping good health, and using it as a medicament when they got ill. The USA Prohibition Act, the 18th Amendment Act of January 16, 1919 proclaimed "that after one year from ratification of this article, the manufacture, sale or transportation of intoxicating liquors within, the importation thereof into or the exportation thereof from the United States and all the territories subject to its jurisdiction thereof for beverage purposes is hereby prohibited" [35, 36]. The US government and law enforcement agencies tried hard to implement this act, but alas after 14 years of prohibition (1920–1933), the 18th Amendment Act was repealed by the 21st Amendment of December 5, 1933 [35, 36]. Alcohol prohibition lost the battle and no attempt to revise the concept of legal prohibition is likely to be tried again in USA or Europe or anywhere in the world except in Islamic countries.

The gradual prohibition of AlKhamr in Medina (3 years) time was amazingly successful, while the USA of the twentieth century miserably failed.

Arnold Toynbee in his book "Civilization on Trial [37]" said: "Islamic spirit… may be expected to manifest itself in…a liberation from alcohol which was inspired by religious conviction, and which was therefore able to accomplish what could never be enforced by the external sanction of an alien law…Here, then, in the foreground of the future we can remark…valuable influences which Islam may exert upon the cosmopolitan proletariat of a Western society that has cast its net round the world."

Even in the US where prohibition of alcohol has failed, Islam has proven capable of solving this intricate problem. Black Americans are maltreated since the time of slavery. In these circumstances insecurity, poverty, ignorance, crime, alcoholism, and drug addiction were rampant among black Americans, and many of them were beyond treatment and labeled psychopaths and sociopaths. However, the light of Islam entered the hearts of some of them, and they were remarkably changed. They stopped alcohol consumption, drug addiction, and crime and were completely resurrected. Baldwin [38], a well-known black American writer who himself converted to Islam wrote in his book, "The Fire Next Time," to his fellow black Americans: "Return to your religion (many of them were originally Muslims when they were snatched from West Africa and brought to the USA). Throw off the chains of slave-master, the devil, and return to the fold. Stop drinking his alcohol, using his dope, protect your women and forsake the filthy swine. I remember my buddies of years ago in the hallways with their wine and their whisky, and their tears, in hallways still frozen on the needle, and my brother saying to me once, if Harlem didn't have so many churches and junkies, there will be blood flowing in the streets."

> And now suddenly people have never before been able to hear this message (of Islam), hear it, and believe it, and are changed…(Islam) has been able to do what generations of welfare and housing projects and playgrounds have failed to do: to heal and redeem drunkards and junkies, to convert people who have come out of prisons and keep them out, to make men chaste and women virtuous, and to invest both male and female with pride and serenity that hang about them like unfailing light.

The miracle had taken place again. The Arabs of Jahiliyyah were changed by the Islamic faith. Similarly, the new converts in USA and elsewhere are changing. The eternal problem of alcohol dependence is being solved today as it was solved 1,400 years ago by a few verses (ayas) of the Qur'an which were revealed in 3 consecutive years, using events that make the effect of the gradual prohibition deep and effective.

If this is called "naskh" abrogation of the Qur'an, then it is a most benevolent and wise order, in order to change and redeem people without need for law enforcement, which fails in the end, as being exemplified by the failure of the Prohibited Act of Alcohol in USA (1920–1933). Now we can understand the advantages of this "naskh" abrogation with this vivid example of alcohol prohibition in the Qur'an. Unfortunately, some Western scholars (called Orientalists) tried their best to criticize the Qur'an for this so called 'Naskh."

The waiting period (the period for which a woman would abstain from remarrying after death of her husband) was mentioned in Surah AlBaqarah 2/240 as one year for which she will have full sustenance. But she was given the choice if she gets out of her deceased husband house, she will lose the sustenance. The repealing verse (aya) was made by the same Surah AlBaqarah Verse 234, which made it only 4 months and 10 days. This explains that the Arab custom for widow idda, was one year, and abrupt change in their custom would cause consternation. Once they had deeper faith, it was changed to the new regulation, which would help the widow to feel for certain if she is pregnant, i.e., quickening which usually occurs at 4 lunar months and 10 days.

Another example of naskh (abrogation, repeal) is the Qur'anic injunction, which orders Muslims to fight their enemy even if the enemy number is 10 times the number of Muslims. Surah AlAnfal 8/65 reads, "O Prophet, urge on the believers to fight. If there be twenty of you, patient men, they will overcome two hundred; if there be a hundred of you, they will overcome a thousand unbelievers for they are a people who understand not."

It was repealed by the next aya (verse) (Surah 8/66), "Now God has lightened it for you, knowing that there is weakness in you. If there be a hundred of you, patient men, they will overcome two hundred; if there be of you a thousand, they will overcome two thousand, by the leave of God; God is with the patient."

Anyhow, the scholar of Islam who can formulate Hokom "rule" should be well-versed and knowledgeable of both Arabic language and Qur'anic studies. He must be also well versed in Sunnah.

II. Sunnah (The Tradition) is divided into

(a) Sunnah Qawliyah the Sayings of Prophet Muhammad (PBUH)
(b) Sunnah Fi'liyiah, i.e., the deeds and acts of Prophet Muhammad (PBUH)
(c) Sunnah Taqririyah, e.g., sayings and deeds of others, which reached the Prophet and he approved of it (approvals).

Whatever the Prophet (PBUH) said, did, or approved, was compiled and collected later on in different books of Sunnah. At the time of the Prophet (PBUH) only a few of the Sahaba (companions) wrote some of the Sunnah, i.e., Ali ibn Abi Talib who wrote the amounts of compensations, Abdullah ibn Amr ibn Al-As who wrote many traditions, and Abdullah ibn 'Umar ibn Al-Khattab who wrote few hadiths.

The Prophet (PBUH) himself was wary not to mix the tradition with the Qur'an. Similarly Abubakr and 'Umar were more worried, lest the Qur'an be intermingled with Sunnah or Hadith. After 30H/650 CE when 'Uthman finalized the compilation of the Holy Qur'an, the danger of mixing Hadith with the Qur'an became less likely. It was only at the time of the pious caliph 'Umar ibn Abd al-'aziz (101H/703 CE) that the collection of Hadith started, since by this time there was no risk of mixing or mistaking the Hadith with Qur'an.

Imam Malik ibn Anas of Medina (93–179H/d777 CE) wrote his famous book al-Muwatta, which contained more than 300 Hadiths plus his rulings (hokom) in many Fiqh questions. In the third century of Hijra the most well-known Sunni compilations of Hadith appeared. Musnad Ahmed ibn Hanbal contained about 30,000 Hadiths. The compilation was according to the narrator of the Hadith at time of Sahaba (companions of the Prophet [PBUH]). This was followed by Sahih AlBukhari (the most authentic book narrators of Hadith. The compilation of Muslim is better organized than AlBukhari). AlBukhari (194–256H died 870 CE) and Muslim (206–261H/d875 CE), were contemporaries; and both travelled widely to investigate meticulously the correctness of the narratives and the authenticity of the chain of transmitters (isnad). The Sunan of Tirmithi, Abu Da'ud, AlNasa'i and ibn Maja appeared in the fourth century of Hijra.

To the Shia the leading compilation is Al-Kafi by Mohammed bin Yaq'ub Al-Kulayni (d329 H). The chain of narrators is different from the Sunni group, usually including Ahl Al-Bait, i.e., the descendants of Ali and Fatima. But there is great similarity in the substance of Hadith (Al Mat'n) in all Islamic sects, viz, Sunni, Zahiri, Zaidi, Ja'fari, and Ibadi. There are of course some differences in the substance, but they are usually minor ones, especially regarding Fiqh (jurisprudence). The differences are more salient in some aspects of dogma (already discussed in the previous chapter). The Science of Hadith (Ilm AlHadith) emerged to scrutinize the chain of narrators, i.e., Sanad, and the substance of the Hadith, i.e., AlMat'n. The chain of narrators (4 or 5) from AlBukhari or Muslim or Ahmed ibn Hanbal (and somewhat more by those coming a century later), goes back to the Prophet (PBUH) himself. If the Sahabi (companion) of the Prophet (PBUH) is dropped the Hadith is called Mursal, i.e., of weak narration, unless supported by other Hadiths.

The Musnad Variety Falls into Three Varieties

(1) Mutawatir, i.e., narrated "uninterruptedly" by several narrators on the authority of the Prophet, followed by several narrators down to the compiler, i.e., Al-Bukhari, Muslim, Ahmad ibn Hanbal, and so on. These are considered the most authentic as it is related by a group of narrators in each epoch of time. Accordingly, it becomes certain that the report is from Prophet Muhammad (PBUH), or the act has been done by him, e.g., the five prayers.
(2) Mashhur (well known) which was narrated by more than one narrator, but not reaching in number that of Mutawatir.
(3) Khabar Al-Wahid, i.e., narrated by one of the companions and then by one or two of the following class until it reaches the compiler.

These are also divided into sahih (correct) or hasan (good) or da'if (weak) and refuted. In matters of dogma, the Qur'an and Mutawatir tradition are obligatory to follow, while in jurisprudence and actual verdict, on different subjects, the mutawatir, mashhur, and khabar al wahid are used; but the chain of narrators must be accepted in a khabar al-wahid (narrated by one person in each class of narrators).

III. **IJMA** is defined as the juristic consensus of all competent jurists after the death of the Prophet (PBUH). It was possible to have all Sahaba (companions) scholars in Medina at the time of Abubakr, 'Umar and part of the time of 'Uthman. Afterwards, the Sahaba dispersed in many places, e.g., Egypt, Syria, Iraq, Persia, etc., and some claim that ijma after the time of the Sahaba is almost impossible to reach as the Muslim Scholars were in widely scattered places, and their consensus was difficult to reach. Many jurists including Hanbalis and others accept the agreement of the four righteous caliphs (the Rashidun) as tantamount to binding ijma. Others considered the followed fatwas of the Sahaba (juridical opinions) as ijma. Imam Malik considered the practice of Medina people since the time of Abubakr, the 1st Caliph (Khalifa) to his time, as a legitimate source of Islamic jurisprudence, as the people of Medina, lived with the Prophet and Sahaba, and their practice tallies with this important source. Therefore, Amm-aal Ahl AlMadina "The Practice of Medina People" is a legitimate source for Imam Malik. Other jurists, for instance, Imam Shafi, did not agree to that, and the practice of Medina people should be supported by Qur'an, Sunnah or ijma to be considered as a source. Jurists agreed that an expressed ijma is binding (if there is an expressed agreement of every single qualified jurist). However, Hanafi jurists considered the silence of the jurists to a particular opinion as an effective implied agreement if the silent jurist is acquainted with the issue and sufficient time has passed to research and express his opinion [39].

Both consultation and using juristic reason (ijtihad) are normal preliminaries for arriving to a binding consensus. The Kholafa Rashideen, the four righteous caliphs,

(Orthodox Caliphs) consulted the Sahaba on whatever a novel issue that arose. If they all agree to one opinion, then it is considered ijma that has to be accepted by all coming generations of jurists. However, if ijma is on an issue of war and peace, or of a political situation that is going to change, it is not considered binding for future generations of jurists.

IV. Qiyas (Analogy, Syllogism)

Dr. Isam Ghanem in his concise book "Outlines of Islamic Jurisprudence" [39, 40] discussed the Qiyas lucidly and succinctly. I will quote him here:

In its widest sense, the use of human reason in the elaboration of the law was termed ijtihad ("effort" or "exercise" of one's own judgment) and covered a variety of mental processes, ranging from the interpretation of texts to the assessment of the authenticity of Traditions. Qiyas or analogical reasoning, then, is a particular form of ijtihad, the method by which the principles established by the Qur'an, Sunna, and ijma' are to be extended and applied to the solution of problems not expressly regulated therein. Qiyas (analogical deduction) must have its starting point in a principle of the Qur'an, Sunna, or ijma' and cannot be used to achieve a result which contradicts a rule established by any of these three primary material sources.

When a new case or issue presents itself, reasoning by analogy with an original case covered by the Qur'an, the Sunna or ijma; is possible provided the effective cause of 'illa is common to both cases, e.g., wine is prohibited by the texts, and the 'illa" (cause) is intoxication. Therefore, spirits are prohibited by qiyas because they also cause drunkeness. So the prohibition is extended by analogy.

The majority of Muslims, including the four major Sunni schools, accept qiyas as a legitimate method of deducing rules of law. Indeed Caliph 'Umar in his famous letter to his Judge? Qadi in Kufa (Iraq), Abu Musa al-Ash'ari, wrote "Study similar cases and evaluate the situation by analogy," which is a clear direction to judges to reason by analogy where applicable. The Prophet approved Mu'adh bin Jabal's use of judicial opinion where no text in the Qur'an or the Sunna covered the point in issue.

V. 59, S. al-Nisa' (Women—Chap. 4) reads: "Obey God and obey the Messenger and those in authority among you. If you should quarrel on anything refer it to God and the Messenger". The istidlal or guidance provided is that if no rule obtains, then go back to the texts to deduce a rule.

V. 43, S. al-'Ankabut (The Spider—Chap. 29) reads: "And these similitudes We put forward for mankind, but none will understand them except those who have knowledge (of Allah and His Signs, etc.). (Q. 29:43)

Thus the four pillars of qiyas are:-

(1) An original subject (asl)
(2) The object of the analogy, being a new subject (far')
(3) The effective cause (reason) common to both subjects ('illa)
(4) The rule arrived at by qiyas (hukm)

e.g.,

(a) wine
(b) whiskey
(c) intoxication
(d) prohibition

This is the Hanafi position. Other schools invoke the hadith "all intoxicants are Khamr" (related by Ibn 'Umar and compiled by Abu Da'ud and Ahmad). In other words spirits and beer are prohibited by the hadith as far as most schools are concerned.

The following are leading examples:

The Qur'an (V. 9, S. al-Jum'a—Friday—Chap. 62) prohibits sale transactions after the last call to the Friday prayer. The rule is extended by qiyas to other transactions which distract Muslims from the Friday prayer.

The hadith deprives a killer from sharing in the inheritance of his victim. This rule is extended to the law of bequests. English law developed the same rule by case law.

Jurists also talk of categories of qiyas. Thus where the 'illa is more evident in the new case the rule is more applicable to it than to the original case. Where the cause if less evident, then the rule is extended only if the similarity is sufficient to justify the extension of the rule (hukm). This is simply a matter of degree or relativity, e.g., the 'illa in the case of whisky is stronger than that in the original case, wine, and so the rule is extended and applied a fortiori.

The Zahiri School does not recognize qiyas (analogy) as a source of Islamic Jurisprudence. The Shiite Jaafri School do not accept Qiyas, though they accept a similar source, which they call aql (reason). Similarly the Ibadiyya use what they call ra'y (opinion = reason). Both in fact use Qiyas under a different name. Some of the Mu'tazila, like Ibrahim bin Sayyar, refused Qiyas like the Zahiris (including ibn Hazm of Andalusia).

We have discussed the sources of Islamic religious law above in brevity and now we will discuss the other subsidiary sources for Islamic Jurisprudence briefly.

Subsidiary Sources

These subsidiary sources concentrate on public interest (utility) viz istihsan (Hanafi School) and al-Masalih al-Mursala (Maliki School). Another source is Sadd ul-Dhara'i, i.e., blocking ways and means that will cause change or evasion of Shari'ah rules. Istishab, i.e., accepting what is already there, e.g., the legal presumption of innocence until the proof of guilt is established. All things are halal and allowed in the absence of prohibition, and so forth. Urf is the custom of any group or community; and is accepted unless it violates a clear "nass," i.e., a verse of the Qur'an, or Hadith (sayings of the Prophet (PBUH) or ijma (of the companions of the Prophet (PBUH) or all the scholars of Islam on a certain issue and so forth). Fatwa al-Sahabi is the decision of the companion of the Prophet.

The laws of the People of the Book, which was not abrogated by Islamic teachings, could be used as a source of Islamic jurisprudence. Not all the Schools of Islamic Jurisprudence agree on all these subsidiary sources, but the differences are minor. The Hanafi School use what they call Istihsan while the Maliki use the "AlMasaleh alMursalah," both of which look after public interest and accept utility. All the schools accept al Urf. The Fatwa of alSahabi: (Decision of the Companion) could be chosen from several Fatwa's of different companions. Even then the jurists are not obliged to follow the Fatwa's of the companions, unless the consensus is reached (Ijma) and then becomes obligatory to follow.

Al Maslaha and al-Masalih al-Mursalah*

Al-Maslaha (the public and personal interest) is a major aim in Islamic teachings. It is not limited to this life, but to the hereafter. All the Islamic jurists who wrote on Usul al Fiqh (the principles, bases or fundamentals of Islamic Jurisprudence) wrote extensively on Maslaha. However, Imam Malik (d 179 AH/896 CE) of Medina was the first to write on al-Masalih al-Mursalah which takes care of public interest.

We will first discuss very briefly the Maslaha, and then discuss al-Masalih al-Mursalah (unspecified or unrestricted interests).

Abu Al Ma'ali al-Juwayni (d 478 AH/1085 CE) wrote his book, "al Burhan fi usul al Fiqh" (The Proof in the Fundamentals in Islamic Jurisprudence). "He was the first to introduce the theory of levels of necessity in a way that is similar to today's familiar theory", as Dr. Jasser Auda says in his book "Maqasid alShari'ah as a Philosophy of Islamic Law" [41]. He suggested five levels and the purpose (aim) of Islamic Law which are: The Protection of Faith, Souls (life), Minds (aql), Private Parts (al ourat) and Property (al mal). He also wrote another book called Ghiyath alUmam (The Salvage of Nations) which concentrated on Usul al Fiqh (Fundamentals of Islamic Jurisprudence) and Maqasid AlShari'ah (The Aims of Islamic Teachings) [41].

Abu Hamid al Ghazali (d 505 AH /1111 CE) [41]

Al Ghazali, the student of al-Juwayni was even more prominent than his mentor. He wrote profusely on Usul and alMaqasid in his books, "alwageez, alwaseet, albaseet and alMustasfa (the purified source). He was the one who put the necessities of maqsid (aims of shari'ah) as preservation of (1) faith (2) soul (life) (3) mind (4) offspring (progeny) (5) property, which are similar to his teacher al-Juwayni, except that he replaced alawrat (private parts) with offspring.

Al Ghazali differentiated between the true masalih and the imagined masalih (almawhumah) [41]. AlGhazali said: "Maslaha means fulfilling what Shari'ah was meant for: The purpose of Shari'ah is preservation of (1) Deen (faith) (2) Nafs (soul or life) (3) Aql (mind) (4) Nasl (offspring), (5) Mal (property, wealth). Anything that threatens them is mafsadah (corruption) and warding off is maslaha [42].

Al-Izz ibn Abdul Assalam (d 660 AH /1209 CE) [41] is another great jurist of Islam. His book, "Qaw'id al Ahkam fi Masalih al Anam" is a very important reference on the subject of Masalih, Maqasid, and Mafasid. Besides extensive investigation of the concepts of maslaha (interest) and mischief or corruption (mafsada), al-Izz ibn Abdul Assalam linked the validity of rulings to their purposes. He said, "It is unlawful to overlook any common good or support any act of mischief in any situation, even if you have no specific evidence from the script, consensus or analogy [41]."

Ibn alQayyim (d 748 AH /1347 CE) [41]

Ibn alQayyim is his book, "I'lam alMuwaqqi'in an Rabi alAmeen" [43] said: "Shari'ah is based on wisdom and achieving people's welfare in this world and the afterlife (hereafter). Shari'ah is all about justice, mercy, wisdom, and good. Thus any ruling that replaces justice with injustice, mercy with its opposite (cruelty), common good with mischief or wisdom with nonsense is a ruling that does not belong to Shari'ah, even if it is claimed to be so according to some interpretation" [43].

Abu Ishaq al-Sha'tibi (d 790 AH /1388 CE) [41]

Al-Sha'tibi built on al-Juwayni and al-Ghazali structure of necessities, but he was the most extensive writer on maqasid (aims of Shari'ah) up to recent times. His book, "al Muwafaqat fi usu'l alShari'ah (Congruencies in the Fundamentals of Shari'ah) is the classic reference in this subject. AlSha'tibi considered the maqasid (aims) as an integral part of the Fundamentals of Islamic Jurisprudence (Usu'l al fiqh). He even considered almaqasid as the fundamentals of religion, basic rules of the law, and universals of belief (usu'l aldin wa qaw'aid alShari'ah wa Kulliyat al milhah) [44].

Al-Shatibi considered the purpose (aim) of Shari'ah is to secure the interest (maslaha) of the individual and community, which he put under the three titles (1) Essentials (Dharurat) (2) Needs (Hajayat) (3) Luxuries or complementaries (Tahsinat). We have already discussed these above.

Al-Tufi (d 716 H /1316 CE) a Hanbali jurist who gave Maslaha precedence even over the implication or some understanding of the specific script and defined alMaslaha as what fulfils the purpose of legislation [45]. Many jurists wrote extensively on Maslaha (public and private interest and on unrestricted interest (al-Maslaha al-Mursalah). The search for public interest is given different names in different Mazhab, e.g., Hanafis call it Istihsan, Malikis call it Maslaha Mursala (singular) or Masalih (plural) and the Hanbalis call it istislah (seeking the best solution for the general interest). The Malikis, e.g., Ibn Rushed (Averros) and Hanbalis, e.g., Ibn Qudama occasionally use the term Istihsan (like the Hanafi's) [39].

Al-Shafi'i rejects this source as he takes the view that it could open the door to the unrestricted use of fallible human opinion that many contradict the clear texts of Qur'an and Sunnah. Shafii jurists say that they look after maslaha (public interest) and avoid mafsada, even when the matter is not mentioned either in the Qur'an or

Sunnah, by using Qiyas (analogy, syllogism) especially if they do not stick to the strict regulations and rules of Qiyas [39]. All the rules and regulations put by a Muslim government, which are not arrived at by the studying of the Qur'an, Sunnah, Ijma, or Qiyas could be resolved by resorting to alMasalih alMursalah (the unrestricted, unspecified public interest). For example, the traffic laws are easily brought under the Masalih alMursala.

The Malikis relaxed the degree of moral probity (adala) required of a witness in communities where the strictly desirable degree is exceptionally rare [39]. The hadd (law) of amputation for theft is not applied even if all the evidence and criteria are satisfied provided there was famine which forced people to steal. The Shafii would apply the same rule, because Omar (the 2nd Caliph) ruled not to amputate thieves at the time of famine. The Shafii accepts the Fatwa of Sahabi (Companion of the Prophet (PBUH) but not by way of Istihsan or Maslaha Mursalah [39]).

The important thing in accepting Maslaha Mursalah or Istihsan that it should not in any way contradict an ordinance derived from the Qur'an, Sunnah, or ijma. The eating of meat, which has not been slaughtered in accord with the rules, is only permissible where no other food is available; the extreme example being the eating of animal corpses in dire need and starvation. However, the human corpse is not allowed to eat, as some jurists deemed it a poison [39]. If Muslim prisoners of war are used by the enemy as a shield, then it is allowed to aim at them their arrows, if the enemy is going to cause disastrous defeat for the Muslim community, and if there is no other way of avoiding the Muslim prisoners. But if the Muslim community is not in danger then it is not allowed to kill the Muslim prisoners used as a shield by the enemy.

'Umar ibn al-Khatab ordered the spilling of the adulterated milk, as a punishment that would prevent deceit, and the sale of adulterated milk. 'Umar also erected state prisons. These are clear uses of almasalih almursalah. Malik gave several fatwas which are based on public interest [39], e.g., (1) The Muslim ruler may exact additional taxes from the wealthy in emergencies and time of need (2) the Khalifa (Caliph) does not have to be the most meritorious claimant, otherwise strife will be inevitable.

Murad Hoffman in his book, "Islam the Alternative [46] commented on Maslaha used by Islamic jurists by the following: "It is clear that Islamic Law thus remained flexible enough to take into account the requirements of public interst, but it was also open to reception of some pre-Islamic customs."

Istihasan: is used by the Hanafi School which means equitable preference or seeking the most just solution. It is defined as equitable preference to find a just solution. It is the preference of a ruling other than the one arrived by qiyas (analogy), when the rule is found to be harsh or contrary to the custom [47]. The Istihsan needs not to contravene a text of the Qur'an or Sunnah or ijma.

Examples of Istihsan [39]

Bay' al-Wafa (a sale subject to future redeem was allowed because of the practical need for such transaction). The prospective borrower sells his property back when he repays the price. The borrower gets by way of loan the price (to be repaid) and the lender gets the use of the property as a consideration or a quid pro quo [39]. The physician is allowed to see the private parts even of a woman if there is a need in order to examine her and treat her.

A divorce in death or sickness does not deprive the wife from her share in the inheritance, because the husband is trying to evade his obligation. The divorce is called the divorce of an escapee. The Hanafis maintain that entitlement of the divorcee last during the idda (the husband died before she finished her idda, i.e., the waiting period). The Hanbalis maintain that she will be entitled even after idda, if she is not remarried; while the Malikis accord the right to participate in the inheritance even if she is remarried provided the praepositus (the dying husband) did not recover in between the illness and his ultimate death [39].

Istishab: means legal presumption of continuances or the rule of evidence. The presumption in the laws of evidence that a state of affairs known to exist in the past continues to exist until the contrary is proven. The legal presumption of innocence until the proof of guilt is established is based on Istishab [39]. Things are presumed halal (allowed) in the absence of prohibition. A debt is presumed to subsist until its discharge is evidenced. A marriage is presumed to continue until its dissolution becomes known.

Doubt does not vitiate the validity of ibadat, e.g., if a man is certain that he made ablution, but doubts that he passed a flatus, he can do prayers without redoing ablution. A judge (Qadi) will presume ownership from valid deeds until the contrary is proven. Similarly if a person is missed in war or long travel and no news are coming he is called "mafqu'd," his wife remains tied to matrimonial bond until the court issues a decree to the contrary, namely death after due enquiries. All the Islamic Schools of Fiqh accept Istishab, with minor differences in the details.

Urf and A'da

Urf embodies custom tradition, local habit, and trade or professional code. In litigations over negligence or medical errors, the professional code, and the opinion of the specialists in the field will identify negligence from expected side effects of the medical or surgical treatment. Similarly, when there is a difference of opinion between the expenses of certain operation or medical management, the Urf (custom) in that country and location will be resorted to Urf is also recognized by all Schools of Islamic Jurisprudence. All customary (Urf) are valid as long as there is no provision in the matter in the texts (Qur'an or Sunnah) or other primary sources. The cardinal rule being that urf must not contradict any other clear rule of Islamic Law.

Examples of Urf

(1) Presents by a fiancé to his fiancée do not form part of dower.
(2) In partnership deeds, if the shares are not specified, then there is a presumption of equality.
(3) In the sale of immovable property the title to buildings, trees, etc., on the land passes to the buyer.

Actually in all professions there was a head of that profession (part of muhtasib functions) who would decide what the Urf (custom) decided when there were differences. Contracts to manufacture (fabricate) furniture or build a house will be controlled by the Urf decided, when there is difference, by the guild or the muhtasib (the Supervisor of the markets) or umda (mayor). The Maliki School gives more rope to custom than the other Schools of Fiqh, but all of them accept Urf as a valid source unless it contravenes a clear Islamic Law of the Qur'an, Sunnah, or Ijma.

Sadd al-Dhara'i

Al-Dhara'i literally means causes, reasons, or means. Sadd: means closing the door or removing the cause. The blocking of ways in the face of evasion of the Shari'a rules to prevent the achieving of illegal ends, even if the method involved is legal is the essence of Sadd al-Dhara'i [39]. It is in a way similar to al-Maslaha al-Mursalah which sometimes closes the door and sometimes opens the door to keep Shari'ah Law.

Examples of Saad alDhara'i:

(1) The paying of ransom to free Muslim prisoners of war is permitted and encouraged, even though such payments boost the finance of the enemy.
(2) The paying of specific money annually to the enemy in order to keep peace with him, when the enemy is much stronger than the Muslim government. However, the Muslim government or community must strive to build its forces, so that it can repel the enemy and stop paying levies to him.
(3) The prohibition of the cursing of idols and false gods of other religions that will be retaliated by cursing of Allah.
    This last example is clearly an Islamic, Qur'anic injunction.
(4) An official in the Islamic government is not allowed to receive gifts from the public, as long as he is in office. Any gift is considered as a bribe.
(5) Monopolies of essential commodities is not allowed.
(6) The digging of a well in the way of people without putting walls or barriers on it, is not allowed as it may cause children or animals to fall in it. During night there should be some light so that people do not tumble over it.

There are many other examples such as biya alajal, i.e., buying a certain good (car or house) at a higher fixed price, if it is to be paid in installments over a certain time (1 year or more). The increment of the price may look like usury (interest), but it is not. The owner will lose some benefit if he sells the house or car, and the ownership will be transferred to the buyer.

He will not be able to regain his property, even if the buyer failed to pay the remaining installments. The court will decide on the matter and if the buyer is capable of paying, he will be forced to pay, but if he is not capable of paying he will be helped by the community or government from zakat or other sources.

Shar'min Qablana (The Laws of Previous People of the Book)

The laws of previous People of the Book may be accepted when there is no other source that we can use to arrive at a decision. Most of the laws of Moses in Torah (Nomos) are either accepted clearly by the Qur'an or Sunnah or abrogated [48]. If there is no other source, e.g., Ijma, Qiyas, or the subsidiary sources, then it is allowed to use the law of the People of the Book, if it is not abrogated by Islamic teachings.

Notes and References

1. Ibn Al Qayim: Ilam AlMuwaqeen An Ribbi Al Alameen, vol 3
2. AlJweeny, AbdulMalik: Ghiath AlOmam fi iltiath Az'Zulam Qatar, Ministry of Religious Affairs 1400H/1980, p 253
3. AlGhazali M. AlMustasfa, Beirut, AlMaktaba AlIlmiyah, 1413H/1993, vol 1/172
4. Oudah Jabir (2012) Maqasid AlShariah translated into Arabic by Abdullatif Khiyat. The International Institute of Islamic Thought, Herndon, VA, USA, pp 31–32
5. Oudah, Jabir Vide Supra, p 35
6. Ben A'shoor (AlTaher) (1999) Maqasid AlShariah AlIslamiyah, Kuala Lumpur, AlFajir, p 183
7. Ben A'shoor (AlTaher) (2006) Osool AlNizam AlIjtimayee fil AlIslam, Dar AlNafayes, Ammam, p 256, 286
8. Quoted in Oudah, Jabir Vide Supra, p 37
9. AlQardawi Yousif (1999) Kaif Nata-Amal Ma'al Qur'an AlAzim. Dar AlShorooq, Cairo
10. AlBukhari: SahihAlBukhari, Hadith No. 1
11. Sunan ibn Majah, vol 2/Hadith No. 1329
12. Sunan ibn Majah Vol. 2/1331 and Sahih Muslim, vol 1/69
13. Musnad Ahmed ibnHanbal, vol 1/153, 163
14. Yacoub Ahmed AbdulAziz (2001) The Fiqh of Medicine. Ta-Ha Publishers, London, p 73
15. The Muslim Scholars Prohibited the Commercial Insurance Islamic Jurisprudence Council of Islamic World League 1st Session in 1398H/1977 CE, Majma Al Bohooth Al Islamiyah, Al Azhar, Cairo, 2nd Session, May 1965, and 3rd session 196; 6 and Islamic Jurisprudence Council (OIC) Second Session, December 1985. All of them allowed cooperative insurance in all fields including medicine and reparation for damage and injury
16. Al Irgoza Fi Attib is a lengthy poem of 1337 lines in which IbnSina (Avicinna) summarized his voluminous textbook "AlQanoonfi'Tib"…The Irgoza was published with other books of Ibn Sina, commented by Prof. M. Zuhair Al Baba, University of Halab, Syria 1984, pp 90–194, The line quoted is line 25, p 92
17. IbnSina (1987) Al Qanoonfi'Tib commented by Edward Al Qish, Izu'din establishment, Beirut, vol 1, p 13
18. Rhazi Abu Bak Al (1987) Al Mansoorifi'Tib, commented by Dr. Hazim A. Assidiqi. Publication of Institute of Arabian Manuscripts, Kuwait, p 29
19. Izzudin ibn Abdulsalam: Qaweed Al Ahkam (Basics of Rules) commented by Nazih Hammad and Othman Dharaniyah, Dar AlQalarn, Damascus 2000, vol 1, p 8

20. Vide Supra vol 1, p 8
21. Albar MA (2007) Seeking Remedy, Abstaining from Therapy and Resuscitation: An Islamic Perspective. Saudi Kidney Dis Transplant 18(4):629–637
22. AlBukhari M. Sahih AlBukhari, Dar AlMarifa, Beirut, Kitab Attib, vol 4, p 8
23. AlTirmithi M.I.: Sunan AlTirmithi, Dar AlFikr, Beirut, 1983, vol 3: 258 Hadith No. 2109 and Abu Da'ood SA: Sunan Abi Da'ood, Dar AlFikr, Beirut, Kitab Attib, vol 4:3, Hadith No. 3855
24. AlHakim MA: Al Mustadrak ala Assaheehain, Dar AlKutub AlIlmiyah, Beirut 1990, Kitab Attib vol 4: 218
25. AlKhatib AlShirbini (1978) Mughni AlMuhtaj Limarifat AlFaz AlMinhaj. Dar AlFikr, Beirut 4:188
26. AlBukhari: Sahih Al Bukhari Hadith No. 2363, Musbad Ahmed ibn Hanbal Muslim: Sahih Muslim all narrated by Abu Huraira Hadith No. 1073
27. Sahih Muslim Hadith No. 2245, narrated by Abu Huraira and Musnad Ahmed ibn Hanbal 2/507
28. Narrated by Abdulla ibn Omar in Sahih Al Bukhari, Sahih Muslim Musnad Ahmed ibnHanbal in Al Ajlood (Ismail): Kashf AlKhafawa Muzeel AlIlbas vol 1/484, Beirut, AlRissalah Publication, 3rd ed 1983
29. Albar M (1994) AlMauqif AlSharee min AlTibiqh wa AlTadkeen. Saudi Publishing House, Jeddah
30. Albar M (1995) The Problem of Alcohol Dependence and its solution in Islam in M. Albar: Contemporary Topics. In Islamic Medicine. Saudi Publishing House, Jeddah, pp 13–19
31. Sahih AlBukhari, Cairo, 1376H, Muktabah Al Nahdah Al Haditha, Kitab Fadyel AlQur'an: 66/6
32. Ghanem I (1983) Outlines of Islamic Jurisprudence. Saudi Publishing House, Jeddah, Saudi Arabia, pp 43–44
33. IbnKathir (1980) Tafsir Al Qur'an Al Azim, Dar AlFikr, Beirut, Surah 4/43
34. Sahih Al Bukhari, Kitab Al Ashiribah 74/3
35. Albar M (1986) Al Khamrbain Al Tibwa Alfiqh, Saudi Publishing House, Jeddah, 7th edition, pp 118–121
36. Miles S. Learning About Alcohol, Washington, DC: American Association for Health Physical Education and Recreation/A National Affiliate of the National Education Association 1974, p 23
37. Toynbee A (1976) Civilization on Trial, quoted in Badri M.: Islam and Alcoholism. American Trust Publication Muslim Student Association, USA and Canada, pp 14–16
38. Baldwin J (1962) The Fire Next Time. Penguin Book, London, pp 39–68
39. Ghanem I, (1983) Outlines of Islamic Jurisprudence, Saudi Publishing House, Jeddah, p 57 and 67–77
40. Isam Ghanem is a friend who got his M. Phil Law London. He was a lecturer in Law, Polytechnic of Central London and in Nigeria, and a Magistrate of the Superior Court Aden. He wrote many books and published many papers in Law Journals. He died suddenly after a heart attack in Yemen on the 3rd of August 2012 (15th Ramadhan 1433). His untimely dealth is a loss to Yemeni Scholars. His father was a well known Poet of Aden and a Scholar, his brother Shihab is a well known Poet in UAE who published many diwans of poetry and became famous after translating many poems from Arabic language to English poetry and vice versa. His other elder brother Qais is a Consultant, Pediatric Neurologist in Canada, and also a Poet in both Arabic and English. Nizar his younger brother is a Family Physician and Lecturer in Public Health, but he is well known for his studies of South Arabian-Sudanese-African music and dances. All the family members are brilliant
41. Auda J, (2008) Maqasid alShariyah as a Philosophy of Islamic Law: A Systems Approach. The International Institiue of Islamic Thought London-Washington, pp 17–21
42. Ghazali (2001) Al Mustasfa, vol 1/139 and Ahmed Abdulaziz Yacoub: The Fiqh of Medicine, 2001, TaHa Publication, Ltd., London, p 27
43. Ibn Al Qayyim: Ilam al Muwaqqi'in an Rabbi alAlameen, 1973, Dar al Jeel, Beirut ed Taha AbdulRauf Saad, vol 1, p 333

44. AlSha'tibi: alMuwafaqat, vol 2, p 25
45. alTufi, Najm alDin: alTayeen fi Sharh al AlArba'een, 1419H, alRayyan, p 239
46. Hoffman M (1993) Islam the Alternative, Garnet Publishing, Reading (UK) p 121
47. Yacoub Ahmed Abdulaziz (2001) The Fiqh of Medicine. TaHa Publisher Ltd, London, p 26
48. Good News Bible, Collins, Fontana, Glasgow, UK, 1979 Leviticus 24/17–22

Chapter 4
Virtue Ethics and Moral Character Related to Medical Profession

Although moral values are universal, their application varies in different cultures. In this study we are inclined to choose the following:

(1) Moral values are the result of habitual adherence to them. They become second nature as a consequence of habitually doing what one considers is right. This is what Aristotle maintained in his famous Nicomachian Ethics [1]. According to him all moral values and characters can be changed. Some Muslim writers on ethics accept such view (with some alterations). Tahanooni in his Kashaf Istilahat alFanoon wa alOloom "the lexicon of the terminologies of Arts and Sciences" says that morality "Khulq" is a habituation and nature, which is affected and directed by religion [2].

(2) Others say morality is innate and emanates from within the self, and cannot be changed (except with great effort) (al-Jurjani [3], Miskawayh (Tahzib Al-aKhalaq).

(3) Galen [4] combined the innate nature and temperaments, e.g., sanguineous temperament, which usually appears at young age and youth, but those of sanguineous temperament continue until their old age. All dictators, conquerors, and despots from Nimrod, Pharoes till Hitler, and Stalin have had this bloody temperament. Others have bilious temperament, some have melancholy, and at old age usually the temperament is phlegmatic. The theory of humors, which he proclaimed, controls the temperament and affects the character. These humors are four: the blood, the bile from the gall bladder, the black bile from the spleen, and the phlegm from the brain and lungs. The theory is obsolete, and instead of these four humors, the new sciences replace them with hormones, genes, and myriads of smaller factors from within the body and from outside the body, i.e., environment, which displays the effect of nature and nurture on our characters and morality.

(4) Al-Mawardi [5] divided the origin of morality into two main branches:

    (a) The innate ones, which are part of our nature, which may be good or bad, and is controlled by instincts and humors (of Galen)

    (b) The voluntary character, which emanates from the training and using our faculties. It is of course influenced by one's education and community.

© The Author(s) 2015

M.A. Al-Bar and H. Chamsi-Pasha, *Contemporary Bioethics*,
DOI 10.1007/978-3-319-18428-9_4

It seems that he is combining both Aristotle and Galen, with a strong inclination to Islamic ethos developed by the Qur'an and Prophet Muhammad (PBUH). Other Muslim philosophers tried to combine Aristotle and Galen, e.g., alFarabi in his book "AlJama' bain al Hakimain [6]" (Combining the two philosophers, i.e., Aristotle and Galen). Similarly, Miskawaih in his book Tahzib Al-akhalaq [7] defined morality as being innate, controlled by instincts and humors, but definitely can be changed by training, cultivation, and culture.

Tom Beauchamp and James Childress in their book "Principles of Biomedical Ethics [8] considered virtue as "a trait of character that is socially valuable; a moral virtue is a morally valuable trait of character … communities sometimes disvalue persons who act virtuously or admire persons for their meanness and churlishness." This occurs when the innate good nature of human beings is changed by a system of life that extols power and wealth, which become the most important aspiration for the whole nation.

It happened in Pre-Islamic Arabia (Jahiliyyah). The poets of that epoch extolled the character of doing injustice to others, killing the men, enslaving the women, children and the weak, and appropriating their wealth (herds, money, jewelry, or land). The poet (Zuhair Ibn AbiSalma, a Jahyiliah) said:

Injustice is innate in all persons …
If you find one who refrains from injustice then he has a serious malady.

It seems that many in the present-day civilization have returned to this old PreIslamic morality, which Beauchamp and Childress deplored.

The Motive

Motive and intention play an important role in the formation of moral character. Hence, the act may appear virtuous, even when the intent and motive are bad. According to some ethicists, such acts are to be classified as immoral (Beauchamp and Childress).

In Islam, Prophet Muhammad (PBUH) taught that acts will in accord be with the intention of God. If the motive is good and the act is good, the person will be rewarded by God; however, if the act is good and the motive is bad, the person will be punished for it. There are many traditions to this effect. "Deeds and acts will be judged by the intention and motive" [9].

In another tradition the Prophet is reported to have said that the one who taught the Qur'an and religion would be dragged to Hell. He would exclaim and say: "O God I have taught people your book and your religion, for your sake." God will say: "Nay you did it to be called a scholar (alim) and they did call you so." The other example is of a wealthy person, who donated a lot of money to the poor and needy, but his intention was not for the sake of God, but to be called generous and benevolent by the people, and it was said.

The third tradition is about a person fought for the cause of religion against infidels, but his intention was to show off his bravery and courage, and not for the sake of God. Though he was slain in the war, and the people called him martyr, God ordered him to be dragged into Hellfire, because his intent and motive was people saying that he was brave and courageous [10].

These traditions show how important is the motive and intent in Islam in considering the deeds and acts of humans, which will only be judged by God according to their intent and motive.

On the other hand, a number of philosophers consider a person disposed by a good character with good motives to be more important than another person who acts only because of the strong sense of duty. The right motives and character tell us more about moral worth than do right actions performed under the prod of obligation [11]. The friend who acts only from obligation lacks the virtue of friendliness and the relation lacks moral merit [12].

The obligation-oriented theories which replaced the virtuous judgment of healthcare professionals with rules, codes, or procedures will not produce better decisions or actions. The most reliable protection of subjects in research is by an informed conscientious compassionate researcher [13]. From this perspective, character is more important than conformity to rules, and virtues should be inculcated and cultivated over time through educational interactions, role models, and the like [14]. Nevertheless, rules and regulations are very important to regulate research and health professionals, as only few will reach the high standards of innate benevolent character of the well-informed conscientious compassionate researcher or health provider. Many have to be controlled by rules, regulations, by-laws, and laws.

The person worthy of trust and praise is one who has ingrained motivation with a burning desire to perform the right action, and possessing a caring compassionate sympathetic generous character [8].

The action must also be appropriately done, according to the state of the art (of medicine), and conforming with the relevant principles and rules [8]. If the physician or nurse acts incompetently, he or she will not be praiseworthy, and has to improve himself/herself to the required standard.

Prophet Muhammad (PBUH) said: "Any person who practices medicine without due knowledge of medicine (or that specialty of medicine) is liable" [13].

He also said, "No person is wise without experience [14]." Islamic jurists for more than 1,200 years put the regulation that no one is allowed to practice medicine unless he is given a certificate from the Muhtasib (the controller of physicians) that he is competent. The practitioner has to get consent from those he is going to treat, or get the consent of the guardian if the patient is a child or mentally incompetent [15].

Roles and practices in medicine and nursing embody standard obligations and virtues. The important virtues in medicine and nursing are:

(1) Compassion: showing active regard for the welfare of the patient. It involves both sympathy and empathy with deep mercy and actions of beneficence that attempt to alleviate the misfortunes and sufferings of others [8].

Physicians and nurses who express no emotions in their behavior toward their patients have a moral weakness. The compassion and emotions of the health provider should not cloud his judgment and his rational and effective response. If the patient is his own relative, he/she should abstain from medical management if his/ her decision is going to be affected by the natural emotions.

Spinoza and Kant have advanced cautious approach to compassion, fearing that compassion will blind reason and proper action. This need not be true, if the person is balanced, and the patient is not his near relative or spouse, or close friend.

Contemporary medical and nursing education inculcates detachment of the health provider, in order to avoid emotional involvement that blurs common reason and proper action. There should be a balance struck between the psychological detachment and sympathy and even empathy shown by the health provider to the patient and/or his family.

(2) Discernment: The virtue of discernment brings sensitive insight, acute judgment, and understanding of action [8]. It is related to the above-mentioned discussion of the effect of compassion and psychological detachment.

A discerning physician or nurse will see when a despairing patient needs comfort rather than privacy or vice versa, or when he needs a spiritual support for which the hospital should provide the spiritual healer, if possible. For Muslims, a religious advisor may be a member of the staff of the hospital. Otherwise the patient or his relatives may provide their own advisor and instructor.

(3) Trustworthiness [8]

The physician/nurse should be trustworthy. It emanates from the belief of the patient that his physician/nurse have both technical competence, the required knowledge, and good moral character. Trust is the most important ingredient in the relation between the patient and the health providers. Many of the allegations and litigations against health providers are rooted in mistrust. The media exposing and magnifying physicians' mistakes erodes the trust of the public with the medical profession. In Arab countries the mushrooming private hospitals, run for business and profit, with some graphic and horrific mistakes published in the media (one surgeon alleged to have killed 20 patients in operations to treat obesity), caused public consternation and loss of trust in the medical profession as a whole [16]. The government hospitals are notorious for being overcrowded with long waiting lists unless you have a friend (crony) of some authority in one of these hospitals, or you are of some status and influence to harness any difficulty.

It is unfortunate that "trust is a fading ideal in contemporary healthcare institutions" as Beauchamp and Childress have noted in their textbook: Principles of Biomedical Ethics [8]." For centuries healthcare professionals managed to keep trust at the center stage of their practice, even when they had far less effective treatments to offer patients than today's professionals do. Recently, the centrality of trust had declined, as is evidenced by the dramatic rise in medical malpractice suits and adversarial relations between healthcare professionals and the public. Overt distrust has been engendered by mechanisms of managed care, and by the incentives some healthcare organizations (health insurance companies in USA) create for physicians to limit the expenses and kind of care provided [8]." The loss of intimate contact between physicians and patients, the increased use of specialists, the growth of impersonal medical institutions, and the loss of good communication are all contributing causes to the erosion of trust.

Physicians, on the other hand, also mistrust their patients, and feel that they will be sued if there is any suspicion of any mistake, and hence they take defensive medicine, and ask for investigations (expensive and laborious) in order to ward off any charge of suspected negligence. The expense of medical care is sky rocketing because of these unrequired investigations, and because of the expensive drugs and machinery of modern medicine.

Integrity

Some healthcare professionals refuse to comply with the requests of their patients or with the decisions of their colleagues on grounds that to do so would compromise their core belief. The physician may refuse to do abortion, on grounds of religious beliefs, or he/she may refuse to change the gender of his patient (transsex), which he/she insists to do.

The current system of medical rules allows the physician to abstain from such managements, but he is required to transfer the patient to another physician who will comply with the patient's requests of such operations. The value of moral integrity is beyond dispute. It means soundness, reliability, wholeness, and integrations of moral character and being faithful to moral values and standing up in their defense if necessary. The medical profession and its constant demands may deprive us of the liberty to structure and integrate our lives as we see fit, and that will affect our integrity. Persons may lose their integrity if they lack sincerity and steadfastness in keeping their fundamental moral convictions, especially if the exigencies of their ever-demanding job enforce them to practice things which they do not believe. Such exigencies may be rare in Western countries, but they are not so rare in third world countries. A gynecologist in a third world private hospital may be sacked from his job if he adamantly refuses to perform any abortion, not indicated medically. Such a person usually believes in the sanctity of life and, hence, he may also stand against do not resuscitate (DNR) policy agreed upon in certain codes where any further management becomes futile. The question of euthanasia is definitely beyond these boundaries, as it is still being considered a type of homicide by all governments except Holland, Belgium, and a few states in the USA.

The situations that compromise integrity can be avoided by an institutional policy that realizes the convictions of its staff, and delegates the work that is against the conviction of one physician to another who accepts it. There should be no retribution for such act of conviction, but that does not rule out incitement for those who perform the act. The medical profession nowadays requires that the physician should not in any way impose or even propose any judgment to the patient's beliefs or indulgences. If the patient, for example, drinks alcohol or takes drugs of addiction, or has multiple sexual relations or is homosexual, the physician cannot even advise him against this perilous behavior. This is considered an intrusion in the patient's lifestyle, for which he/she, the physician is not even allowed to advise against.

However, the physician is allowed to advise against smoking and obesity, but the decision of course should be taken by the patient without any instigation or prodding. But why the physician cannot advise against fornication, adultery, sodomy, drugs of addiction and alcohol is beyond our comprehension in the Muslim world. The physician should be a sincere advisor to the patient in matters that would affect his/her health, and if he fails to advise accordingly, he is failing in fulfillment of his duty.

This attitude is considered paternalistic in modern medical ethics and interfering with autonomy. Let us agree that enforcing a certain point of view is definitely encroaching on autonomy, but there is no point in allowing the physician to strongly advise against smoking and obesity and provide the means to help the patient overcome these problems, and at the same time refusing to allow the physician to strongly advise against sodomy, adultery, fornication, drug addiction, and alcohol drinking.

Conscientiousness

"An individual acts conscientiously if he or she is motivated to do what is right because it is right, has tried with diligence to determine what is right, intends to do what is right, and exert an appropriate level of effort to do so [8]." In a nation where 50 million citizens have no medical insurance, the duty of all conscientious persons is to strive hard to remove that injustice. It is not right to condone the prevailing system and relegating such an issue to the politicians and congress.

Beauchamp and Chiildress in "Principles of Biomedical Ethics" fifth edition stressed the fact that Afro Americans were without medical insurance and found to suffer from hypertension when they attend Casualty Department, should not be treated, as many researchers found that such poor patients will not be able to continue medication or follow-up, as they have no family physician nor medical insurance, and hence consider treating them as a waste of time, effort, and money. In fact, Beauchamp and Childress in the seventh edition (2013) of their book criticized the American health system and considered it unjust to all those citizens without any health insurance or health coverage; without saying it, they agree to let them suffer and die with their hypertension and its sequelae , e.g., strokes, heart attacks, heart failure, and kidney failure [17].

It is unbelievable to find that neighboring Cuba, which suffers from poverty and American sanctions have better health indices, e.g., infant mortality rate, 5 years mortality rate of children, longevity. Cuba provides free health services not only to its citizens, but even to the visitors of Cuba. Definitely the standard of health of Cubans is much higher than the 50 million US American citizens without any health insurance.

The authors praised the ethical moral stance of a recent Ph.D graduate in chemistry, who refused to take a job in a laboratory that pursues research in chemical and biological warfare, though he is in dire need for the job to support himself and his family. If this chemist refuses this job, it will be taken by another young man who will pursue the research with greater vigor. Despite all these circumstances, George, the chemist, refused this job and accepted all the sufferings to himself and his family because his conscience stood in the way of accepting it [8].

There is no doubt that George's decision is praiseworthy from an ethical and moral stance. But if the suffering of his family is great, and the wife with the children might leave him, the decision of George needs reconsidering. The research will go on in chemical warfare with or without George; the sequelae (consequences) may be worse with another chemist. The family of George will disintegrate and the harm is so great that he should reconsider his position. An Islamic point of view would advise George to balance the two evils, and accept the lesser one, which is in this case working in the chemical laboratory. His refusal in not going to change anything in the lab research of chemical warfare will definitely result in disintegration of his family and great suffering to all its members. The axiom in Islamic jurisprudence of accepting the lesser evil when faced with two evils will solve the dilemma of George or anyone in a similar situation.

This shows the pragmatic sequential Islamic point of view, which agrees in this case with utilitarian consequentialist philosophy.

In other situations, where a clear cut encroachment on Islamic dogma or laws occurs, the consequentialist utilitarian philosophy will be refuted. For example, opening of a brewery or wine factory may benefit the owners, the workers, their families, and the vendors and make the consumers happy. Nevertheless, it will not be allowed by Islamic Law (Sha'riah), as there is clear prohibition both in the Qur'an and the Tradition. The cumulative harm to the society may be much more than the apparent benefit. The Qur'an says: "They ask you about wine and gambling. In them is a great sin and some benefit for people. But their sin is greater than their benefit" (The Qur'an 2:219).

People with conscience feel that they are obliged to take a certain action even if harm is going to befall them or their family. Such a person will resist the temptation to set aside what he or she believes to be right. Prophet Muhammad (PBUH) when he started to preach against idolatry in Makkah, the elders of his tribe tried their best to dissuade him from this course. They offered to make him their chief, collect money for him to be the wealthiest person in Quraish (his tribe), and to marry him with the most beautiful girls. He refused all these offers and said to his uncle: "I swear by God, if they put the sun in my right hand and the moon in my left hand, to leave this message, I will not leave it" [18] .

The physician should not contravene his conscience and will not be lured by temptation or by threats. Prophet Muhammad said: "You should not obey whoever may be, if he orders you to disobey God's commanments and laws" [19]. The physician can withdraw from any action that contradicts his conscience, e.g., gender selection in gynecological practice, both prior to conception as in test tube babies, or after conception by chorionic villus sampling or amniocentesis. If the conceptus proves to be a girl, the parents may ask for abortion. The physician may refuse certain operations as sex transfer or beauty operations or hymnography (closing the hymen of a girl in order to marry as a virgin). These objections should be respected and the conscientious physician should be allowed to withdraw from such management. The hospital may direct the client to another health provider. If the country upholds the Sha'riah, such practices should not be allowed by law. The principle of autonomy entails respecting the others, their decisions, and their free will, which needs veracity (truthfulness), fidelity (faithfulness), respecting the privacy of others, and confidentiality. There are a lot of virtues required in the health provider, such as compassion, concern, caring, sympathy (and sometimes empathy), modesty, patience, and courage. All these virtues and many others have no norms of obligation.

Moral Ideals [8]

There are two levels of moral standards: ordinary and extraordinary moral standards. The ordinary form requires adhering to the minimum moral requirement, which include honesty, trustworthiness, and faithfulness. Others of high standard will include self-sacrifice in certain situations, e.g., saving a person from drowning, or from fire or in a battlefield to save his comrades and exposing himself to real danger and even loss of life. Such a person feels that he is only doing his duty, and nothing more. These actions however are supererogatory and praiseworthy.

In Islam it is incumbent on every Muslim to give 2.5 % of his wealth annually to the poor and needy. That is obligatory, but if a person gives much more than that fixed amount, then it is supererogatory. Similarly, if a physician or nurse does much more than his/her obligatory duty, then he/she is performing a supererogatory action which is praiseworthy.

Any action or even intent in Islam will be under one of the following moral categories:

(1) Actions that are right and obligatory (wajib), e.g., truth telling.
(2) Actions that are wrong and prohibited, e.g., lying, cheating, and the most heinous, killing an innocent person.
(3) Actions that are allowed and are optional. They include normal activities of eating, drinking, wearing clothes, habits, and working. They are usually neither wrong nor obligatory and hence called Mubah, e.g., allowed, and the person can choose to do or not to do.

(4) Supererogatory: which include actions commendable, praiseworthy but they are not obligatory. In Islam it is called Mandub or Nafil.

(5) Actions which are not obligatory nor prevented, but is recommended to avoid, for example, wasting time without any good effect. This is called Makrooh in Islam, and if it is done no punishment is expected, and if it is avoided, reward from God is expected.

Many duties in the medial practice and nursing are profession-related rather than obligation. A physician or nurse who cheers his patient and brings hope to him is doing an obligation in certain situations or a supererogatory action in other situations. To care for patients with communicable diseases, e.g., Ebola virus, tuberculosis, typhoid, typhus fever, plague, and even severe influenza epidemic is definitely an obligatory moral action for health providers. If the health provider exceeds his duty then it is supererogatory. HIV patients and Hepatitis B and C patients are not infectious except by contact of blood, blood products, body fluids, and sexual contact. The health providers and lab technicians should be careful not to come into direct contact with blood and body fluids. They should wear gloves and be careful with needles.

As John Stuart Mill said: "The contented man, or the contented family who have no ambition to make any one else happier, to promote the good of their country or their neighborhood, or to improve themselves in moral excellence, excite in us neither admiration or approval" [20]. Virtues beyond obligations are needed for the whole community, but more so for health providers. The virtues of courage, patience, hospitality and tactfulness, and so forth are needed to give example of moral excellence. Morally exemplary lives guide and inspire us to higher goals and morally better lives.

Each individual should aspire to a level as his or her ability permits. Persons vary in their moral life, as they differ in their athletic performance or their academic performance, but there should be a level that no one goes below it. This is the obligatory level, but there are those who excel and are exemplary models in moral performance. The best of these are the Messengers of God, e.g., Abraham, Moses, Jesus, and Muhammad. They are the shining stars which every human should aspire to emulate.

Aristotle maintained that we acquire virtues as much as we do skills. Surely virtues can be built up by training and by exemplary characters, but persons differ by their innate nature. Some are easily trained to build up moral values and virtues, while others are less fortunate. The important thing is that whatever their abilities are, they should not go beyond the standard minimum of morals and virtues through self-cultivation, guidance, and aspiration. Everyone should aspire to improve and strive to climb up the ladder of virtues and morality.

The Aristotelian model does not expect perfection, on that persons strive toward perfection … the ideals motivate us in a way that basic obligations may not set out a path we can climb in stages, with a renewable sense of progress and achievement [18]

Notes and References

1. Nassar J (2004) Makanat AlAkhlaq fi al fiker alIslami. Dar alWafa alMansoorah, Egypt., pp 10–20
2. alTahanooni: Kashaaf istilahat alFanoon wa alOloon
3. alGirgani A: Kita alTaarifat, Dar alKutob alIlmeyiah, Beirut, Kholoq and Akhlaq
4. Galen Theory of Humors in M. Albar: alAkhlaq: Osoolaha Addeeniyah wa Gothooraha alFalsafiyiah, King Abdulaziz University, Jeddah, Chair of Medical Ethics 2010, pp 36–40
5. alMawardi A (1987) Tasheel alNadhar wa Ta'geel alDhafar, Dar alOloom alArabia, Beirut. pp 101–106
6. alFaraby Tarkhan (1986) Al Jama bain alHakeemain, Dar alMashriq, Beirut, p 95
7. Miskawaih A (1966) Tahzeeb alAkhlaq, commented by Constantine Zuraiq, Beirut, pp 31–32
8. Beauchamp T, Childress J (2001) Principles of biomedical ethics, 5th edn. Oxford University Press, New York, pp 27–51
9. AlBokhari M: Sahihu alBokhari, kitab alShaab, Cairo(nd), vol 1/1, Hadith no. 1
10. AlBokhari M: Sahihu alBokhair, kitab alShaab, Cairo(nd), Kitab al Imarah, and Sahih Muslim bishareh AlNawawi, Dar AlFiker, Beirut, and Sunan alTirmithi, all through Abu Huraira and Omar ibn alKhattab
11. Philippa F (1986) Virtues and vices (Oxford, Basil Blackwell), 1978, and Trianosky, Gregory: Superrogtion, wrongdoing and vice. J Philos 83:26–40
12. Beecher H (1966) Ethics and clinical research. N Engl J Med 24:1354–1360
13. Abu Da'ood: Sunan Abi Daood, Kitab alDiyat, bab man tatabab, Dar alFiker, Beirut
14. Al Baihaqi: Shuab alIman
15. Abdulmalik ibn Habib AlIlbeiri (1993) Tibbi Nabawi, commented and explained by Dr. Mohammed Albar, Dar alQalam, Damascus, pp 165–174
16. The Saudi Papers published many horrific stories in the Spring of 2012 about surgeons and anesthetists in private hospitals
17. Beauchamp T, Childress J: Principles of Biomedical Ethics (ref. 8), pp 347–348
18. Narrated by ibn Ishaq in his book "Al Maghazi", and ibn Asaaker and ibn Abi Yaala. Al Albany said it has two narration, one is weak and the other is strong, and that is why he put each in a different book of his ahadith (one in the weak hadith and the other in the strong hadith)
19. This hadith was narrated by both alBokhari and Muslim the most authentic books of Hadith (Sayings of the Prophet Muhammad [PBUH]). "No obedience for anybody if it entails disobeying Allah". It is also narrated by Ahmed ibn Hanbal (Al Musnad). Al Tabarani (Al Moojam al Kabeer wal Awsat), ibn Abi Shaiba and alBazaar; all through Imran ibn Hussain. Al Albani in his Al Jamee Al Sahih Hadith no. 7520 commented that is a strong Hadith (sahih)
20. Mill JS (1977) Considerations on representative government, in the collected works of John Stuart Mill, vol 19, chapter 3. Tronto University, p 409

Chapter 5
Regulation of Medical Profession and Medical Research

The Medical Oaths and Codes

Medicine as a Profession

Professional virtues and codes of conduct were historically associated with the philosophy and ethos of each community. The medical profession, in particular, was esteemed by all nations and cultures. Imam Shafi [1] (767–820 CE) said: "There are two kinds of persons who are indispensable for people. The scholars (of religion and law = ulema) for dealing with their matters of religion, and physicians for dealing with their bodies. Abubaker AlRhazi [2] (864–925 CE) said: "The physicians possess traits that are not found in others, among such is the unanimous view of the followers of religion and authority, of the preference of their occupation, and the acknowledgement of both kings and laymen for the exigent need for their services; for their everlasting strive to discover the unknown in the field of knowledge, of their pursuance to improve their profession, and of their persistent concern of introducing happiness and comfort to others."

The medical profession should be practiced with efficiency and honesty. Prophet Muhammad (PBUH) said: "Allah likes when any one does a work, to do it with perfection" [3]. The physician should observe good conduct and fine character in both his acts and behavior. The manual guide for medical practitioners in Saudi Arabia [4] claims that: "The ethics of morals of profession mainly stem from the teachings of Islam which call for nobility of character, perfection of performance and fear of God in every act. The Prophet Muhammad said: "I have been sent to call for and complement high moral standards" [5].

Every nation and culture has its morals, mode of conduct, and ethics. The old Egyptians, Chinese, Indians, Persians, Babylonians, etc., had a mode of conduct for the medical profession, requirement for the priest physicians, and laws regulating the profession.

The Greeks were probably the most elaborate since the time of Hippocrates. The oath they promulgated and proclaimed became the cornerstone of medical ethics,

© The Author(s) 2015
M.A. Al-Bar and H. Chamsi-Pasha, *Contemporary Bioethics*,
DOI 10.1007/978-3-319-18428-9_5

which should be taken by anyone who contemplates to be involved in this noble profession.

The Hippocratic Oath: is part of a collection of writings known as the Hippocratic Corpus. The oath is generally believed to have been written a hundred years after the time of Hippocrates who lived in the Island of Cos in ancient Greek, in the fifth century B.C. (460–350) [6]. Ludwig Eldestein (1967) thinks that the Hippocratic tradition arose from the Pythagorean Cult, which was interested in Science, Philosophy, Medicine, and Religion [7].

The oath starts with a pledge to Greek gods and goddesses Apollo, Asclepius (a deified physician) the god of Medicine, and his two daughters Hygeia (from which hygiene is derived) and Panacea (the drug that cures all maladies). When the Muslim physicians adopted the Hippocrates Oath, they omitted these pledges and pledged to God [8]. Similarly, early Christians were at odds with these idol worshippers, and hence destroyed the Hippocrates temple in the Island of Cos [9].

The oath of Hippocrates then pledges loyalty to the teacher and his posterity, and to keep the profession of medicine secret except to those who deserve it by their character, or being the children of previous physicians.

The oath then applied dietetic measures for the benefit of the sick, in order to keep the patients from harm and injustice. "I will never give a deadly drug to anybody if asked for it, and will not give a woman an abortive drug. In purity and holiness I will guard my life and my art. I will not use the knife, not even on sufferers from stone (in the urinary bladder which was amenable to treatment), but withdraw in favor of such men as engaged in this work."

The cause of abhorring surgery is religious, as holiness and purity implies not being contaminated by blood and waste products, which are religiously defiling [10].

Keeping Virtuous: The oath pledges: "Whatever houses I may visit, will come for the benefit of the sick, remaining free of all intentional injustice, of all mischief and in particular of sexual relations with both female and male persons, be they free or slave."

Keeping Secrets: "What I may see or hear in the course of the treatment, or even outside of the treatment in regard to the life of men, which on no account one must spread abroad, I will keep to myself such things shameful to be spoken about."

The Hippocratic Oath extolled the following principles:

(1) **Beneficence** [11]: in English language connotes acts of mercy, kindness, and charity. It includes all forms of action intended to benefit other persons.

Benevolence refers to the character trait or virtue of being disposed to benefit others.

The Principle of Beneficence: refers to moral obligation to act for the benefit of others.

Nonmaleficence

"Above all do no harm" or Primum non nocere is entwined with beneficence; it says: "I will use treatment to help the sick according to my ability and judgment, but I will never use it to injure or wrong them".

It clearly guards life, "I will never give a deadly drug to anybody, and will not give a woman an abortive drug and even will not use the knife," as surgery was hazardous at his time, and also for purity and religious reason avoiding blood and defiling religiously. The Hippocratic Oath is pro-life and vehemently against abortion, suicide, and any type of killing including Euthanasia. Doing harm in whatever way is abhorred, and should be avoided, even unintentionally. The physician should be careful in prescribing drugs and should take a detailed history of drug allergies, lest one of his drugs cause harm to his patient. More care will be needed in cases of surgery.

Confidentiality

Keeping the secrets of the patient, his family and even his servants and slaves, whom the physician comes across while visiting the patient at his home, should be kept secret "I will keep to myself such things shameful to be spoken about." This attitude is also part and parcel of benefiting the patient "Beneficence" and not doing any harm to him "Non Maleficence." However, if divulging the secret may be of benefit to the patient, as considered by his physician, then it should be exposed, as far as it is beneficial to him or warding off harm thwarted against him.

Paternalistic Attitude

The physician in the Hippocratic Oath is obviously paternalistic who is looking after his patient, as if he is his son or daughter, trying his best to benefit him, and prevent any harm that would befall him/her, and keeping all the secrets he comes across during his treatment of the patient, unless exposure is going to benefit the patient or ward off harm befalling him.

The Hippocratic Code endorsed the virtues of modesty, sobriety, patience, promptness, and piety. The physician must be upright and pure in character, diligent, and conscientious in caring for the sick.

The paternalistic attitude should be praiseworthy. But as changes occurred in the West, the enlightenment era approached and the liberal attitudes appeared, this attitude was disregarded and considered obsolete.

In the late eighteenth century an epidemic of typhus and typhoid fevers broke out in Manchester, England, and the Manchester infirmary staff were overworked. The medical practitioners were divided into dieticians, apothecaries (working with drugs), and surgeons and were blaming each other of negligence, as nobody exactly knew his duty in this epidemic. Percival, a well-educated retired physician wrote for them a medical code of conduct in 1803. It was in the Hippocratic tradition, which stressed the duty of the physician to benefit the patient, and placed no emphasis on the rights of patients in matters such as informed consent or open disclosure.

This duty to benefit the patient with absence of any recognition of the rights of patients is the hallmark of the Hippocratic tradition. It is one of the major differences between medical ethics that is Hippocratic and many of the other religious and secular ethics [10].

The American Medical Association (AMA) of 1847 turned to Percival's Code, taking whole sections of it and incorporating in the 1847 Code of Ethics. Both Britain and USA have Codes of Ethics that are essentially Hippocratic. However, both mention the duties of physicians to benefit the society, which was never mentioned in Hippocratic Code of Ethics.

The American Medical Association (AMA) Code (1957–1980) endorsed the virtues that Hippocrates commended: modesty, sobriety, patience, promptness, and piety. However, in contrast to the first code in 1847, the AMA over the years has deemphasized virtues in its codes. In 1980, it eliminated all traces of virtues except in the admonition to expose those physicians deficient in character or competence [12].

The paternalistic virtues of benevolence, nonmaleficence, and compassion were extolled, while in recent attitudes of autonomy, these virtues are not called for; instead the virtue of respectfulness is more prominent and important. The contractual natures of medicine and health profession as a whole, became a business, ruled by contracts, mistrust, and litigations, which needed changes in medical codes, its by-laws and ethics.

However, the Hippocratic Oath remained with minor alteration in the World Medical Association Declaration of Geneva 1948 and 1956 [10].

Post-Soviet Russia constructed an oath for the Russian physician in 1993, which replaced the previous Marxist oath, and adopted the World Medical Association of 1956, which is Hippocratic [10].

But gradually the Hippocratic attitudes were replaced by autonomy and respect for the individual and his wishes. From 1970, the Hippocratic tradition started to collapse. The rights of the patient became more important, and the ethics of respect for persons (duty-based principles) were dominant. These included fidelity, autonomy, and veracity.

Not all the old codes of ethics were paternalistic like the Hippocratic Oath. Hinduism, Buddhism, various Chinese traditions, and Islamic teachings all differ from the paternalistic approach of the Hippocratic Oath.

Islam is considered as the religion of all the Prophets and Messengers of God. Islam means submission to God. Since monotheism is the true religion of Allah (God) from primordial times, as Adam, Noah, Abraham, Moses, Jesus, and all the Messengers of Allah were all of them monotheists, then Islam should be defended, expounded, and proclaimed. However, there is no compulsion in religion. "There shall be no compulsion in (the acceptance of) religion. The right course has become clear from the wrong" (Surah AlBaqarah 2/256).

And say: The truth is from your Lord, so whoever wills let him believe; and whoever wills let him disbelieve (Sura AlKahf 18/29).

Are you going (O Mohammed) to compel the people to believe (Sura Yunus 10/99).

You are not in control of them (Sura AlGhashiya 88/22).

The Qur'an is replete with such verses, which orders freedom of faith and human personal responsibility.

Verily God does not change men's condition unless they change their inner selves (Sura Ar-Rad/The Thunder 13/11).

Every soul will be held responsible for what it had done (Sura AlMuda'ththir/The Cloaked One 74/38).

If there is no compulsion in accepting religion (which is the most important thing for humans), then there is no compulsion in accepting medicine by drugs or surgery.

The consent of the person to be treated should be obtained if he/she is adult and competent. If he is a minor (a child) or mentally incapacitated then the consent of the guardian should be obtained. Only in life saving situations that consent may be ignored. Otherwise, it is imperative to obtain the consent prior to any medical or surgical intervention. If the guardian refuses to give consent for the child or incompetent person under his guardianship, and the physicians think it is very important to operate or give kidney dialysis or whatever medical intervention, then the magistrate can appoint another guardian who will give consent. There are many ways in implementing this treatment immediately, and in cases of emergency and life saving situations there will be no need for the consent.

The Islamic jurisprudence considers seeking remedy depends on the situation.

Seeking remedy in Islamic jurisprudence may be obligatory (mandatory) in certain life saving situations or may be preferred or encouraged (Mandoob) in other situations. It may be facultative or optional and may be Makrooh, i.e., not preferred and in some situations and with certain type of treatment may be Haram, i.e., not allowed.

Ibn Taimyiah said: "seeking remedy may be Haram (not allowed) or Makrooh (not preferred), may be facultative i.e. optional (Mubaah), it may be preferred (Mandoob) or may be obligatory when it is life saving" [13]. He also said: "seeking remedy is not obligatory in the opinion of majority of Ulema (religious law experts), they however differed which is better: to seek remedy or not, for those stoics who can forebear" [14]. During that time, almost all modes of therapy were of doubtful results and many involved certain dangers, especially when surgery was contemplated.

Seeking Remedy: Obligatory (Mandatory)

It is incumbent that everyone should seek remedy in life saving situations. In such cases, if the person is unconscious or he is a minor, there is no need to wait for obtaining consent from proxy or guardian. The physician (or nurse) should do his/her best to save the life, organ, or limb without waiting for due consent. He/she would be liable otherwise. In case of infectious diseases that will endanger the health of the community, the government has the power to enforce treatment on a patient, irrespective of his will [15]. However, in cases like appendicitis, the doctor cannot enforce treatment if the patient refuses, except in case of a minor; then the court will appoint another guardian to give consent for treatment [16].

If the patient requires a caesarian section, the consent of the lady is sufficient and there is no need for consent of her husband, a practice common in many Arab countries where the consent of the husband is thought imperative [17].

In case where the life of the fetus is endangered, e.g., prolapsed cord, many jurists would advise caesarian section even without the consent of both parents [18].

The governments impose mandatory immunization schemes for children and in case of epidemics such as meningitis; vaccination is required for many Hajj seasons. Such actions have been supported and encouraged by many Fatwas (decision 67/5/7 of Islamic (jurisprudence 7th meeting) [15].

Seeking Remedy: Encouraged and Preferred

a. In all cases where therapy is likely successful and harm from that mode of therapy is most unlikely.
b. In all cases where the ailment is going to hinder the activities and duties of a Muslim to himself, his family, and his community.
c. The mode of therapy is "Halal." In case of "Haram" medication, it will be allowed if there is no alternative, if it is deemed necessary to cure the ailment and/or it is prescribed by Muslim physician [19].

Prophet Muhammad (PBUH) said: "O servants of Allah seek remedy, for Allah has not put an ailment except that he puts its remedy except one ailment. They asked: what ailment? He said: old age". And in another Hadith he said: death.

Seeking Remedy: Facultative (optional)

a. Where benefit is not proved or even doubtful.
b. Where ill effects of that mode of therapy are uncertain.
c. The person should have autonomy and decide for himself, whether to accept or refuse that modality of treatment.
d. Informed consent is mandatory except in emergency situations.

Abstaining from Remedy Is the Better Option

Seeking remedy may be **Makrooh** (not preferred) in the following conditions:

a. When therapy is unlikely to bring benefit.
b. Where harm or even inconvenience from therapy may exceed its benefit.

Some jurists from the Hanbali School thought that abstaining from remedy is the better option in the following conditions:

a. Non-life threatening conditions.
b. No danger to the health of the individual.
c. Not encroaching on other's health.
d. In terminal cases.

There are two hadiths of Prophet Muhammad (PBUH), which encourage abstaining from remedy. They are:

a. "There are 70,000 of my people will enter paradise without being questioned; they are the ones who do not seek remedy by ruqia, the ones who don't consult talismans, the ones who don't allow themselves to be cauterized; and they leave the matters in the hands of their Lord and completely depend on His grace" [20].

b. A black lady complained to the Prophet (PBUH) that she got convulsions and got naked during these attacks and asked him to pray for her to get cured. He said: "If you persevere and be patient you will enter paradise". She said: "I will be patient but I don't want to get exposed (i.e. naked); he said: "I will pray for you that you might not get exposed."

She had attacks but never got exposed after that incident. (Narrated by AlBukhari) [21].

Many companions refused therapy in their last illness, as they felt it would be futile e.g. Abubaker Assidiq-The First Caliph, Muath ibn Jabal and Abu Darda'a.

Seeking Remedy is Prohibited

a. If it involves amulets, (other than Qur'an), sorcery, divination, or talisman. It encroaches on creed [22, 23].
b. Any medication made of liquor or any intoxicating drink [23, 24].
c. Use of pork or porcine material [25].
d. Killing animals, e.g., frogs, etc., and using them as medicine [26].
e. Using blood [27].

Only in conditions or situations, when it becomes life saving that these substances will be allowed. It will also be allowed to use these substances if there is no alternative medication. A competent Muslim physician should prescribe it [19].

The Oath of a Muslim Physician

Many oaths were presented in the First International Conference on Islamic Medicine in Kuwait, January 1981, which were similar, and Hippocratic with minor differences. The one adopted was that presented by Dr. Hassan Hatout. Many Schools of Medicine adopted it in a shorter version.

The Oath of a Muslim Physician

In the name of Allah, Most Gracious, Most Merciful.
Praise to Allah, the Sustainer of His Creation, the All-Knowing.
Glory to be Him, the Eternal, the All-Pervading.
O Allah, Thou art the only Healer, I serve none but Thee, and, as the instrument of Thy Will, I commit myself to Thee.
I render this Oath in Thy Holy Name and I Undertake:
To be the instrument of Thy Will and Mercy, and, in all humbleness, to exercise justice, love and compassion for all Thy Creation; To extend my hand of service to one and all, to the rich and to the poor, to friend and foe alike, regardless of race, religion or color; To hold human life as precious and sacred, and to protect and honor it at all times and under all circumstances in accordance with Thy Law; To do my utmost to alleviate pain and misery and to comfort and counsel human beings in sickness and in anxiety; To respect the confidence and guard the secrets of all my

patients; To maintain the dignity of healthcare, and to honor the teachers, students, and members of my profession; To strive in the pursuit of knowledge in Thy name for the benefit of mankind and to uphold human honor and dignity; To acquire the courage to admit my mistakes, mend my ways and to forgive the wrongs of others; To be ever-conscious of my duty to Allah and His Messenger (PBUH), and to follow the precepts of Islam in private and in public. "O Allah grant me the strength, patience and dedication to adhere to this Oath at all times".

New Codes and Oaths Breaking with Hippocratic Tradition

The Nuremberg Code 1946 appeared after Nuremberg Trials of the Nazi Physicians (World War II) who experimented with prisoners of war, gave them lethal drugs, caused pain and suffering to all of them and ended in death of many. All the experiments were not serving any benefit to those researched and of course, were done without any consent. The physicians claimed that these experiments were advancing knowledge and science, while in fact they did very little in this aspect. They were sadistic brutal experiments.

The Nazi physicians had abandoned the traditional ethical commitment of the physician to the individual patient welfare. They were committed and found guilty.

The appearance of Nuremberg Code is considered a landmark in the history of medical ethics research, which emphasized the importance of consent of those to be researched with their own free will.

The Nuremberg Code is a public document of International law, not one written by the medical profession. The Nuremberg Code is grounded in liberal political philosophy and henceforth changed gradually the medical ethics codes and philosophy, which refused the paternalistic attitudes and gave all its attention to the respect of human being, which became dominant. These included autonomy, fidelity, veracity and care for the rights of patients.

Ethical Codes

Nuremberg Code
1947 and 1946

- "The voluntary consent of the human subject is absolutely essential."
- Research Subjects "should be so situated as to be able to exercise free power of choice."
- Research Subjects "should have sufficient knowledge and comprehension of the elements of the subject matter involved as to make an understanding and enlightened decision."

Nuremberg Code 1947
10 Rules for "Permissible Medical Experiments"

(1) Voluntary consent without coercion.
(2) Results must benefit society and must only use human subjects when there is no alternative.
(3) Should be based upon non-human studies with justifiable expected results.
(4) Avoidance of all unnecessary physical and mental suffering.
(5) No experimentation where death or serious disability is foreseen unless performed on the medical provider as a subject.
(6) Degree of risk less than potential benefit.
(7) Proper preparations must be made to minimize injury.
(8) Experiment should be conducted by only scientifically qualified person.
(9) Subjects can cease their participation at any time.
(10) Experimentor must stop if it is believed it will result in death or serious disability.

This was followed by many codes, which regulated Bioethical Research. These codes stressed not only consent but informed consent and made many requirements for accepting or allowing biomedical research e.g. the research should be approved by Institution Review Board (IRB). The National Commission for the protection of Human Subjects of Biomedical and Behavioral Research instituted the National Research Act in 1974 in USA. It required the formation of institution Review Boards (IRB) in order to evaluate any research proposal.

This was followed by Belmont Report 1978 and World Medical Association: Declaration of Helsinki, which was amended several times since it was declared in 1964.

The prominent features of these two codes are given here.

The main issues in Medical Research are as follows:

The Belmont Report—Department of Health, Education and Welfare, April 18, 1978

The Belmont Report summarizes ethical principles and guidelines for research involving human subjects. Three core principles are identified: respect for persons, beneficence, and justice. Three primary areas of application are also stated. They are informed consent, assessment of risks and benefits, and selection of subjects.

World Medical Association—Declaration of Helsinki 1964–Present

(1) Physician's responsibility to protect the life, health, privacy and dignity of the human subject.
(2) Research must follow accepted scientific guidelines.
(3) The welfare of the environment and animals must be respected.
(4) A protocol must be submitted to an ethical review committee

- Ethical considerations must be explained
- Prediction of risks, burdens and benefits should be enunciated

(5) Conducted only by scientifically qualified persons
(6) Each potential subject must be informed, understand and consent after being told of all the material facts
(7) Consent must be given without coercion

- Legal guardians must provide consent for those that cannot give consent
- Minors must assent to the research

(8) Researchers must utilize scientific integrity in reporting.

Consent

Consent should be informed. The research should be fully explained to the participants in simple language, which he could fully comprehend. Any questions should be answered. A written document in simple language should be given to the participant. He should be given enough time to review it, ask questions and have free choice to accept or refuse participation; alternatives (in case of refusal) should be explained.

Refusal of Participation

Refusal of participation will not in anyway affect his/her right to full treatment and management.

Participant Withdrawal

The participant can withdraw at any time frame. The researched person even then, will not affect his right to full treatment and management.

Risks to Participants

1. The foreseeable risks, discomforts, and hazards should be explained, indicating the probability, magnitude, and duration.
2. The risks should include the physical, psychological, social, legal, and economic risks.
3. If any hazard occurs during research, the research should be stopped immediately and the participants should be informed, treated of any injury, and compensated duly.
4. All the consent documents in Saudi Arabia declare that no compensation will be paid in case of injury or even death. (This should be changed, and some IRB's do not accept the research until the sponsors agree to treatment and compensation).

Consent of Minors

Children should not be exposed to nontherapeutic clinical research. The consent of the minor is invalid and hence it is obligatory to obtain the consent of the guardian. Children under seven cannot comprehend the intricacies of medical research. However, children who can comprehend and understand should be informed in simple language and their consent obtained. If they refuse, no research should be done on them, despite the consent of the guardian.

Consent of Incompetent Adults

Incompetent adults should not be exposed to any nontherapeutic research. The consent of the guardian is imperative. The research should be useful to the person (patient) or his group. There should be no other alternative to obtain that information.

Consent of Prisoners

Prisoners and incarcerated persons should not be exposed to research unless it is going to help the person or group. The consent of the prisoner is legally invalid, however it should be obtained without duress.

Research on Pregnant and Lactating Ladies

1. Ladies should be scrutinized for pregnancy prior to any research. If there is any harm expected to the mother or fetus no research should be carried on. The lady should avoid pregnancy, if the research period is prolonged and contraception should be used.
2. The informed consent of the lady should be obtained. The consent of the husband or any other member of the family is not enough.
3. The consent of the husband may be essential in research involving reproduction.

Benefit of Research

1. The research should benefit the pregnant lady, her fetus, or the group.
2. The clinical research should in no way expose the pregnant lady, nursing mother, her fetus, or baby to any harm.

Monitoring Research

1. Provision to monitor data for the safety of the participants should be available.
2. Potential benefits to the participants, his group or community should be explained to the participant.
3. Protection of privacy and confidentiality of the participant /patient should be assured.
4. Medical care and compensation for injury. If the research involves more than minimal risk of the participant (discomfort during medical exam) provisions for medical care and compensation should be explained to the participant prior to carrying the research. Pharma companies in developing countries declare that they will not compensate for any harm caused by the experiment.

Holding No Responsibility

1. The researcher should not obtain from the researched subject, any agreement that makes him irresponsible for any injury that can accrue from the research. Even if he gets a written consent, it is considered invalid legally. The subject has the right for proper compensation for any injury.

2. Costs and payments to the researched subjects should be explained prior to starting the research. The amount should be appropriate to compensate the subjects for their lost time.

Research on Embryos and Fetuses

1. Research on embryos and fetuses is not allowed unless the research is going to benefit the embryos or fetus.
2. Left over pre-embryos (fertilized ova) in IVF projects could be used in stem cell research after obtaining the consent of the parents.

The Fatwa of the Islamic Jurisprudence Council of the Islamic World in Makkah Al-Mukarama in its 17th session (19-23-10-1424H 13-17 December 2003G)

Stem Cell Therapy

Decision

First: It is permissible to obtain stem cells to be grown and used for therapy, or for permissible scientific research, if its source is legitimate, as for example:

1. Adults if they give permission, without inflicting harm on them.
2. Children provided that their guardians allow it, for a legal benefit and without inflicting harm on the children.
3. The placenta or the umbilical cord, with the parent's permission.
4. A fetus if spontaneously aborted, or when aborted for a therapeutic reason permitted by Sharia'a, with the parent's permission (be reminded of decision 7 of the council in its 12th session about abortion).
5. Leftover Zygotes remaining from in vitro fertilization, if donated by the parents, when it is ascertained that they will not be used in an illegal pregnancy.

Second: It is forbidden to use stem cell, if their source is illegal as for example:

1. Intentionally aborted fetuses (that is, abortion without a legal medical reason).
2. Intentional fertilization between a donated ovum and sperm.
3. Therapeutic human cloning.

Bioethics Research Without Control Despite Ethical Codes

Despite the fact of many local and international ethical codes, there were many irregularities, deceits, and unethical practices which were exposed by Western physicians, moralists, and media. The occurrence of blatant unethical procedures is disappearing in the West. The drug companies pushed their experiments and unethical procedures in third-world countries. But even there, the international codes are exposing them.

Despite all these codes and regulations medical research is replete with horrendous stories of cheating, maiming and even killing many innocent persons, both prior to Nuremberg Code and after. The Nuremberg trials of the Nazi Physicians opened the eyes for what was happening both in the democratic countries of the West and the heinous experiments of the Nazi Germany.

Here are some examples of what happened in the USA and International drug companies up to 2012.

1915

The U.S. Public Health produced Pellagra in 12 Mississippi inmates to find a cure for the disease. In 1935, after millions died from the disease, the director of the U.S. Public Health Office said that they had known Niacin as a cure for this disease for some time, but withheld it as it affected NEGROES, as he called them.

1941

- Dr. William Black infected a 12-month-old baby with herpes as part of a medical experiment.
- Doctors infected children to produce Vincent's angina.
- Doctors gave 800 poor pregnant women radioactive Iron, to study requirements in pregnancy.

1945

- Col. Safford Warren, of the University of Rochester, injected plutonium into patients of the University Hospital without their knowledge.
- 3 patients at the University of Chicago's Billings hospital were similarly injected with plutonium.

1950 Experiments

- Dr. Josef Strokes of Pennsylvania infected 200 female prisoners with viral hepatitis.
- Doctors in Cleveland Hospital studied cerebral blood flow by spinal anesthesia, inserting needles in jugular veins and brachial arteries, causing blood loss and paralysis.

CIA Trials 1947–1953

- CIA and U.S. Navy trials on LSD, Scopolamine and Mescaline involved military and civilians who were given these hallucinating drugs without their knowledge.

1950–1953 U.S. Army released chemical clouds on 6 American and Canadian cities that resulted in increase of respiratory illness.

1950 U.S. Navy Trials

- U.S. Navy sprayed a cloud of Bacillus globigii over San Francisco shoreline. Many residents developed pneumonia like illness.

1953

- U.S. Atomic Energy Commission gave 200 pregnant women high doses of I-131 and then aborted them at different stages to learn at what stages the serious effect occurs.

1952–1953 Experiment

- Ohio State Prison inmates were injected with live cancer cells to study the progress of the disease by Dr. Chester Southam, of Sloan-Kettering Institute.

Post-Awareness Research

Cincinnati Radiation Experiment

1960–1972

- Mostly African American cancer patients with lower than average intelligence were exposed to large doses of whole body radiation.
- None of the patients consented to the experiment or had any idea of the potential side effects.
- This experiment was sponsored by the United States Military. Subjects experienced severe burns and some died prematurely as a direct result of the experiment.

Post-Awareness Research

Jewish Chronic Disease Hospital, 1963

- 22 chronically ill and debilitated noncancer patients were injected with live human cancer cells.
- Patients were not told of the cancer injection. Hospital covered up the lack of consent and tried to fraudulently obtain consent.
- 2 years after the investigation, the American Cancer Society appointed the principle investigator as a Vice President.

Experimentation
Tuskegee Syphilis Experiment
1932–1972

- Targeted 600 poor and illiterate African American males (399 with syphilis and 201 without).
- Told they were being treated for "bad blood."
- Followed their progress without providing penicillin, which was a known antidote as of 1943.
- Conducted painful lumbar punctures under the fraudulent precept of "free treatment" to test the progression without providing any benefit to the researchees.
- Provided no beneficial treatment and admittedly shortened the lives of the researchees.

- 29 men died directly from syphilis and 100 others died of illnesses related to syphilis.

Pfizer Company Deceived Nigerians 1996

- Pfizer agreed to pay 75 million dollars as compensation for the death of 11 Nigerian children, used as guinea pigs in nonconsensual unlicensed trial in 1996.
- The company deceived them and distributed a new drug "Trovan" as a proven useful drug for meningitis.

USA Today September 2, 2009 Published the Following

Pfizer to Pay $2.3 Billion Fine

Pfizer was ordered to pay $2.3 billion to resolve criminal and civil allegations that the company illegally promoted 4 drugs: Pain Killer Bextra, antipsychotic Geodon, antibiotic Zyvox and antiepileptic Lyrica, which were promoted in off label uses.

Porcine H1N1 Influenza Vaccine
2010 Hoax

- Alarmed people all over the world.
- WHO experts received money from big Pharmaceutical companies.
- Drug companies gained billions.
- Governments and nations lost billions.

2012: GlaxoSmithKline to pay $3B in Largest Healthcare Fraud Settlement in US History (Published in the Media and Internet):

- British drugmaker GlaxoSmith Kline will pay $3 billion in fines—the largest healthcare fraud settlement in U.S. history—for criminal and civil violations involving 10 drugs that are taken by millions of people.
- The Justice Department said that GlaxoSmithKline PLC pleaded guilty to promoting popular antidepressants Paxil and Wellbutrin for unapproved uses. The company also pleaded guilty to failing to report to the Government for seven years some safety problems with diabetes drug Avandia, which was restricted in the U.S. and banned in Europe after it was found in 2007 to sharply increase the risks of heart attacks and congestive heart failure.
- In addition to the fine, Glaxo agreed to resolve civil liability for promoting Paxil, Wellbutrin, asthma drug Advair and two lesser-known drugs for unapproved uses. The company also resolved accusations that it overcharged the government funded Medicaid program for some drugs, and that it paid kickbacks to doctors to prescribe several drugs including asthma drug Flovent and herpes medicine Valtrex.
- Thorpe (who works with Glaxo) said in a statement that he was penalized after he reported kickbacks being paid to doctors and sales reps encouraging doctors to promote drugs for unapproved uses, including using Paxil and Wellbutrin in children.

Merck Vaccine Fraud Exposed by Two Merck Virologists; Company Faked Mumps Vaccine Efficacy Results for Over a Decade, Says Lawsuit

According to Stephen Krahling and Joan Wlochowski, both former Merck virologists, the Merck Company engaged in all the following behavior:

- Merck knowingly falsified its mumps vaccine test results to fabricate a "95 % efficacy rate".
- In order to do this, Merck spiked the blood test with animal antibodies in order to artificially inflate the appearance of immune system antibodies. As reported in CourthouseNews.com: Merck also added animal antibodies to blood samples to achieve more favorable test results, though it knew that human immune system would never produce such antibodies, and that the antibodies created a laboratory testing scenario that "did not in any way correspond to, correlate with, or represent real life … virus neutralization in vaccinated people", according to the complaint.
- Merck then used the falsified trial results to swindle the U.S. Government out of "hundreds of millions of dollars for a vaccine that does not provide adequate immunization".
- Merck vaccine fraud has actually contributed to the continuation of mumps across America, causing more children to become infected with mumps.
- Merck used its false claims of "95 % effectiveness" to monopolize the vaccine market and eliminate possible competitors.
- The Merck vaccine fraud has been going on since the late 1990's, says the Merck virologists.
- Testing of Merck's vaccine was never done against "real-world" mumps viruses in the wild. Instead, test results were simply falsified to achieve the desired outcome.
- This entire fraud took place "with the knowledge, authority and approval of Merck's senior management."
- Merck scientists "witnessed firsthand the improper testing and data falsification in which Merck engaged to artificially inflate the vaccine's efficacy findings," according to court documents.

The exposure of the big Pharma (drug companies) continues, and the media every now and then brings horrific stories. The above examples are sufficient to give an idea of how these companies are implicated in fraudulent activities. The latest one exposed by a BBC report on 2nd November 2012 where Western companies are carrying out trials on ignorant people, without taking consent and telling the patients that they are provided by charities of important expensive drugs. More than 500 persons were reported dead because of these new experimental drugs. The companies bear no responsibility at all.

The Royal College of Physicians Journal (Clinical Medicine) (2002, 2, (2): 116-18) published a charter of medical professionalism project announced by American and European Medical Associations.

The fundamental principles were:

(1) Principle of Primacy of Patient Welfare: based on a dedication to serving the interest of the patient with altruism from the side of the treating physicians, when needs arise.
(2) Principle of Patient Autonomy
(3) Principle of Social Justice

A set of professional responsibilities involve the following:

(1) Commitment to Professional Competence with life long learning and teamwork.
(2) Commitment to Honesty with Patients including reporting to the patient of medical error that resulted in his injury. Reporting and analyzing medical errors provides the basis for appropriate prevention and improvement strategies.
(3) Commitment to Patients Confidentiality especially that access to patients data, genetic makeup, and secrets are becoming easier with electronic information and computerization.
(4) Commitment to Maintaining Appropriate Relations with Patients. Physicians should never exploit patients for any sexual advantage, personal financial gain, or other private purpose.
(5) Commitment to Improving Quality Care: Increasing medical competence, reducing medical errors, increasing patient's safety, and optimizing the outcome of medical care.
(6) Commitment to Improving Access to Care. (Equity) Physicians must individually and collectively strive to reduce barriers to equitable healthcare aiming to eliminate barriers based on education, laws, finances, ethnicity, and social discrimination. Commitment to equity entails the promotion of public health and preventative medicine.
(7) Commitment to a Just Distribution of Limited Resources.

   • Guidelines for cost-effective care
   • Appropriate allocation of resources
   • Avoidance of superfluous tests and procedures

(8) Commitment to Scientific Knowledge

   • Prompting research
   • Creating new avenues of management of disease and their prevention
   • Appropriate use of new knowledge

(9) Commitment to Maintain Trust

   • Avoiding conflict of interest, private gain or personal advantage
   • Management and supervision of medical and pharmaceutical industries whose aim is profit and profit alone. Exposure of any misconduct of these giant corporations involving the medical trials the effect of drugs or

procedures or equipment's, is a responsibility of the physicians along with appropriate bodies of licensing and censure.

(10)   Commitment to Professional Responsibilities

- Collaborative work
- Self-regulation
- Discipline of members of the profession when required.
- Education and standard setting of current and future members of the medical profession.
- Accepting internal and external scrutiny of all aspects of professional performance.

Notes and References

1. Imam Shafii is a great Islamic Scholar who founded "a separate school of Sunni Islamic Jursiprudence" and was the Pioneer and Founder of "The Fundamentals (osool) of Islamic jurisprudence"
2. AbuBaker Rhazi is a great Islamic Physician and Philosopher who wrote profusely in Medicine, Pharmacology, Chemistry, Ethics and Philosophy
3. Hadith narrated by alBaihaqi, Abu Yaala and alTabarani
4. Saudi Council for Health Specialities (2003) Ethics of the medical profession: a manual guide for medical practioners, 2nd edn. Riyadh, Saudi Arabia
5. Narrated by Imam Malik in AlMuwata'a, and Imam Ahmed ibn Hanbal in AlMusnad
6. Veach R (2003) The basics of bioethics, 2nd edn. Prentice Hall, New Jersey and Pearson Education New Jersey, London. etc., p 13
7. Eldestein L (1967) The Hippocratic oath: text, translation and interpretation. In: Temkin Owsei, Temkin Lilian (eds) Ancient medicine: selcted papers of Ludwig Eldestein. The John Hopkins Press, Baltimore, pp 3–64
8. Ibn Abi Ousaibi-a (1965) O'yoon al anba fi Tabagat al Attiba (Arabic). Muktabat alHyat, Beirut, p 45
9. Veach R, Mason C (1987) Hippocratic versus JuedoChristian medical ethics: principles in conflict. J Religious Ethics 15:86–105
10. Veach R (2003) The basics of bioethics, 2nd edn. Prentice Hall, New Jersey and Pearson Education New Jersey, London. etc., pp 15–18
11. Beauchamp T, Childress J (2001) Principles of biomedical ethics, 5th edn. Oxford University Press, New York, p 166
12. Beauchamp T, Childress J (2001) Principles of biomedical ethics, 5th edn. Oxford University Press, New York, p 31
13. Ibn Taimyiah: Al Fatawa, Maktabat alMaarif, AlRibat (Morrocco) sponsored by King Khalid ibn Abdulaziz AlSoud, vol 37, p 471
14. Vide Supra, vol 24, pp 272–276
15. Islamic Jurisprudence Council (OJC) (1992) Book of decisions, 4th edn, Jeddah 1423H/2003 CE, Decision No. 67 (5/7) of 1992, pp 226–230

16. Fatwas Regarding Medicine and Patients. Department of Religious Sciences, Research and Fatwa Riyadh. Supervised by Saleh Al Fawzan, 1424H / 2004 CE, Fatwa No. 119, dated 26/5/ 1404, p 182
17. Vide Supra, Fatwa No. 140, dated 20.6.1407, pp 182–183
18. Islamic International Jursprudence Council, Fatwa 184 (19/10), 30 April 2009, 19th Session, UAE
19. AlKhatib AlSherbini (1978) Mughni AlMuhtaj Limaritat AlFaz AlMinhaj. Dar AlFiker, Beirut 4:188
20. AlBokhari, MI: Sahih AlBokhari, Dar Al Ma'rifah, Beirut, Kit Attib, vol 4, pp 11, 12, 18 and Kitba Alibas, vol 4, p28
21. Vide Supra, Kitab Attib, Kitab AlMardha (the sick persons), vol 4, p 3
22. Ibn Taimyah: Al Fatawa Maktabat alMaarif, AlRibat (Morrocco) sponsored by King Khalid ibn Abdulaziz AlSoud, vol 19, p 13
23. Abu Da'ood: Sunan Abi Da'ood, Dar AlFIker, Beirut, Kitab Attib, vol 4, p 6, Hadith No. 3869
24. Muslim AlQushairi: Sahih Muslim Bishareh AlNawawi, Dar AlFiker, Beirut, Kitab Attib, vol 4, p 6, Hadith No. 3869
25. Glorious Qur'an: Sura AlBaqara 2/173
26. Abu Da'ood Al Fatawa Maktabat alMaarif, AlRibat (Morrocco) sponsored by King Khalid ibn Abdulaziz AlSoud Kitab Attib (Book of Medicine), Chapter: The Abhorred Medicines, vol. 4, pp 6–7, Hadith No. 3870 and 3871
27. Glorious Qur'an: Sura AlAnaam 6/14

Part II
The Four Principles of Biomedical Ethics with an Islamic Perspective

Chapter 6
Autonomy

Autonomy is a Greek word, autos: self, nomos: govern, rule, i.e., self-rule or self-government in the political sense, but it took a wider meaning as liberty rights, privacy, individual choice, freedom of the will, causing one's own behavior, and controlled by none except himself [1].

Personal autonomy means self-rule free from being controlled by others and from inadequate understanding that prevent meaningful choice. If the ability of free choice is curtailed by imprisonment, duress, or prodding (circumstances and environment) or by limitation of mental capacity or being a minor, we cannot speak of autonomy. Even if the person is addicted to alcohol or drugs his autonomy will definitely be curtailed.

In order to have autonomy two conditions are essential:

i. Free will: being independent from controlling influences from without (incarceration, threatening, duress, effect of the media, friends, and comrades or from within due to mental deficiency, disease, or age being minor or very old, or due to drugs of addiction or alcohol).
ii. Capacity of intentional action by an adult competent individual.

A person may be unable to comprehend financial matters, and hence needs a true advice, but he can comprehend many other things, e.g., buying a car or even a house. He may be able to decide about his treatment or being enrolled in medical research.

Informed Consent and Transparency

In order to have autonomy he should be well informed on the subject. The consent obtained is invalid if he is not informed, even if there is no coercion. In financial matters it is called transparency, and if there is no transparency the deal or contract can become invalid.

In Islam, if there is concealment of some facts or worse there are some lies, the deal or contract becomes invalid because of "Gharar" [2], i.e., being deceived by withholding important information. In pre-Islamic Arabia, some of the deals and contracts were so ambiguous that Prophet Muhammad (PBUH) considered these deals invalid. Any deceit or concealment of important information about the house you are going to buy or the land you are going to till or the machine you are going to work with makes the contract invalid.

© The Author(s) 2015   107
M.A. Al-Bar and H. Chamsi-Pasha, *Contemporary Bioethics*,
DOI 10.1007/978-3-319-18428-9_6

Similarly, any coercion makes the contract invalid. The pre-Islamic Arabs had slave girls, whom they forced them into prostitution to gain money. Islam emancipated them from this slavery and they were declared by the Qur'an to be forgiven, as they were driven into this dirty business without their will (Surah al Noor 24/33).

We have already alluded to the many verses of the Qur'an which declared that there is no compulsion in religion (Surah 2/256) and that each person has the full will to accept Islam or refuse it (Surah 18/29). The Qur'an said to the PBUH "Are you going (O Mohammed) to compel the people to believe" (Surah 10/99) and "You are not in control of them" (Surah 88/22). The Qur'an is replete with verses that orders freedom of faith and human personal responsibility [3].

Therefore there should be no intrusion, coercion, or even prodding to accept or refuse any modality of medical intervention. The exceptions are:

a. In an emergency where there is a life-threatening situation whereby action and intervention should be immediate in order to save life and ward off serious consequences.
b. In a situation, where the patient is a minor or mentally deficient, and the guardian adamantly refuses the treatment, which may be essential for the person under his custody. The magistrate should appoint another guardian or give authority to the treating physicians to implement the necessary required treatment, e.g., blood transfusion to the child of Jehovah witness parents, or an operation for appendicitis or hemodialysis required for a child or for a mentally retarded person.
   If the patient is a competent adult then the situation and dangers should be explained to him/her but the decision is his or hers.
c. In immunization schemes decided by the government to protect children and in cases of infectious diseases the treatment, if available becomes imperative.
d. In cases where a woman is in labor and there is a prolapsed cord that strangles the baby, this needs immediate caesarian operation. If the woman refuses to consent to the operation, the baby might die or suffer from serious sequelae in his mental capacity or nervous system or both.

The Islamic Jurists of the International Islamic Jurists Council (OIA) passed a ruling allowing the caesarian operation even if the lady and her husband refused the operation as it is an emergency to save a human life from death or serious sequelae [4]. Apart from these situations the decision of the patient should be respected if he/she is competent (mentally), and is an adult, not under the effect of alcohol or drugs. If there is misunderstanding of the seriousness of his/her medical condition, it should be carefully explained, but the final decision is his or hers. The volition and autonomy will definitely be curtailed by alcohol, drug of addiction, and the psychiatric condition of the person.

Advanced directives may be required, where a person is suffering from a chronic disease, or when he had cancer. He should be offered choices of what he/she wants to be done if for example his heart stops suddenly. Do not resuscitate (DNR) policy should be decided by the treating physicians, and it should remain a medical decision, though the situation could be discussed pre-hand if the patient is competent and wants to discuss this matter. He/she could appoint a proxy to act in his name, if he becomes incompetent because of the disease.

For an action to be autonomous it needs freedom from constraints and ability to comprehend its situation. "People's actions are rarely, if ever fully autonomous" [1], however they should have a fairly good knowledge of the modality of treatment or research, its side effects along with its presumed advantages, in order to give an informed consent.

The Role of the Family

In Asia, Africa, and the Middle East the family plays a major role in medical decisions. The patient whether he is elderly or a young person, has to listen to the opinion of his close family to the mode of treatment he/she is going to accept. In some places in Africa, the elders of the tribe, will decide in serious matter of life and death.

The Western attitude of individualism it is not accepted in many societies. In most countries of Asia, Africa, and the Middle East there is no health insurance for the public at large. Usually the family bears the burden of any cost of medical intervention.

Similarly there is no welfare state, and hence the breadwinner takes care of the elderly, the children, and ladies. Though females and children may be working at home, and in the field, or looking after the cattle and sheep of the family, they are usually not the breadwinners.

The role of the family and close friends should be respected in places where they have different philosophies and cultures that differ greatly from Western liberal, individualistic patterns. Even in the West itself, different minorities, e.g., Chinese, Indians, Pakistanis, etc., the role of the family should be respected, as the patients themselves agree to this role, and health providers have to understand that there are different cultures that do not give priority to autonomy, as it is understood in the West.

Advice and Waiver

Sometimes that patient will say to his doctor: "What is your advice in my condition? What would you do if your parent was in my situation? The physician may feel embarrassed, but he/she should be honest and give the sincere advice [5]. The matter may be more complicated when the patient relegates the decision making to the doctor saying: "Look I have trust in you, and whatever you decide I will accept." The physician should be tactful and try to explain the situation and give information to the patient and/or his family, and reach with them the course to be taken. As far as he can make it, the physician should explain that the decision should be in the hands of the patient (plus his family). He might help by giving all the required data, and even may give his personal advice.

In cases where the patient does not want to know the diagnosis, the physician should discuss the condition fully with the family, and let them try to persuade the patient, at least to take part in the decision-making.

The question of confidentiality will crop up here, if the family gets to know the details of the ailment and its management. If the patient agrees to divulge the intricacies of his medical condition to the family or proxy, then there is no breaking of confidentiality, as it is done after getting the consent of the patient himself.

Even in the West, there are many patients who do not want to know about their medical condition, or take part in decision-making. Dr. Schneider [5] said "While the patients largely wish to be informed about their medical circumstances, a substantial number of them (especially the elderly and the very sick) do not want to make their own medical decisions or perhaps even to participate in those decisions in any significant way."

Beauchamp and Childress [1] defended the right of the patients to choose whatever they find appropriate. They can delegate the decision making to a member of the family, a proxy or even to the treating physician himself.

In one study, researchers (UCLA) examined the different attitudes of 800 elderly subjects (65 years or older) from different backgrounds toward [1] disclosure of diagnosis and prognosis of a terminal illness [2] decision making at the end of life [6]. Only 47 % of Korean Americans agreed to be told of metastatic cancer, while 87 % of European Americans agreed to know the diagnosis and a similar figure of African Americans (88 %).

Similarly, in questions about decision of life support only a minority of Korean American and Mexican Americans agreed to decision-making in these matters while 60–65 % of European and Afro Americans agreed to decision-making in this terminal illness [6].

The investigators in this study stress that "belief in the ideal of patient autonomy is far from universal." A family centered model places higher value on the harmonious functioning of the family than on the autonomy of its members. Even in cases where family relations are strained, the family becomes furious if one of its members enters a hospital without prior consultation with family elders.

The physicians should ask their patients if they wish to receive information and make decisions, or if they prefer that their families handle such matters. The choice is rightly the patient's [1].

Traditional Navajo (Red Indians of USA) regard the discussion of negative information of a disease with the patient as potentially harmful. Any talk of the potential complications would result in the appearance of these complications, whether true or imagined [7].

A Navajo nurse reported that her father refused a bypass operation, as the cardiac surgeon explained so many complications of the surgical procedure [7]. A similar situation is found in many Arab countries. The physicians and surgeons usually give minimum information of the complications to the patient, if the patient is not accepting any such information, and would give more information to the family. The PBUH ordered the physician and visitors of the patient to give him hope, as it will improve his psychological condition, which may help in cure. Even if it did not help it will do no harm.

Many physicians in Arab and Muslim countries try to implement the Western standards of medical ethics; and especially in the field of autonomy, face many difficulties with at least some of their patients especially the elderly and those suffering from serious diseases. They have to adopt a softer attitude and give more hope to the patients [8], or at least abide by the patient's wishes if they do not want any further information. It may be more suitable to discuss the details with a responsible person/persons of the family. The norms are changing rapidly and with expansion of education and globalization, the Western attitudes toward autonomy, privacy, and personal liberty are going to be more acceptable especially to the young educated generation.

"There is a fundamental obligation to ensure that the patients have the right to choose, as well as the right to accept or to decline information. Forced information, forced choice and evasive disclosures are inconsistent with this obligation" as Beauchamp and Childress say [1].

The health providers should inquire whether their patients wish to receive information and make the decision or whether they would prefer to delegate these matters to certain members of their family. These wishes should be respected; and in fact represent respect of autonomy.

<u>Therapeutic Privilege</u>

The Hippocratic Oath gives the physician the privilege to decide whether to tell the patient of the diagnosis, prognosis or the side effects or conceal whatever he feels is going to harm the patient. The physician should tell the patient all the relevant data that will help the patient in his malady or ward off certain side effects. If the physician prescribed a drug that may cause drowsiness (e.g., diphenylhydantoin for epilepsy, diazepam anxiolytic drug or antiallergy drug) he should warn the patient not to drive a car or operate dangerous equipment until he is sure he knows how he responds to this drug.

This is engrained in beneficence and nonmaleficence, which is cornerstone of Hippocratic ethics.

The therapeutic privilege is when holding certain information that the physician believes would be harmful or upsetting to the patient. If the cancer patient knows that radiotherapy may cause severe burns, he or she may refuse the required treatment. Many patients refuse essential management or operative intervention, when they are told of the serious side effects that may occasionally occur. In such a case, the physician or surgeon may not divulge the information that he knows will disturb the patient and cause him to refuse an important mode of therapy.

The therapeutic privilege came into question in the USA in the 1960s, when litigations against physicians went to court. A lady Irma Natanson suffering from breast cancer needed radiation after mastectomy. The radiation caused severe burns and she sued her doctor, as she was not told about this side effect (the signature of consent was considered invalid as she was not informed). Her doctor defended himself that he withheld the information, as he felt, she would not agree to the required treatment , i.e., radiotherapy, if she knew about the possibility of severe burns. This is called Therapeutic Privilege [9].

The Judge Schroeder declared that "Anglo American law starts with the premise of a thorough going self- determination. It follows that each man is considered the master of his own body, and he may, if he be of sound mind, expressly prohibit the performance of life saving surgery or other medical treatment" [9].

In the 1970s the informed consent became well entrenched in Bioethics and any deviation needed the consent of the patient himself to waiver his responsibility and delegate it to others.

The problem was what would be considered an informed consent, and how much to tell. "Telling the patient everything about a procedure is an impossible task. All that is being called for is adequate information" [9]. However, the limits of adequate information may differ from case to case, and from culture to culture. A young man (19 years) suffering from ruptured disc in his backbone had laminectomy. Afterwards he fell from bed, which resulted in paraplegia (lower body paralysis). He sued his doctor, as he did not warn him about the seriousness of falling out of bed. The doctor's answer was that everybody (adult competent) should be careful not to fall out of bed; and this incident is so rare, that he did not mention it. Doctors are not expected to tell about the very rare complications [9].

In Islamic jurisprudence the consent of the patient is essential. When Prophet Muhammad, in his last illness, asked his wives not to force medicine if he gets stuporosed, through the side of his mouth, they did., When he came around, he ordered them to take the same medicine in the same way given to him. Each one of them did the same with the other [10]. This illustrates that the consent of the patient is essential, even if his condition is serious, and even if his refusal is by his hand [10]. All the books of Islamic jurisprudence for the last 1,000 years agree that in order to practice medicine (or surgery) there are two conditions [1] the physician is qualified and has been given permission to practice medicine (or surgery) by the responsible authority [2] he should obtain the consent of the patient if he is a competent adult [11]. If he is a minor or incompetent then the consent of his guardian should be obtained (unless in emergency).

For veterinary medicine, the veterinary physician should obtain the consent of the owner of the cattle (camels, cows, sheep, or goats). Otherwise, he may be liable and pay the compensation of any harm.

If the physician is not known of practicing medicine and he has not obtained permission to practice, then he is liable to another punishment (may be corporal or incarceration); and he is prevented from practicing medicine until he gets the required license [12].

The Ministry of Health of Saudi Arabia distributed regulations to all health providers in 1404H (1984 CE) ordering physicians not to practice any mode of treatment unless there is consent from the patient, if he is competent, or his representative, if he is incompetent, except in emergency cases. There is no difference between male or female in this respect. The physician/surgeon should give sufficient information to the patient or his/her representative, if incompetent, so that his/her consent is informed [12].

Prior to this regulation, many patients were operated on without consent. The surgeon agrees with the family to operate without informing the patient. Newspaper AlMadina Issue No. 5495 on 10/6/1402 Hijra (1982 CE) published that the surgeon in AlKhubar Hospital (Eastern Province of Saudi Arabia) operated on a competent adult patient without his consent or even knowing that he is to be operated. The surgeon collaborated with the family to operate on the patient, as he was afraid of all surgical interventions, without his knowledge. The newspaper commended this approach, for which one of us (M. Albar) responded by writing a long letter, which was published condemning such act, and that it is illegal and the patient can sue the surgeon, even if the operation was successful.

Even after the circular of Ministry of Health was published, many hospitals continued to ask the patients just to sign that he/she agrees to have an operation and anesthesia, without even mentioning the type of anesthesia or the name of the operation, let alone getting an informed consent.

Fortunately, this unethical practice is disappearing. In China, at the time of the Cultural Revolution (Mao Tse Tong era) 100 million Chinese men and women were sterilized without any consent. Indira Ghandi of India in the seventies of twentieth century sterilized 11 million men and women by force.

In Egypt, at the time of President Jamal Abdul Naser, the doctors of government hospitals were ordered to insert I.U.D.s (intrauterine devices) whenever they examine the female genital system, without even informing the lady, if that lady has a certain number of children. This was witnessed by one of us (M. Albar) who was working as an intern in Cairo Hospitals in 1964–1965.

Such horrendous actions were not uncommon in third world countries, which were unfortunately supported by Western Governments in order to curb explosion of World population. China was encouraged since early sixties to adopt one child policy. If a woman was pregnant for the second time, then she had to abort by force of law.

Female infanticide became rampant both in China and India; and when ultra-sound became available late pregnancy abortion was carried on whenever the pregnancy was assured of being female, which is still happening up to this moment (2014).

The informed consent and human rights are limited to the democratic countries of the West, but may be absent in many third world countries. If a country is lacking the essential food and clean water for a major sector of its population, then any talk of informed consent, autonomy, and human rights is superfluous, unless the basic needs of food, clean water, shelter, and basic rule of law is first established.

The Change of Attitude of the Physicians in Telling Bad News in USA [9]

Donald Oken published a study in 1961, in which he asked US physicians what was their policy of telling the truth to terminally ill cancer patients. 84 % said it was their policy not to tell the patients the true diagnosis, in order not to cause more distress to their suffering patients.

However, in the late 1960s and early 1970s, the community was changed. Respect of persons emerged as a dominant principle in medical ethics—the time of Roe versus Wade involving abortion (1973), the Natanson Case involving informed consent (1960), and the Karen Quinlan Case involving the right to refuse life support. In 1979, Dennis Novack published a study in which he replicated Oken's question (about the policy of physicians in telling the patients the diagnosis of their terminal cancer); 98 % of the physicians declared that they tell their patients the true diagnosis of their terminal illness. The change is dramatic in less than 20 years.

The changes in the community at large, and the libertarian movement and philosophy became predominant, and respect of autonomy and human rights became an integral part of medical ethics, i.e., an ethic of respect for persons. There is also a practical consequential pragmatic need to tell the patient of his/her true diagnosis. The treatment of malignancy involves operative intervention, chemotherapy and radiotherapy, and each of these has many complications. It is impossible that any competent person would consent for these drastic procedures, unless he/she knows exactly the true diagnosis, and its seriousness.

The veracity of the physicians (telling truth) is important in the medical profession as it (a) engenders fidelity: the physician by telling the truth is actually showing fidelity to his patient, which will be reciprocated by trust of the patient and fidelity from his side (b) it engenders better relations between the physician and his or her patients. It will definitely be reflected in better management of diseases. The patient will be more attentive to the advices of the physician, e.g., losing weight, stopping smoking or drugs or alcohol, dangerous sexual practices, etc. He or she will be more amendable to suggestion of changing his/her lifestyle, or taking his antihypertensive or diabetic drugs regularly as advised and prescribed... (c) it fulfills the autonomy of the patient.

The respect of persons is interweaved with (i) autonomy; (ii) veracity; (iii) fidelity, each one of these leads and supports the other.

Limits of Autonomy

The freedom of one person cannot in anyway interfere with other people's freedom; otherwise it will be a hegemony or dictatorship. The limit of the freedom is respect of others freedom, faith and conduct as long as it is not going to disturb the community or sects in that community.

The rights of any one are reciprocated by duties. Those who speak of woman's rights to abortion, as the fetus is part of her body, and she, according to their point of view, can remove that part if she wishes.

There is a fallacy here; the baby in her womb is another life (formed from both parents), and it is an independent new life though still needing the mother's placenta and womb for its growth. Killing that fetus (baby) is killing another life or at least (in its early stages) a prospect of another life.

The human being according to the Islamic dogma is created by God and he/she should obey the orders of God, as revealed by his Messengers.

God himself gave human beings a degree of autonomy to choose between things and hence he/she will be held responsible for their actions.

Van Bommel also says: "For a Muslim patient, absolute autonomy is very rare, there will be a feeling of responsibility toward God, and he or she lives in social coherence, in which influences of the relatives play their roles". Consequently, personal choices are only accepted if they are the "right" ones [3].

A person cannot kill himself (suicide), as he is not the giver of life. It is Allah (God) who gives life and take life, and hence transgressors will be held responsible for all their actions in the final Day of Judgment.

The human being in Islamic teaching is entrusted with his body, his faculties, his youth, his fortune, and so on. He/she can only act in the way already prescribed by God. He cannot mutilate himself, or do harm to himself by smoking, taking drugs or imbibing alcohol. His sexual relations should be through marriage alone. Extra or premarital sex is not allowed. Sodomy is worse than fornication and is no less than adultery.

We, all of us, will be called to answer why did we transgress these clear teachings, even if the harm does not involve any one else except the perpetrator.

If we have traffic laws, and we have to obey these laws, even if breaking the law did not cause any harm to others or even to ourselves; then we have to obey the laws of God, of respecting life and not purposely endangering it otherwise we will be judged by Him on resurrection day.

Many philosophies and religions put limit to autonomy, e.g., Marxism, Socialism, Judaism and Christianity. Robert Veach says: "Early Judaism and Christianity had no principle of autonomy any more than any other ancient culture did...Jewish Talmudic ethics has no principle of autonomy" [9].

Bleich [13] (a well-known Jewish ethicist Rabbi) said that in the Talmudic teachings, the patient has no right to refuse treatment. Early Christianity had no principles of autonomy, and only when John Wycliffe and John Hus in the four-teenth century recognized the importance of the individual, it became more evident with appearance of Protestantism in the sixteenth century and clearly accepted as the cornerstone of ethics by the German Philosopher Immanuel Kant (1724–1804), one of the greatest philosophers of Europe and Enlightenment. His comprehensive and systematic work in the theory of knowledge, ethics, and aesthetics greatly influenced many subsequent philosophers and thinkers [14].

He refused to be ordained as a Lutheran Minister, and preferred the humble job of a private tutor and lecturer. His chief works were "critique of pure reason," "critique of practical reason," and "critique of judgment." He extolled duty (deontology) and refused utilitarian consequentialist philosophy. He built his philosophy on respect of every human being; his free will (autonomy), veracity (truth telling) and keeping promise. Lying or breaking promise is not allowed whatever may be the excuse. If truth telling is going to harm an innocent person, it is not allowed in Kantian Philosophy to lie, and if we gave a promise to our children to have a picnic or travel in vacation, but one of the parents fell ill and needs our help, to Kant it is imperative to fulfill the promise especially if we gave the parents no promise of help in their need. All religions especially Judaism, Christianity, and Islam order us to be kind to our parents, and whatever they need we have to fulfill first. In Christianity, it is claimed that Jesus refused his mother (Mathew 1/18-25). In Islam, the Qur'an says that Jesus was obedient and very kind to his mother, and always praised her [15]. Islam considers being kind and good to your parents takes precedent of anything else. You have to obey them except when they order you to worship idols or to transgress; only then you should not obey them. Nevertheless, continue to be kind and generous with them [16].

Deontologist (Kantian Philosophy) hold that some choices cannot be justified by their effect no matter how morally good their consequences are. The right has priority over good, no matter the amount of good it will produce. It also stresses the importance of good intention in order that the act be considered moral. Both Christianity (Aquinos: Summa Theologica) and Islam stress the importance of good intention and nonreprehensible means.

In Islamic teachings, though the intention is of paramount importance (niyah), the means to fulfill such an intention bear the same value. However, Islamic teachings look to the consequences and if we can predict an evil or bad result then that action should not be taken.

Lying is one of the worse sins in Islam, but if lying is going to save an innocent person (e.g., a Jew hiding in your house followed by the Nazi as happened in Morocco during World War II), lying in this case can become a virtue instead of being a vice. The categorical philosophy of Kant will never accept such attitude, as principles should be kept whatever may be the consequences.

Letting a patient die by not putting a ventilator and doing cardiopulmonary resuscitation (CPR) is not tantamount to killing. In fact, physicians order DNR, in terminally ill patients where CPR and putting a ventilator will only increase the suffering of the patient and his family, and is considered futile.

The Fatwa No. 12086 dated 30/6/1409 (1989) of the High Council of Scholars and Ifta'a (issuing religious decisions) of Saudi Arabia, Riyadh, allowed "Do Not Resuscitate Policy" if three competent physicians decided it, as it is futile. The decision of these specialists and competent physicians of integrity should be respected [17].

The subject should be discussed with the patient prior to his final illness or if there is advanced directives. It should be discussed with the family (usually there is no advanced directive in third world countries).

Mercy killing (euthanasia) is not allowed even if the patient insistently request it and his family agree to it. Killing is a crime whatever its name (mercy killing) and is not allowed in Islam and by the law. The perpetrator will be punished; the type of punishment may be reduced from capital punishment to imprisonment, as the perpetrator did it on demand of the person himself. Even if the law exonerates him from retribution, he is morally wrong and will be judged by God on the final Day of Judgment.

The Deontological Kantian Categorical Philosophy is rights based. They proscribe using of another's body, labor, and talent without consent. Several philosophers of this school, e.g., Robert Nozick, Bernard Williams, and Thomas Nagel have developed the doctrine regardless of consequences [18]. The heinous examples of biomedical research carried out in USA and elsewhere, without consent (let alone informed consent) which exposed those researched to serious harm and sometimes death, should be considered as nefarious crimes that should never be condoned or allowed. The utilitarian consequential philosophy allowed such horrendous experiments and research, on the presumption that great good would occur to whole communities, was proved to be a fallacy. Even if there are good consequences; that will not in any way allow such nefarious heinous so called biomedical research, which ended in killing and harming many. Deontological constraints cannot justify serious harm done to few to ward off greater harm to many.

The deontologists will abide by the moral law of autonomy giving those to be researched full information with all the bad consequences, and letting them decide freely without any coercion or incitement to accept or refute participation in such research. It also abides by the moral law of nonmaleficence.

The researcher or the physicians treating patients should never do harm to patients or those to be researched intentionally. However, if research or treatment ended in unintentional harm (not due to negligence) then the question of compensation will be raised. If however, there was an intention to harm; or even harm due to blatant negligence then the case should be under criminal and not civil law.

Kantian philosophy is important in changing the Western countries to the importance of autonomy, veracity, fidelity, and human rights. It has a great moral effect in improving the standards of medical management and bioethical research.

Notes and References

1. Beauchamp T, Childress J (2001) Principles of biomedical ethics, 5th edn. Oxford University Press, New York, pp 57–104
2. Gharar means a kind of deceit which makes the contract invalid. There are many Hadiths admonishing Muslims not to deceive or conceal any defects. The Prophet (PBUH) found somebody selling wheat; he found the inside of the heap of wheat wet. He asked the vendor "What is this?" He said, "It was raining and made it wet". The Prophet said: "Why did not you expose it and put it on top of the heap. That who deceives us is not from us (i.e. not from the Muslim community)". It is not allowed even to deceive that who had already deceived you. There should be not deceipt whatsoever in any dealing with any body, Muslim or non Muslim. If a person knows he is sterile and wants to marry a woman, then he should tell her the fact. Otherwise, she can repudiate the marriage, even after consummation, the dowry (mahr) will be hers and she will not have to repay it back to him
3. Chamsi-Pasha H, Albar MA (2013) Western and Islamic bioethics: How close is the gap? Avicenna J Med 3(1):8–14
4. Fatwas and Decisions of the International Islamic Jursiprudence Council (OIA: Organisation of Islamic Countries): Decision No. 7/5/67 on Consent of the Patient, in 7th session, held in Jeddah 9–14 May 1992 and Decision (Fatwa) No. 171 (10/18) held in PutraJaya, Malaysia, 18th Session 9–24 July 2007, and Fatwa (Decision) on Consent in urgently needed operative intervention; and Decision No. 184 (10/19) in the 19th session held in Sharja, UAE 26–30 April, 2009 on Consent in Urgently Needed Operative Intervention which was started in the previous meeting (18th Session 2007) but not finished. Book of Decision. International Islamic Jurisprudence Council, Jeddah
5. Schneider C (1998) The practice of autonomy: Patients, Doctors and Medical Decision. Oxford University Press, New York, p xi

6. Blackhall L, Murphy S, Frank G (1995) Ethnicity and attitudes towards patient autonomy. JAMA (J Am Med Assoc 274:820–825

7. Carrese J, Rhodes L (1995) Western bioethics on the navajo reservation: benefit or harm? JAMA 274:826–829

8. The Prophet Muhammad (PBUH) said: If you visit the patient, give him hope of recovering and living. That will not change his fate, but it will improve his psyche. SunanalTirmithi (Kitab Attib). Sunan ibn Maja (Kitab AlJanayiz) narrated through Abu Saeed AlKhodri, the Companion of the Prophet (PBUH). Ibn AlQayim commented in his book Tibbi Nabawi that improving the psychological condition of the patient and giving him hope, improves his own defenses against disease, and gives him power to overcome the disease

9. Veach R (2002) The basics of bioethics, 2nd edn. Prentice Hall, New Jersey, pp 74–84

10. This Hadith (Saying of the Prophet) is narrated by Aisha bint Abibaker (the favorite wife of the Prophet (PBUH) in Sahih AlBokhari and Sahih Muslim, and by Om Salama (another wife of the Prophet [PBUH]) with more details e.g. Constituents of the medicament: Ood hindi (costos), worse [a yellow plant like curcumine] and olive oil. Everybody in the house was ordered to take the medicament in the same way as they gave to the Prophet Muhammad (PBUH); except his Uncle Al Abbas who did not participate with them

11. Chamsi-Pasha H, Albar MA (2013) Islamic medical ethics a thousand years ago. Saudi Med J 34(7):673–675

12. Albar M (1995) Al Ma'sooliya Attibiya wa Akhlaqiat Attabib (The liability of physicians and bioethics). Jeddah, Dar AlManarah, pp 67–76

13. Bleich D (1979) The obligation to heal in the judaic tradition: a comparative analysis. In: Rosner F, Bleich D (eds) Jewish Bioethics. Sanhedrin Press, New York, pp 1–44

14. Encyclopedia Britannica, 15th edn, 1982. Micropedia vol 5/695

15. Surah Maryam 19/32, Jesus said (talking in the cradle after his birth): "And God made me dutiful and kind to my mother, and He has not made me a wretched tyrant"

16. Sura Luqman 31/14, 15, "And We enjoined upon man (to care) of his parents. His mother carried him in weakness upon weakness, and his weaning is in 2 years. Be grateful to Me and to your parents; to Me is the final destination. But if they endeavor to make you associate with Me that of which you have no knowledge do not obey them, but accompany them in this world with appropriate kindness". The Qur'an is full of many verses ordering Muslims to be kind with the parents especially in their old age. He/she should be grateful to Allah and to his/her parents e.g. Surah 2/83, Surah 4/36, Sura 6/151, Surah 17/23, 24, Surah 19/32. There are also many Hadiths (Sayings of the Prophet [PBUH]) ordering Muslims to worship God and be kind and grateful to parents. Being unkind to parents is one of the worst sins in Islam. It comes next to associating God with deities (Shirk) i.e. polytheism

17. Appendix No. 5 in Dr. M. Albar book: Alhayata AlInsaniyah alDonyawiah: Mata Tabda wa Mata Tantahi (Human life in this world: when it starts and when it ends), Dar Al Qalam, Damascus, 2004

18. Beauchamp T, Childress J Principles of biomedical ethics (reference no. 1), pp 352–354

Chapter 7
Nonmaleficence

This is an important obligation in morality and medical ethics (doing no harm). It is associated with the maxim "primum non nocere," above all do no harm. In Islamic teachings Prophet Muhammad (PBUH) said, "Doing harm and reciprocating harm is not allowed" [1]: "La Dharar wa la Dhirar."

In Islamic jurisprudence axioms: "Avoiding harm takes precedence over bringing good." It simply means if a certain action end in both good and harm, then it is preferable first to thwart off harm. However, if the benefit is much greater than the harm, then that action could be applied. Al Izz ibn Abdul Salam (d660H/1262 CE) a renowned Islamic jurist in his book "Qawaeed AlAhkam" "Basics of Rulings" said "The aim of medicine is to preserve health, restore it when it is lost; remove ailment or reduce its effect. To reach that goal it may be essential to accept the lesser harm, in order to ward off a greater harm, or lose a certain benefit to procure a greater one" [2].

He also said, "Medicine in the Sha'riahis regarded as a field that brings the benefits of health and wards off the harms of disease and ailments" [2].

The axioms of warding harm in Islamic jurisprudence are:

(1) Doing harm and reciprocating harm is not allowed.
(2) Harm should be warded and avoided as much as possible.
(3) All that is harmful is prohibited in Sha'riah. That will involve medicines made from porcine material, alcohol, carrion (dead animals) or seeking remedy by amulets, sorcery, and divination. Any mode of treatment that causes harm without any good is not allowed. Similarly if the harm is more than the benefit, or even if the expected harm is equal to the expected good, it is not allowed. However, if the expected benefit is greater than the harm, then it is allowed. If a patient is having a gangrenous foot or limb, and the gangrene might increase and even kill the patient, then it is allowed to amputate the limb. Similarly if a woman is pregnant and continuation of pregnancy is threatening her life, then she is allowed to abort. If the continuation of pregnancy is going to endanger her health, but not her life, or the fetus is grossly malformed, then abortion is allowed prior to ensoulment, i.e., in the first **120 days** computed from time of fertilization of the ovum (i.e., conception) which is equivalent to **134** days from last menstrual period

© The Author(s) 2015
M.A. Al-Bar and H. Chamsi-Pasha, *Contemporary Bioethics*,
DOI 10.1007/978-3-319-18428-9_7

(LMP) which is used by obstetricians, and that is equivalent to **19 weeks + 1 day** [3]. But it is not allowed to have abortion after that date. Yet it is possible to have preterm delivery, e.g., 36 weeks or even less if deemed necessary.

(4) If there is certain harm, then it should be removed.

(5) Harm should not be removed by another harm, which is equivalent to the previous harm; or worse if it is removed and replaced by a worse harm. However, if the harm cannot be removed except by accepting a lesser harm, then the lesser harm is accepted. This follows the next axiom.

(6) The greater harm could be replaced by a lesser harm. Examples of this in medicine is amputation of a limb, if gangrene is spreading; or accepting to use narcotics to relieve pain, even if morphine and its derivative have a double effect, i.e., the debilitated patient suffering from pain due to metastasis and chronic pulmonary disease where morphine and its derivatives is going to depress the respiratory center in the medulla in the brain stem, and therefore may end in respiratory failure. The serious side effect in such a patient would be accepted if the pain was not relieved except by the narcotic. The dose should be the minimum required to alleviate pain. Muslim jurists in the past brought the case of a man who adopted Islam. He was required to circumcise his prepuce, but if that was going to harm him (there was no proper anesthetic), then he was allowed to pray and do all the required worship of Islam without circumcision.

The balancing of harms is important in Islamic jurisprudence, and if it is impossible to thwart harm, without causing another harm, then the lesser harm should be accepted.

(7) The prohibited things would be allowed if there is necessity. If a person is lost in the desert and he is thirsty and he finds only alcoholic beverages, e.g., wine, then he is allowed to drink it to quench his thirst. Similarly, if he has no food, and only finds pork or carrion (dead meat), or blood, then he is allowed to eat it to save his life. But he is not allowed to kill another human being (a child or diseased weak person) in order to save his life. He can kill any animal that he finds or even eat the corpse of an animal or, worse, the corpse a human if there is no alternative.

In medicine the same rules may apply. Taking medicine made of porcine material or alcohol or poisonous snakes is allowed if there is no alternative medicament.

Similarly, autopsy and dissection of human bodies would be allowed in

   (i) Coroners' cases, i.e., medicolegal cases ordered by the magistrate in order to reveal the cause of death or help in identifying the perpetrator

   (ii) To teach anatomy, physiology, and pathology which are needed to bring up physicians and health providers [4].
       It is allowed to take an organ from a living donor if such donation is not going to harm the donor seriously. The donor should be adult competent and donating by his free will [5].

If the person is deceased (brain dead), then organs could be taken if he had agreed during his lifetime to donate, or his family has agreed to donate after his death [5]. The consent should be informed and no selling or bargaining is involved. The government can encourage donation by giving medals, free medical services, or even a fixed amount of money. This is still debatable in the West, but it is practiced in Iran and Saudi Arabia [5].

(8) As long as harm continues, it cannot be ignored. So long as the harmful effect is there, then it should be removed. Whatever system is there that involves harmful effects, then that harm should be removed out of the system. Otherwise the whole system should be changed. If in a certain community all foreigners officially residing in a country are not covered by health insurance or health services, that system should be changed.

(9) The harm befalling a whole community is worse than the harm falling an individual. The general harm should be warded off first. If the general harm cannot be prevented unless it affects few, then the general harm should be prevented, even if it involves one or few individuals.

(10) If there are two harms, then the lesser harm could be done if it is impossible to ward off both harms.

(11) If there are two benefits, then the higher benefit should be obtained, even if it involves losing the lesser one.

(12) If both harm and benefit are involved, then try to get the benefit and refuse the harm. If that is not possible and the benefit is much greater than the harm, then accept the lesser harm. However, if the harm is equal or even more than the benefit, then refuse the harm even if it means loss of the benefit.

(13) "Legal permission negates tortious liability," except in cases of flagrant negligence. These rules have great bearing in medical practice from both the ethical and legal points of view. The law differentiates between crime and tort.

Crime is a legal wrong, the remedy of which is the punishment of the offender at the instance of the state. It can be defined also as a legal wrong that can be followed by criminal proceedings, which result in punishment [6].

Tort is the law of damages; the civil law of liability is not designed to punish anyone, punishment is the function of the criminal law, compensation is the function of civil law (tort) [7].

The Sha'riah combines both the civil law (tort) and the criminal law. An act can be either a civil wrong or a crime, or can be both [8].

Similarly, an act may be morally wrong but is not punishable by law.

Some moral philosophers combine nonmaleficence with beneficence in a simple principle. "William Frankena, for instance, divides the principle of beneficence into four general obligations, the first of which we identify as the obligation of nonmaleficence and the other three of which we refer to as obligation of beneficence" as Beauchamp and Childress say in "Principles of Biomedical Ethics" [9]. These are:

(1) One ought not to inflict evil or harm
(2) One ought to prevent evil or harm
(3) One ought to remove evil or harm
(4) One ought to do or promote good

Frankena arranges these elements serially, so that other things are equal in a circumstance of conflict. The first takes precedence over the second, the second over the third, and the third over the fourth [9].

It is amazing to find a saying of Prophet Muhammad (PBUH) ordering Muslims to:

(i)   Do and promote good
(ii)   Remove evil or harm
(iii) Prevent evil or harm and enjoin doing good and preventing harm, and
(iv)   The least thing one can do is not to inflict harm [10].

In another tradition, he told his companions not to stay in public way (roads or lanes), they said we have to stay there. He said if that is so then give the public way its rights. They exclaimed, "What are the rights of the way?," he said: "Not to stare at people (passing by); do no harm, greet people, enjoin right and forbid wrong; guide those who lost their way and help those who are in need [11]."

Muslim jurists, as already mentioned, put thwarting harm, removing harm, and not doing harm as more important than bringing benefit (good), unless the benefit is so great that the harm could be accepted in order to obtain this great benefit.

Beauchamp and Childress [9] said: "Obligation not to harm others (e.g. those prohibiting theft, disablement and killing) are distinct from obligation to help others."

"Obligation not to harm others are sometimes more stringent than obligations to help them, but obligations of beneficence are also sometimes more stringent than obligations of nonmaleficence." The obligation to rescue an injured or dying person is definitely more important than giving alms to the needy or even if it involves doing a minor harm to a person.

Generally, nonmaleficence is more important than beneficence.

The authors (Beauchamp and Childress) put the following arrangement:

Nonmaleficence: [1] one ought not to inflict evil or harm.

Beneficence: [2] one ought to prevent evil or harm, [3] one ought to remove evil or harm (both 2 and 3 could be also included in nonmaleficence), [4] one ought to do or promote good

The Glorious Qur'an is full of verses ordering Muslims to enjoin what is right and forbidding what is wrong, e.g....

Surah 3/104: "And let there be from you a nation inviting to good, enjoining what is right and forbidding what is wrong; and those will be the successful."

Surah 3/110: "You are the best nation produced for mankind. You enjoin what is right and forbid what is wrong and believe in Allah."

Surah 3/114: Describes the believers, "They believe in Allah, and the Last Day, and enjoin what is right and forbid what is wrong and hasten to do good deeds. And those are among the righteous."

Surah 16/90-91: "Indeed, Allah orders justice and good conduct, and giving to relatives and forbids immortality and bad conduct and oppression. He admonishes you that perhaps you will be reminded. And fulfill the covenant of Allah you have taken and do not break oaths after their confirmation, while you have made Allah, over you, a security (i.e., witness). Indeed Allah knows what you do."

Surah 2/177: "Righteousness is not that you turn your faces toward the East or West (in prayers), but (true) righteousness is one who believes in Allah, the Last Day, the Angels, the Books, and the Prophets and gives wealth in spite of love for it, to relatives, orphans, the needy, the traveler (way farer), those who ask (for help) and for freeing slaves; who fulfill their promise when they promise, and who are patient (i.e.. forebear) in poverty, hardships and during battle. Those are the ones who have been true, and it is those who are righteous."

Surah 31/17-19: "O my son, establish prayer, enjoin what is right, forbid what is wrong, and be patient over what befalls you ... and do not turn your cheek (in contempt) toward people, and do not walk through the earth exultantly. Indeed Allah does not like every one self deluded (conceited) and boastful. And be moderate in your pace, and lower your voice; indeed, the most disagreeable of sounds is the voice of donkeys." Many other verses/ayas order enjoining the right and forbidding the wrong, e.g., Surah 7/157, Surah 9/71, Surah 29/45.

Preventing evil or harm and removing it when it is there can also be considered as a type of beneficence. Beneficence is not limited to doing or promoting good, but definitely will involve preventing or removing harm.

Harm is not limited to physical harm; it involves harm to reputation, property, privacy, and liberty. Omar ibn AlKhattab (the 2nd Caliph) ordered a poet called alHutta'ia to be imprisoned as he in one of his poems inflicted harm on alZubraqan by saying, "Do not travel and toil to do the magnanimous act, but stay in your locality for food, drink and dress." This was considered libel, and hence he was imprisoned. The Arabs considered libel worse than killing if it was said in poetry, as the Arabs were fond of poetry and learning it by heart; and the whole nation will know about it.

Negligence and the Standard of Due Care

"Obligations of nonmaleficence are not only obligations of not inflicting harms, but also include obligation of not imposing risks of harm. A person can harm or place another person at risk without malicious or harmful intent" [9].

Unintended harm should be compensated in both Sha'riah and Civil Law, though there is no punishment. If a person aims at animal (game), but the bullet or arrow struck unintentionally a human being, then the perpetrator should pay a blood fine (100 camels or its value plus freeing a slave. If that is not available he should fast for two consecutive months). The blood fine should be paid by the Aqila, i.e., the male members of the tribe, as it is almost impossible to be paid by the perpetrator, unless he is wealthy. This system of Aqila changed at the time of Omar ibn alKhatab, the second Caliph, as whole tribes were dispersed in different places fighting the Roman and Persian Empires. He created the Diwan, i.e., the registry, taking note of the people who live together and get their pay from one government source. The jurists of today accepted the insurance, as both the Aqila and Diwan are no more in existence [12].

Health providers should pay compensation if their actions of medical or surgical treatment resulted in harm. However, if side effects of the management occur, then the competent physician should be considered not liable. The legal Islamic axiom "Legal Permission negates tortuous liability." Ibn alQayim in his book "Tibbi Nabawi" (The Medicine of the Prophet) [13] said: The Practitioner (attabib) who is well trained, alert, and keen is the one who has done his job well. He was authorized by the state and had the consent of the patient. Despite that his patient succumbed or there was damage to a part or to one or more of his senses, such a practitioner is not liable. This is the view of almost all jurists (fuqaha) of all the schools of Islamic fiqh (jurisprudence). Ibn AlQayim then brings the position of the person who claims to be a physician, but he neither had proper training nor had been authorized to practice medicine. Then he should be liable according to the saying of the PBUH. "That who practices medicine without due knowledge is liable." But if the patient knew that he is not authorized to practice and gave him consent, then the patient himself is responsible of the outcome. However, if the patient thought he is an authorized physician then that person (the quack) is liable. AbdulMalik ibn Habib alBeiri (Andalusia) said: "Not only he should be liable and pay the compensation but he should be punished for practicing without due knowledge and not being authorized" [14].

If the person is qualified to practice medicine, but he did not obtain consent from his patient or his guardian (if he is incompetent or a minor), then he may be liable unless it is an emergency to save a life or a limb or thwart a serious damage. However, ibn alQayim thinks it may be said he is (i.e., the practitioner) is only trying to do good and God says, "There is no blame for those doing good (or intending to do good)," [Surah 9/91] as God is Forgiving and Merciful.

However, the other jurists agree that if the practitioner caused harm (unintentionally), then he is liable and should compensate. If the compensation is 1/3 of the Diyah (blood fine: the value of 100 camels), then it should be paid by the practitioner himself, but if it is more than 1/3 of the Diyah, then it should be paid by the Aqila, or if not available, then it should be paid from the public funds. Jurists of today agree to a type of insurance [12].

All jurists agree that if there is blatant negligence, even if the practitioner is a highly qualified and well-known physician, then he will be liable.

Negligence is the absence of due care. In the profession of medicine, it involves a departure from the standard care. The more senior the person, the more responsible he becomes and if a minor mistake is forgiven from a junior, such a mistake may not be forgiven for a consultant. Negligence usually occurs due to lack of proper care, and therefore, considered unintentional (inadvertent). However reckless, blatant negligence is considered in the civil law as intentional (advertent). Thus, for example, the mistake that occurs in the case of operating on the normal limb instead of the diseased one, or operating in the normal eye or ear instead of the diseased one. Forgetting surgical instruments, cotton, or swabs in the wound without removing it and stitching over it resulting in serious sequelae. Such practices are not very rare and hence the perpetrator is liable and compensation (indemnity) is required. Other disciplinary measures may be taken, e.g., suspension of the authorization of practice, or even canceling it completely if the horrible mistake is repeated by the same person. Surgeons who perform surgery after drinking alcohol are more liable to succumb to these horrendous mistakes.

Professional malpractice is an instance of negligence. If the physician does not follow the professional standards, he may be considered liable. However, if there is harm despite the health provider following the standard care required by his profession, then he is not liable. Negligence cannot be imputed because a cure is not affected. The practitioner should put his effort and knowledge to cure the disease, if possible, but he cannot guarantee cure, or even improvement of the malady, even if the disease is known to be curable. The patient's immune system may be weak, the microorganism may be more virulent, or the drug used caused an unexpected side effect or allergic reaction.

The practitioner has to do his duty by providing required care, and by following the standards of the profession. The implied contract with the patient does not include a promise to effect a cure; and negligence cannot be imputed because cure is not effected [9].

To win a negligence case it is necessary to prove the duty of care, the standard of care given (should be acceptable by professional peers), and the injury that was caused by the failure to practice properly [15].

Beauchamp and Childress [9] put the following essential elements to prove negligence:

(1) The professional must have a duty to the affected party.
(2) The professional must breach that duty.
(3) The affected party must experience harm.
(4) The harm must be caused by the breach of duty.

The question of end-of-life treatment will be discussed in a separate chapter in detail. The salient points in this regard are:

(a) It is not imperative on a Muslim to seek remedy except in life-saving situations, and where the illness is due to infectious bugs (microorganisms) for which treatment is available. The patient should be treated, even against his will, if he is going to infect other people.
(b) Stopping (withdrawing) or not starting (withholding) certain types of management are allowed in the following cases:

   (i) Brain dead cases firmly diagnosed;
   (ii) If the treating physicians find a certain modality of treatment useless (futile), or going to increase the suffering of the patient;
   (iii) Stopping certain measure that support life (withdrawing) or not starting these measures (withholding), e.g., Do Not Resuscitate or Do Not

Intubate measures are accepted if the decision is reached by at least three competent specialist physicians as ordered by the Fatwa of the Permanent Commission for Research and Endowment No. 12086 dated 28/3/1409 (1989) which allowed withholding and withdrawing life support if decided by at least three competent specialist physicians. This medical decision should be fully explained to the family, but it remains a medical decision [16].

The question of artificial feeding of comatose or persistent vegetative states, by intravenous or by nasogastric tube, is a point of contestation in the West. There are many who considered it as a type of treatment, and hence could be futile. Many courts allowed stopping sustenance technology (i.e., nutrition and hydration by artificial means). The first one was the New Jersey Supreme Court in 1976 that it was permissible for a guardian to disconnect Karen Ann Quinlan from respirator and allow her to die. However, she lived for 10 years after disconnection of respirator, but continued her sustenance (nutrition and hydration) by tubes [9].

Several Roman Catholic moral theologians advised the relatives that they were not morally required to continue medically administered nutrition and hydration (MN & H) or antibiotics to fight infections.

The New Jersey Supreme Court allowed withdrawal of MN & H in 1985 from an 84-old person in a nursing home suffering from debilitated disease who had been on artificial feeding for many years.

A Massachusetts court reached a similar decision in Brophy case, a 49-year-old man who was in persistent vegetative states for 3 years in 1986 [17]. Courts since then viewed MN & H as a medical procedure subject to the same evaluative standards as other medical procedures, and thus allowed stopping sustenance (nutrition and hydration) and letting the patient die.

It is a horrible type of death as it takes 10 to 14 days to die suffering from hunger and thirst. These poor patients do not die in peace, as alleged by the perpetrators, and it would be less painful by injecting drugs that would end the suffering in a few minutes.

We are not endorsing euthanasia, but this type of dying is worse than euthanasia, as they will not suffer the agony of being deprived of nutrition and hydration.

In Islamic jurisprudence preventing nutrition and hydration, is a clear case of murder, that would be punished by Qisas (capital punishment unless the awliya agree to pardon or take blood fine, i.e., diya).

The case of Theresa Schiavo (Born December 1963 and died by stopping nutrition and hydration March 31, 2005). She was married to Michael Schiavo in 1984, suffered cardiac arrest in 1990 and as sequelae suffered from brain damage (persistent vegetative state). The court appointed Michael Schiavo her husband as Terri's guardian. Michael Schiavo received $250,000 in an out of court settlement with a physician for malpractice. A trust fund was set up for her treatment $750,000, and Michael Schiavo received another $300,000 for loss of consortium.

The Schindlers, her parents, attempted to remove Michael Schiavo as Terri's guardian, but failed (1993). Michael Schiavo filed a petition with the court to have

PEG (for feeding and fluids) tube removed. The Schindlers (the parents) opposed the petition.

After a long battle in which President Bush and his brother Jeb Bush (the Governor of Florida) and the Pope tried hard to continue hydration and nutrition of Terry Schiavo; the court insisted on removing the feeding tube and Terry Schiavo died after 2 weeks. Her death was announced on March 31, 2005.

Michael Schiavo got 1 million dollars in life insurance of his deceased wife.

On January 26, 2006, Michael Schiavo married his girlfriend with whom he had two children.

The ethical, moral, and legal problems are mounting due to this policy of stopping hydration and nutrition to patients in persistent vegetative state, or terminally ill patients.

They will soon find that euthanasia is less painful and less harmful than this drastic inhumane death by stopping nutrition and hydration, and they will resort to it.

Notes and References

1. This Hadith (saying of the Prophet [PBUH]) is narrated by Abu Saeed alKhoder. (The companion of the Prophet). It is in Sunan ibn Maja, and Sunan alDarqutni, and Abu Daood. The chain of narrators is good. Imam Malik ibn Anas narrated it in AlMu'wata without mentioning the companion of the Prophet (PBUH) (Abu Saeed alKhodri)
2. al Izz ibn AbdulSalam (2000) Qaweed al Ahkam commented by Nazih Hammad and Othman Dhamariyah. Dar alQalam Damascus 1:8
3. Fatwa of Islamic Jurisprudence of Makkah on abortion 12th Session 10–17 Feb 1990 Decision No. 4 on Abortion of Congenitally Malformed Fetus
4. Fatwa of Islamic Jurisprudence of Makkah on Autopsy 10th Session 17–21 Oct 1987. Decision on Dissection of Dead Bodies. Book of Decisions. Majma alFiqh alIslami. Makkah AlMukaramah
5. Fatwas on Organ Transplantation. Corneal transplantation was allowed by Sheikh Hasson Ma'amoon (Grand Mufti of Egypt) in 1959 followed by Fatwa of Sheikh Hureidi (Grand Mufti of Egypt) in 1966, allowing taking organs from cadavers. All the Fatwas were discussed in: Mohammed Albar: Organ Transplantation A'Sunni Perspective. Saudi Journal of Kidney Diseases and Transplantation 2012, 23(4):817–822
6. Williams G (1983) Textbook of criminal law, vol 2. Stevens and Sons, London, p 27
7. Winfield: Textbook of the Law of Tort, 1948, p1 and Atiyah: The Damages Lottery, 1997, pp 3–6
8. Ahmed Abdel Aziz Yacoub: The Fiqh of Medicine, 2001, Taha Public, London, p 64
9. Beauchamp T, Childress J (2001) Principles of biomedical ethics, 5th edn. Oxford University Press, New York, p 114
10. There are many Hadiths in this issue, He ordered his companions to give alms daily. They said, "Who can do that?" He said, "Removing thorny tree or bone or dirt from the way (street), show the right path for those lost, enjoin right and forbid wrong, help those who are inefficient in their work". The companion said, "What if I did not do any of these?" He said, "At least do no harm to others". Narrated by AlBokhari and Muslim, and ibn Hibban and by alHaitham in

Majuna AlZawayed, p 31107. The Hadith is authentic narrated by Abu Huraira, (the companion of the Prophet PBUH)

11. Sunan Abu Da'ood, vol 7/160, 161
12. Fatwa of International Islamic Jurisprudence Council on Medical Insurance, Decision No. 149 (7/16): 9–14 Apr 2004, Session 16, Dubai
13. Ibn alQayim: Attib alNabawi, Dar al Torath, Cairo 1978, pp 202–214
14. Ibn Habib alAlbairi aTibbi Nabawi, commented by M. Albar, Dar alQalam, Damascus 1993, pp 165–174
15. Montgomery J (1997) Healthcare law. Clarendon, Oxford, p 166
16. Albar MA (2007) Seeking remedy, abstaining from therapy and resuscitation: an Islamic perspective. Saudi J Kidney Dis Transplant 18(4):629–637
17. Brophy V (1986) New England Sinai Hospital, Inc., 398 Mass 417 NE, 2nd edn. 626

Chapter 8
Beneficence

Beneficence connotes acts of mercy, kindness, and charity. It includes all forms of action intended to benefit or promote the good of other persons. The principle of beneficence refers to a normative statement of moral obligation to act for the benefit of others, helping them to further important legitimate interests, often by preventing or removing possible harms. As we have mentioned in the previous chapter on nonmaleficence both are interconnected. Preventing harm and removing harm (or evil) are both considered a type of beneficence.

Prophet Muhammad (PBUH) ordered his companions to do charity daily. They said: Who can do that? He said: Removing a thorny bush, or bones or dirt from the way (street) is a charity; showing the right path for those lost is a charity, enjoining right and forbidding wrong is a charity; helping those who are inefficient in their work is a charity." One of the companions said, "What if I didn't do any of these?" He said, "At least do no harm to others." Narrated by AlBokhari, Muslim and Ibn Hibban [1]. Doing Harm and Reciprocating Harm is Not Allowed [2].

The Qur'an and the Tradition are full of passages and sayings of the Prophet enjoining good and refraining from doing harm. We will quote here a few ayas of the Qur'an:

(1) Have you seen the one who denies the religion (hereafter)? That is the one who drives away harshly the orphan. And does not encourage the feeding of the poor. So woe to those who pray, (but) who are heedless of their prayers. Those who made show of their deeds and withheld their assistance to their neighbors (Holy Qur'an 107/1-7).

(2) Woe to every scorner and mocker. Who collects wealth and (continuously) counts it. He thinks that his wealth will make him immortal. No. He will surely be thrown into the crusher (Hellfire which crushes their bones) (Holy Qur'an 104/1-4).

(3) Whoever does an atom's weight of good will see it and, whoever does an atom's weight of evil will see it (Holy Qur'an 99/7, 8).

(4) And they were not commanded except to worship Allah; (being) sincere to Him in religion, inclining to truth, and to establish prayer and give zakat (obligatory alms giving) and that is the correct religion (Holy Qur'an 98/5).

(5) Did he not find you (O Muhammad) an orphan and gave you refuge? And He found you poor and made (you) self-sufficient. So for the orphan do not oppress him and for the petitioner do not repel him (Holy Qur'an 93/6-10).

(6) And the righteous one will avoid it (hellfire). He who gives his wealth (to the needy) to purify himself. And not giving in return for favor but only seeking the countenance of His Lord, Most High (Sura alLayl 92/17-20).

© The Author(s) 2015
M.A. Al-Bar and H. Chamsi-Pasha, *Contemporary Bioethics*,
DOI 10.1007/978-3-319-18428-9_8

(7) Does he (i.e., Man) think that never will anyone overcome him. He says, "I have spent wealth in abundance. Does he think no one has seen him?... But he has not overcome the difficult obstacle (steep incline). It is the emancipation of a salve, or feeding on a day of famine an orphan of near relationship, or a needy person in misery. And being among those who believe and advised each other to be patient and compassionate. Those are the companions of the right" (Sura alBalad 90/5-18).

Karen Armstrong in her book "A History of God" [3] says: In practical terms Islam means that Muslims had a duty to create a just equitable society where the poor and vulnerable are treated decently. The early moral message of the Qur'an is simple: It is wrong to stockpile wealth and build a private fortune, and good to share the wealth of society fairly by giving a regular proportion of one's wealth to the poor" (Holy Qur'an 92/18, 9/103, 63/9, 102/1).

Prophet Muhammad (PBUH) said: "I swear by God, that a person who inflicts harm to his neighbor is not a [full-fledged] believer of God" [4].

In another hadith, he said, "A woman entered hellfire, because she incarcerated a cat until it died of hunger and thirst [5]".

These two hadiths admonish against maleficence , i.e., doing harm to humans or animals. The following hadith recommended beneficence to a dog: "A prostitute of Bani Israel (Children of Israel) was thirsty, so she came to a well and got water for her to drink. As she finished, she found a dog very thirsty licking the ground from thirst, so she went back to the well and got him water in her shoes until she quenched his (its) thirst. God was pleased with her and let her into paradise [6]".

AlGhazali said: "If you cannot reach the level of angels, then do not fall into the level of beasts, scorpions and snakes. If your soul is content to come down from the highest heights, at least do not let it be content into the lowest depths (to the rank of beasts, snakes and scorpions). Perhaps you will be saved by the middle way where you have neither more nor less than what suffices" [7], i.e., not doing harm and doing some good.

David Hume's moral psychology and virtue ethics makes motives of benevolence all-important in moral life, and maintains that benevolence is an original feature of human nature. He, like AlGhazali, recognizes egotism and selfishness can mask the inherent good in human psyche, and he uses the metaphors of the dove (angel with AlGhazali) wolf (beast) and serpent (snakes and scorpions) to illustrate the mixture of elements in our nature. Hume regards persons as motivated by a variety of passions, both generous and ungenerous, i.e., good and bad [8]. He maintains that these elements vary by degree from person to person. Each person should strive hard to uplift himself from the level of beasts and snakes to the level of doves (peaceful and doing no harm), if he cannot reach the level of angels doing good (as AlGhazali maintains).

The Holy Qur'an says: "We have indeed created man in the best stature, then we abase him to the lowest of the low" (Holy Qur'an 95:4–5).

Man can be almost like an angel, but he also can be like snakes and scorpions.

And those who strive in Our (cause), We will certainly guide them to Our path, for verily God is with those who do right (Holy Qur'an 29/69).

And by the soul and He who proportioned it and inspired it with discernment of its wickedness and its righteousness. He has succeeded who purifies it, and he has failed who instills it in (corruption) (Holy Qur'an 91/7-10).

Islam recognizes that the true nature of man (alFitra) is good, but it can be lured by egotistic desires and the luring of Satan and human devils. Those who strive to purify themselves, abstaining from harming others (humans, animals or environment), performing good and enjoining others and the whole community to do the right things and abstain from evil acts, are the true believers and those will succeed in the Day of Judgment.

Nonmaleficence and Beneficence is the cornerstone of morality and ethics through out history in different nations and cultures.

In the book of dead in the old Egyptian civilization the dead person was brought in front of the Chief God Oziris. He defended himself saying: "I did no crime in all my life. I never assaulted anybody. I never assassinated anybody. I always forwarded sacrifices to the Gods. I never destroyed a cultivated land or do mischief on earth. I never committed fornication or adultery and I never refused to hear the truth, and abide by it. Never I made false promises or deceive anybody in weights, selling or buying or in any way. I never throw dirt into the water (used for drinking or cleaning). I never prevent a baby from suckling (from his mother or his wet nurse) I never close or change the course of water canals (very essential in irrigation in Egypt). I never ignore the voice of God in my heart. I always abstained from doing harm; and aspired to doing good. I am pure!! I am pure [9]"!!

He of course is found, unblemished and ordered to live forever in Heaven.

All other nations had clear rules and orders for abstaining from harm and doing good, e.g., the laws of Hamurabi (Hamurapi) of Babylon (1792–1750 BCE) who ruled a great country in Iraq for 42 years; established a great empire noted for its justice and laws. Hamurabi Code [10], the most complete and perfect extant collection of Babylonian Laws (282 laws). They included economic provisions (prices, tariffs, trade, etc.), family law, criminal law (assault, theft) and civil law (slavery, debt). It also included laws on practice of medicine and surgery. The law established peace and justice in the country, allowing it to develop greatly. Doing good was extolled and doing evil was degraded and punished. The laws of retribution (Qisas), which was later found in Torah, were all there: an eye for an eye, a tooth for a tooth, and a soul (life) for a soul (i.e., murder crimes being punished by slaughtering the offenders).

The Hamurabi Code established nonmaleficence and beneficence in the whole community by establishing the law of justice. It also paid great attention to health, cleanliness, and a proper drainage system for dirty and soiled waters. It was considered a crime to throw dirt in canals and potable water.

The background of the law goes even further in history to Sumerian Law, under which civilized communities lived for many centuries (almost 6000 years from our time). They enjoined doing good and avoiding doing harm to humans, animals or even to the environment (throwing dirt into canals and potable water was a punishable crime). They particularly enjoined being good to parents, especially the mother. The highest goddess was Po; and the King Judea made many poems and songs for her sake, as he considered her his mother and the mother of all men and women in his Kingdom, where she was caring for them all [11].

The Buddhists, the Indians, and the Chinese had different civilizations, but all of them stressed doing good and shunning and avoiding evil, to man, animal and environment. The Greek Philosophers similarly laid down the Philosophy of morality, which was built on the principle of nonmaleficence and beneficence. Hippocratic Oath and writings stressed, "Primum non nocere" "Above all do no harm," and Beneficence. It was already discussed in detail.

The Old Testament (Torah and other books) stressed these important principles.

The Ten Commandments (Exodus 20/1-17) starts by "Worship no God but Me," monotheism, observing the Sabbath and then "Respect your father and your mother. Do not commit murder (thou shall not kill). Do not commit adultery. Do not steal. Do not accuse anyone falsely and do not desire another man's house; do not desire his wife, his slaves, his cattle, his donkeys or anything that he owns" [12]. It is a clear message of nonmaleficence.

Treatment of Slaves. (Exodus 21/1-11 and Deut 15/12-18) [12]. They should be treated fairly. If the slave is a Hebrew then he should be freed on the 7th year. If he is not Hebrew, then he should pay for his emancipation. The laws about violent acts are harsh by today's standards. "Whoever hits his father or his mother is to be put to death. Whoever curses his father or mother is to be put to death" (Exodus 21/15, 17). Lending money to Jews should be without interest, but lending money to non-Jews, should be with usury. (This is definitely put by the Rabbi's).

Premarital, extramarital sexual practices, sodomy, and bestiality are all punished by killing those who practice it (Leviticus 18/1-30) [13].

The respect of parents is repeated several times. "Do not steal or cheat or lie. Do not make promise in my name if you do not intend to keep it (that allows breaking promises if not under oath in God's name" [13].

Do not take advantage of anyone or rob him. Do not hold back the wages of someone you have hired, not even for one night. Do not curse a deaf man, or put something in front of a blind man so as to make him stumble over it. Be honest and just. Do not bear a grudge against anyone, but settle your differences with him so that you will not commit a sin. Do not take revenge on anyone or continue to hate him, but love your neighbor as you love yourself (Leviticus 19/11-18) [13].

That is clear beneficence, and not only nonmaleficence. The Israelites generally didn't keep these commandments and betrayed God, worshipped idols, did all the crimes they were told to avoid, and disobeyed their prophets and killed many of them and when Jesus, the last Prophet who came to them they called him a quack, a magician and accused his mother with adultery. They tried to kill him and crucify him (the Muslims believe that he was saved from crucifixion and raised to Heaven, while Christians believe that he was crucified, buried and raised from the grave on the third day and then raised to Heaven).

Jesus warned against the teachers of the law and Pharisees and called them hypocrites: "How terrible for you teachers of the Law and Pharisees. You hypocrites. You lock the door of the Kingdom of Heaven in the people's faces, and you yourselves don't go in, nor do you allow in those who try to enter" (Mathew 23/13-27, Luke 11/39-42, 52, 20/47) [14].

Jesus had many sermons to his followers in which he asked them to give all their property to the poor and needy, and to forgive all who wronged them. He said in the Sermon on the Mount (Mathew 5/3-12): "Happy are those who are humble…Happy are those who are merciful to others…Happy are the pure in heart…Happy are those who work for peace…" [15].

Love for enemies (Mathew 5/43): "Love your enemies and pray for those who persecute you."

Teachings about revenge (Mathew 6/38, Luke 6/29-30) [15]: "You have heard that it was said: an eye for an eye, and a tooth for a tooth. But now I tell you: do not take revenge on someone who wrongs you. If anyone slaps you on the right cheek, let him slap you on the left cheek too…when someone asks you for something, give it to him."

He warned against performing religious duties in public as hypocrites do. (Mathew 6/1-17) [15]. "Do not store up riches for yourselves here on earth, where moths and rust will destroy it and robbers break in and steal. Instead, store up riches for yourselves in heaven" (Mathew 6/19-20) "You cannot serve both God and money" (Mathew 6/24) [15].

The teachings of Jesus were very hard to follow. Only very few could raise themselves to this high standard of beneficence, charity, and nobility. All through Christian history only saints were capable to fulfill what Jesus ordered his followers to practice. The rich young man came to Jesus asking to receive the eternal life. He ordered him to worship and love God (the 10 commandments), but the young man asked for more Jesus said, "Go and sell all you have and give the money to the poor and you will have riches in heavens then come and follow me. The young man went away as he was very rich and the disciples said: "Who then can be saved? Jesus answered: This is impossible for man, but for God everything is possible" (Mathew 19/16-26) [16].

The beneficence ordered by Jesus was considered by his followers as supererogatory as it can never be reached and practiced except by saints. However, Jesus gave a very good example of beneficence that could be done by ordinary person. This is the parable of the Good Samaritan (Luke 10/25-37) [17]. The Samaritans were considered nonbelievers by Jews. They had their own temple in Mount Gerzim in Samaria (near Nables today), and refused to go to Mount Temple in Jerusalem. They only acknowledged the Torah and refused the other books of Old Testament. They also refused the Talmud.

Jesus said: "There was once a man who was going down from Jerusalem to Jericho when robbers attacked him, stripped him and beat him up leaving him half dead. It so happened that a priest was going that road, but when he saw the man, he walked on by on the other side. In the same way a Levite (the tribe of Moses and Aaron) also came along, went over and looked at the man, and then walked on by, on the other side. But a Samaritan who was travelling that way came upon the man, and when he saw him, his heart was filled with pity. He went over to him, poured oil and wine on his wounds, and bandaged them; then he put the man on his own animal and took him to an inn, where he took care of him. The next day he took out two silver coins and gave them to the innkeeper: "Take care of him," he told the innkeeper, and when I come back I will pay you whatever else you spend on him."

Jesus concluded: "In your opinion, which one of these three acted like a neighbor towards the man attacked by the robbers."

The teacher of the law answered: "The one who was kind to him". Jesus replied: "You go then, and do the same."

This parable of the Good Samaritan is quoted by anybody who speaks about beneficence. It is an important illustration of what we can do to fellow humans in such circumstances. It is certainly a praiseworthy act, but definitely not an extreme ideal that is only done by saints and heroes.

Beauchamp and Childress [18] after quoting the parable of the Good Samaritan agreed that the Samaritan's motives and his actions were beneficent, but considered the parable as an ideal and not an obligation. "Only ideals of beneficence incorporate such extreme generosity." Definitely, the actions of the Samaritan are commendable but they are not of extreme generosity and should be done by any decent human being.

It may be almost obligatory to help in such a case, but the action definitely deserves praise and will be rewarded by God in Heaven. It cannot be considered supererogatory as these authors claim; as it should be done by any kind-hearted man. Saving human life takes precedent over any other argument in Islam, unless such a person is incriminated by murder or doing great mischief on earth. "We decreed upon the children of Israel that whoever kills a soul unless for a soul, or for corruption (done) in the land it is as if he had slained mankind entirely. And whoever saves one (life), it is as if he saved the whole of mankind" (Holy Qur'an 6/32).

What the Samaritan did should be emulated by every human being, if there are no real obstacles to fulfill it.

Traditionally acts of beneficence are done from obligation (like the case of the Samaritan), but may be supererogatory (optional moral ideals where things are done more than required).

"Not all supererogatory acts of beneficence are exceptionally arduous, costly or risky e.g. generous gift-giving, uncompensated public service, forgiving another's costly error and complying with requests made by other persons for benefit when these exceed the obligatory requirements of ordinary or professional morality" as Stanford Encyclopedia of Philosophy say [8].

Beneficence is a continuum starting with obligatory morally, and sometimes legally, as in saving a life, when one can do it without any hazard to himself. Professionally things which are considered as supererogatory for the public become obligatory for the professional, e.g., a physician or nurse in a hospital where he is tending patients with highly infectious diseases, e.g., Ebola virus, tuberculosis, epidemic of influenza, etc. He or she cannot abstain from treatment of these patients as it is one of his/her duties. In emergency the physician/nurse may work extra hours forgoing his other duties to his family and friends.

All cultures, religions and philosophies considered non maleficence-beneficence as the cornerstone of morality and ethics.

In modern times Hume considered motives of benevolence all important in moral life, and the origin of morality [8].

John Stuart Mill (the utilitarian English Philosopher) considered the principle of utility, or the greatest happiness principle as the basic principle of morality and ethics. Actions are right if they bring happiness and wrong if they bring pain and suffering. It is a straightforward principle of beneficence (though it may cause harm to few) [8].

Mill holds that the concept of duty, obligations and rights are subordinated to, and determined by, that which maximizes benefits and minimizes harms, i.e., utility based on beneficence and non maleficence. Kant rejects the utilitarian understanding of beneficence. He calls for beneficence and non maleficence from the point of view of duty. Any other motive is not really moral or ethical, though it may be commendable in itself. The motive of benevolence, so admired by Hume is morally unworthy in Kant's theory unless the motive is that of duty.

Some philosophers like Gert maintains that there are no moral rules of beneficence, only moral ideals. In Gert's theory, the general role of morality is to minimize evil or harm. Rational persons can at all times act impartially and abstain from doing harm (evil), but they cannot impartially promote good for all persons at all times. Gert considers non maleficence (doing no harm) as obligatory [19]. He accepts moral rules such as "Do Not Kill" don't cause pain or suffering of the others and so forth. Rules of nonmaleficence are negative prohibitions of actions. That must be followed impartially, while beneficence actions are positive actions which are usually non obligatory except in life saving situations, and the person can easily save the others without any risk to himself.

It is definitely laudable and supererogatory if saving others involves high risk to the benevolent rescuer. But it is obligatory to save others if it does not pose any risk to the rescuer. It may be also obligatory even if it involves risks to those health professional, firefighters, and ambulance workers. What may be supererogatory to the public may be obligatory to those professionals whose jobs and duties entail rescue operations.

Beneficence played a major central role in the practice and ethics of medicine since AmHotib (deified Egyptian physician who lived 4000 years from our time). Hippocratic Oath is wholly dependent on non maleficence and beneficence.

Only in the 1970s that autonomy, patient's rights, and contractual procedures replaced gradually beneficence from its throne in medical ethics.

Benefit in medicine is limited historically to healing. Nowadays medicine is used for other purposes, e.g., gender selection, transsexualism, preventing fertility by pills or operations, providing purely cosmetic surgery and genetic manipulation to improve posterity, and nonmedical abortions.

All these types of medical interventions, surrogacy, and new methods of procreation are outside the boundaries of classical medicine which treats patients.

These are no longer patients and hence called customers (clients); and doctors and nurses are now called health providers.

New problems are also arising both in medicine and biomedical research. End of life issues, withholding or withdrawing life support measures, e.g., do not resuscitate (DNR) policy, do not intubate (using ventilator) and using morphine and its derivatives to control pain whereby it has "a double effect," i.e., alleviating pain and may depress respiratory center of the brain, especially in patients suffering from chronic pulmonary disease, or patients suffering from diseases affecting the brain, or phrenic nerve that supplies the diaphragm (the main muscle for respiration).

Medical practice became more complicated and decisions are not only built on the old rules of nonmaleficence and beneficence, but should involve the patient and/ or his family in all decisions pertaining to life and death. Many cases are not solved except by the intervention of the law and court decisions, especially in cases where ventilation or nutrition and hydration are withdrawn and stopped. Physician hastened death by the request of the patient ± request of the family is highly debatable in the West. It is not accepted in Muslim countries and to Muslim patients anywhere. Euthanasia is still considered a crime in the majority of the world countries.

Organ transplantation has been accepted as a modality of treatment that improves the patient's suffering from end stage organ failure and may be life saving. It has been accepted in Islamic countries (with some resistance from some jurists and even some physicians). Many Fatwas (decrees) of Islamic Jurisprudence Council's have been issued since 1959 till 2003. It allowed organs to be donated from living adult competent donor, without any form of compulsion; and from deceased (decedents, cadavers) provided that they have agreed to donate or their families have agreed to donate after their death (usually these are brain dead cases). In all these cases, informed consent is essential without any duress or any type of compulsion or entrepreneuring.

The scarcity of organs have prompted new policies in Europe, which is called "presumed consent or opt out system" (sometimes called opt in) whereby every patient in Government hospitals is presumed that he agrees to donate his organs, if the brain death is firmly diagnosed. He can during his life time object to this rule and it will be accepted. But if there is no such objection then he is presumed consenting and organs will be taken from his body without any need for the consent of the family.

Islamic countries, USA, UK, Canada, and Australia are still requiring a clear consent from the person during his lifetime, or/plus consent of the family. The routine retrieval of organs from all dead candidates is not justified on the traditional grounds of respect of autonomy. The advocates of the new policy are reverting to the rule of beneficence, which they have in many aspects refused and called it paternalistic medicine. Now, because of shortage of organs, they are going back to the old regime, i.e., paternalistic medicine built on the principle of beneficence.

Breaking confidentiality to prevent harm, e.g., if a psychiatric patient tells his doctor that he is going to kill a person (due to delusions and hallucinations), then the psychiatrist has a duty to inform the police, and also to inform the person to be attacked, so that he may take steps to avoid being attacked. Similarly if a consort is having HIV, then the physician has a duty to inform the other consort of the true diagnosis (i.e., HIV). He should take the permission from the infected person, or require him to tell his consort in his presence of the true diagnosis; otherwise he would be allowing harm to occur. If the health authorities require reporting infectious diseases, then it should be reported, so that measures could be taken to protect the whole community; and breaking confidentiality in such cases is allowed. If the magistrate ordered the physician to divulge the true diagnosis, in most cases he has to obey, lest he would be accused of obstructing justice.

Social Beneficence

Some ethicists like Singer suggested taking 10 % of the income to provide services of the poor. This is not new as the Torah ordered Israelites to pay tithe which was 10 % of whatever they earn, or produce in the fields.

In Islam, it is obligatory to pay 2.5 % of all your wealth annually to the poor and needy. It is also highly recommended to pay more, but that is supererogatory. It is incumbent on every adult male to support himself, his wife, his children and his parents if they are in need. If he is wealthy enough then he should support the poor members of his family which will involve grandparents, grandchildren, brothers and sisters, aunts and uncles. It may extend to cousins, nephews, and nieces, or may even involve other members of the tribe depending on his ability and their condition. It becomes obligatory and could be enforced by the law, provided he is the only one capable of supporting them, and they are in real need of his support. It is not supererogatory in such cases but becomes obligatory.

This rule differs greatly from secular systems especially in the West, which extol autonomy, and the societal obligations are kept at minimum. However, these countries usually provide a type of welfare state, and hence individuals are relieved from these duties. Beauchamp and Childress talked about "specific beneficence and obligations in families, friendship or special commitments, such as explicit promises and roles with attendant responsibilities, e.g., physicians and nurses caring for contagious patients. Promoting the welfare of the patients—not merely avoiding harm—expresses medicine's goal, rational, and justification. As the American Nurses Association puts it: "The nurse primary commitment is health welfare and safety of the client." Likewise, in the Hippocratic Oath, physicians pledge that they "will come for the benefit of the sick, will apply treatment for the benefit of the sick according to their ability and judgment, and will keep patients from harm and injustice." Preventative medicine and active public health interventions have also long embraced concerted social actions of beneficence, such as vaccination programs and health education as obligatory rather than optional [18]".

This is of course paternalism which was decried since 1970s and replaced by autonomy, patient's rights, and informed consent. Only in cases of an incompetent minor or mentally incompetent adult that paternalism (parental guidance and control) is allowed.

Paternalism is defined as the intentional overriding of one person's known preferences or actions by another person who overrides it, justifies the action by the goal of benefiting or avoiding harm to the person whose preferences or actions are overridden [18].

The tendency is to refuse this type of paternalism, and consider it unjustified except in certain specified cases [18] viz:

(1) A patient is at risk of significant preventable harm
(2) The paternalistic action will probably prevent the harm
(3) The projected benefits to the patient of the paternalistic action outweigh its risks to the patient
(4) The least autonomy-restrictive alternative that will secure the benefits and reduce the risks is adopted.

However if a Jehovah witness patient needs blood to save his life, but he refuses blood, then his refusal should be respected. In fact, any modality of treatment could be refused, even if it is essential to save life if it is done by a competent adult person without duress and with information about the dangers of his decision to his health and life [18].

Notes and References

1. The Hadith is authentic narrated through Abu Huraira (the Companion of the Prophet [PBUH]) in AlBokhari, Muslim and Ibn Hibban. AlHaithami: Majma AlZawayed, p 31107
2. Sunan Abud Da'wood, Sunan Ibn Maja, Sunan alDarqutin and Mu'wata Malik (fairly good chain of narrators up to Abu Saeed AlKhodri (the Companion of the Prophet [PBUH]))
3. Armstrong K (1993) A History of God. Baltimore Books, New York, pp 142–143
4. Narrated by Sahih AlBokhari, Sahih Muslim, Musnad Ahmed in AlAjlooni (Ismail) Kashf AlKhafa was Muzeel AlIlbas, Beiruty (1983) AlRisalah Publication 3rd edn, vol 2/450
5. Narrated by Abdullah ibn Omar. Sahih AlBokhari, Sahih Muslim in AlAjlooni, Kashf AlKhafa (vide supra) vol I/484
6. Muslim S. Hadith No. 2245 and Musnad Ahmed ibn Hanbal, vol 2/507
7. AlGhazali M (n.d) Ihya Oloom alDeen, Kitab Ajayib AlQalb, vol 3/9, Beirut Dar AlMarifa (n.d)
8. Stanford Encyclopedia of Philosophy: The Principle of Beneficence in Applied Ethics through Google Search 1st published January 2, 2008, pp 3–12
9. Albar M. AlAkhlaq: Osoolaha Addyinyah wa Gothooraha alFalsafiya (2010) Chair of Medical Ethics, King Abdulaziz University, Jedah, (Konooz AlMarifa Distribution) pp 62–63
10. Encyclopedia Britannica (1982) Micropedia, 15th edn, vol IV, p 878
11. Albar M. (reference No. 9), pp 67–69
12. Good New Bible with Apogrypha/Deuterocanonical Books. The Bible Societies, Collins/ Fontana, 1979, Glasgow, 1979, pp 80–82
13. Good News Bible (vide supra), pp 119–120
14. Vide Supra, The New Testament, Mathew (23/39-40), pp 34–35
15. Vide Supra, (Mathew 5/3-12), pp 7, 9–10

16. Vide Supra, (Mathew 19/16-26), p 28
17. Vide Supra, (Luke 10/25-37), pp 92–93
18. Beauchamp T, Childress J (2001) Principles of Biomedical Ethics, 5th edn, Oxford University Press, New York, pp 167, 173, 178–187
19. Gert B (2005) Morality. Oxford University Press, New York

Chapter 9
Justice: The Lost Value

All nations and cultures extolled justice, at least to a certain class of the community. The Indians had a strict caste system, which resulted in complete injustice to the lower castes. Similarly, the Greek and Romans had a strict system which excluded the slaves, and limited citizenship to a minority of the population. The old Egyptian Civilization had also a class system, which was not closed and persons with their ability and hard work could go up the ladder. Still in China, the class system was less obvious. Hamurabi of Babylon (1792-1750 BCE) was probably the first ruler who put a complete code (Hamurabi Code) which aimed at establishing peace, justice and prosperity to the people of Babylon. It succeeded to a great deal in fulfilling its aspirations, with the strong and just hand of Hamurabi who ruled for 42 years. However, the slaves were not included in the system, though they were treated relatively kindly. The Egyptian and Chinese systems allowed brilliant salves to be ministers and hold great responsibilities in these empires. Joseph was a slave but was raised to the highest post in Egypt under the King. Similarly many slaves in China were the generals of the army or admirals of the navy or ministers in the administration.

The Indians had a strict caste system and it was not allowed to move up the ladder. Similarly the Greco-Roman system was against slaves. Still worse was the European attitude in the sixteenth−eighteenth centuries. The slaves snatched from Africa and deported to the Americas, West Indies, and other colonies were brutally treated. More than 100 million Africans were taken from the black continent during two centuries. More than 70 million died in the hazardous journeys, the diseases that cropped, the stifling of mutinies, in the mines and fields of the white colonialists of both Americas (North, South, and Central America), and the many islands in the Caribbean (West Indies). They were maltreated all through those horrible times. Unfortunately, it is still there, though in a much smaller scale in USA, the world champion of democracy and human rights. There are about 50 million citizens with no health insurance, or partial on and off insurance, in the USA until the beginning of the twenty-first century (CE). Although the Afro-Americans constitute about 17 % of the population, they form more than 70 % of the prison crime population; and 90 % of those who received capital punishment in the twentieth century were blacks. Despite the tremendous improvements in the status of blacks since Martin Luther King cried, "I have a dream," in the 1960s of the

© The Author(s) 2015   141
M.A. Al-Bar and H. Chamsi-Pasha, *Contemporary Bioethics*,
DOI 10.1007/978-3-319-18428-9_9

twentieth century, there are still many blacks suffering from degradation, crime, instability, and inequality, both in education and health services.

It is amazing to find USA spending the greatest amount of money ($7285 on each individual health in 2010) [1] while in Finland they only spent $2840 on each individual; but the infant mortality rate in USA was double that of Finland [1]. In fact all the health indices put by WHO viz Infant Mortality Rate (the numbers of babies under 1 year that die in a certain year out of 1000, 1-year-old babies) or the 5-year mortality rate (the number of children under 5 who die in a certain year out of 1000 five-year olds) or longevity rate…or the number of women who die in parturition (delivery) or post partum in 100,000 deliveries in a certain year, or the number of persons who die in traffic accidents per 100,000 in a certain year in a certain country and so forth.

In all these indices, USA is the worst of all industrialized 28 nations. Beauchamp and Childress in "Principles of Biomedical Ethics" [2] say: "More than 40 million US citizens (approximately 18 % of the nonelderly population) lack health insurance of any kind. Inadequate insurance affects those who are uninsured, uninsurable, underinsured, or only occasionally insured. Although each year USA spends more resources on health care than any country in the world (double or almost triple any industrialized country, and 20 times what Cuba spends), it is the only industrialized nation with less than half of its population eligible for public health insurance" [2, 3].

"More than 50 million non elderly adults in the US—approximately 1/3 of that population—experience a gap in coverage within a 2-year period, approximately 2/3 of these have no insurance for at least one year [2].

"Many uninsured persons are employed, but by companies offering no health benefits. This situation is common with employees of small firms for whom the costs of maintaining insurance are much higher than for large employers. Many employee benefit packages also provide no coverage for dependents or part-time employees" [2, 4].

"Other US citizens are uninsurable, although many of them are employed by firms offering health coverage. The problem for them is that they are required to give full family and personal medical histories and to be examined fully prior to being eligible for insurance. Those with poor health or pre-existing conditions or family history of certain diseases are denied coverage or offered inferior and more expensive coverage. Many persons suffering from diseases that could need expensive medical management in the future are denied coverage. People who have HIV positive tests are also denied any coverage" [2].

It is strange to find some big firms in the USA denying their employees or some of them, any medical insurance. The law in the USA allows employers to offer or deny medical insurance coverage for their employees. The companies that offer medical insurance to its employees find it difficult to compete with the companies that offer no insurance benefit. This is partially redressed by reducing taxes of those offering insurance benefits. The system in the USA serves the wealthy, the big firms and companies. The taxes paid by the most wealthy constitute only a very small percentage of their income, while the less wealthy, the middle class, and even the poor bear the brunt of the taxes and pay a much higher percentage of their income as taxes (direct and indirect taxes). This is an unfair and unjust system. "The US pays 3.5 billion US dollars a day on health services; still the health of many Americans is in a sorry state. It is far from the top in life expectancy at birth. Infact mortality is 60 % greater than in Sweden. In 2000, about 14 % of the US population had no health insurance at all. Still others were covered only part of the year or were woefully under insured. There are dreadful differences in health based on income, education and race. Enormous International differences exist as well" [5–7].

We conclude here the following points:

(1) 50 million USA citizens are uninsured or only partially insured on and off. The majority of these are Afro Americans, or of Hispanic origin.

(2) In USA, the companies are not forced by law to insure their employees or their dependents.
Most countries even in developing countries require from big companies health insurance or bear the responsibilities of providing health services to their employees and their dependents. In Saudi Arabia, all companies even very small businesses and shops have to provide some type of health services (sometimes the bare minimum).

(3) The insurance companies can refuse any person or group of people to be insured, if they have the possibility of being affected by a chronic disease or liable to acquire a hereditary disease that may appear at the age of 40 or 50. All those suffering from congenital or hereditary diseases since childhood are not covered. Patients suffering from chronic diseases that may end, for example, in end organ failure (kidney, heart, liver, etc.) are denied health insurance. These companies are after easy profit and are similar to blood sucking vampires or blood sucking insects. They provide services only to gain more money. Otherwise, they may let you die or have long suffering before you die.

(4) USA spends on health per capita double or triple all the 28 industrialized countries; nevertheless it is behind all these countries in the health criteria put by WHO viz: infant mortality rate, 5 year old mortality rate, longevity rate, mortality rate during parturition (delivery) and post partum (after delivery) for every 100,000 deliveries. It is amazing to find Cuba (and many third-world countries) having much better indices than the 50 million US citizens uninsured or partially insured. Cuba has better figures than the USA in term of longevity and infant mortality rates. Cuba is a poor developing country suffering from strict US blockade for many years (since the 1960s of the twentieth century) until now (2014).

(5) There is a huge waste and inefficiency in the management of health services in USA evident by the huge difference between the expenditure of USA (on Health) and the other countries (developed and developing), and the end result is the worst in certain indices set by WHO among the industrialized (28) countries; and almost similar in some indices to Cuba, Malaysia, Thailand, etc.

The WHO figures of Infant Mortality Rate in 2000 (WHO):

In 1000 live births		
USA	7.2	
Australia	5.2	
Canada	5.2	
Denmark	5.2	
Finland	3.9	
France	4.6	
Singapore	2	The best figure
Japan, Norway	4	
Switzerland	4.7	
UK	5.9	

These figures improved remarkably by 2010, but still USA is at the bottom.

In the developing countries (third world), the worst figures are in Somalia, Afghanistan, sub-Saharan African countries, and Yemen. Iraq before US invasion of 1991 and 2003 was ranking high among Arab countries, but became almost like Yemen, Somalia, and Jibouti, after US invasion (2003). The Gulf Arab countries showed a remarkable improvement in health indices and made fairly good use of its oil revenues. Although Saudi Arabia is the richest one, all others performed much better, because of:

(i) Inefficiency and waste emulating the US system in a worse way.
(ii) Much higher population than the others (28 million). By 2010, the infant mortality rate in Saudi Arabia came down to 12 per 1000 live births (was 27 in 2007 figures) but Malaysia infant mortality rate was only 3 per 1000 live births (better than USA figures and much better than Saudi Arabia figures) [1].

Malaysia spent US$ 604 in 2010 on health services. Saudi Arabia spent $768 while USA spent $7285 [1]. Malaysia spent 1/12 what USA spent and nevertheless had better indices than USA. Similarly Singapore spent a small fraction of what USA did; nevertheless, the infant mortality rate was 2 since 2000 and a little above one in 2010. How amazing!!!

It does not require a high IQ to discern that it is the blatant system of capitalism and avarice that brought these poor indices and high expense in USA. The financial debacle of 2008 and its sequelae will make things worse, unless egalitarian attitudes take the upper hand and enforce equity and justice in the market economy, seeking only profit by whatever means.

(6) The health system should move from only curative medicine to preventative medicine and health promotion, as well. Most of the diseases nowadays are due to:

(a) Junk Food—inducing obesity, which contains a lot of fat, many additives ,e.g., mono amino glutamate which gives good taste, increases insulin secretion, and ends in obesity and diabetes. Of course, there are other factors such as: more sedentary lifestyle, and in many third world countries including Saudi Arabia, opening more supermarkets, restaurants, and shops instead of playgrounds, walking stretches, and greenery.
(b) Lack of Exercise
(c) All types of Pollution
(d) Smoking Tobacco
(e) Drinking Alcohol
(f) Sexually Transmitted Diseases, including HIV.

In developing countries, lack of clean water, sanitation, drainage system, malaria, tuberculosis, high infant mortality rate due to early stopping of breast feeding, malnutrition, and multiple childhood infections, all play havoc and cause shortened life span.

If the major effort in these countries is spent on primary healthcare, health education, and supplying villages with clean potable water and good drainage system, providing the minimum requirements of healthy food, the health of these countries will improve dramatically.

(g) Wars

Unfortunately wars never ceased in Africa, Middle East, Iraq, Afghanistan, and so forth. Ethnic cleansing in Bosnia, Burma (Myanmar), and Fatani (Southern Thailand), sectarian violence in many other places, brought havoc to many countries. The worst sufferers were, as usual, children, women, and civilians.

Wars and Health

In an article by Victor Sidel under the title: "War, Terrorism and Public Health" in Medicine, Conflict and Survival (April–June 2008, Vol. 24, Nos.: 13–25), he exposed the dangers of wars on health. I will quote here the abstract:

War and terrorism, which are inseparable, cause death and disability, profound psychological damage, environmental destruction, disruption of the health infrastructure, refugee crises, and increased interpersonal, self-directed and collective violence. Weapons systems such as weapons of mass destruction and landmines have their own specific devastating effects. Preparation for war and preparedness for terrorism bring constraints on civil liberties and human rights, increase militarism, and divert resources from health care and from other needed services. War and terrorism may be best prevented through addressing their causes, which include limited resources, injustice, poverty and ethnic and religious enmity, and through strengthening the United Nations and the treaties controlling specific weapons systems, particularly weapons of mass destruction. In particular, the United States should cease its interference in the internal affairs of other nations and its advocacy of unilateral pre-emptive war.

After starting with the horrors of World War II, he commented on war on terror that it elevated fear, engendered hate, and increased militarilism even among people far removed from the attacks…with loss of liberties, discrimination against groups and individuals who are not terrorists, and diversion of resources better used to deal with problems in health, education, and other social services.

Wars in the twentieth century killed 200 million people, more than half of them were civilians. During each year of the last decade of the twentieth century there had been 20 wars, mainly civil. Millions died, many millions were maimed, still more millions were refugees (Total refugees in the world are about 50 millions). The whole infrastructure of many countries was in shambles after these wars. Rape was rampant in all these wars. In Bosnia-Herzegovina (in former Yugoslavia) more than 10,000 Muslim women were raped by the Serbs militias and army. Children are particularly vulnerable during and after the wars both physically and psychologically.

Land mines killed and maimed many millions in the last three decades of the twentieth century and many millions were widowed and orphaned. With wars, millions are driven from their homes and become refugees. Many areas of Africa suffered also from drought; famine spread several times in Somalia, Ethiopia, and the Horn of Africa in the last three or four decades.

The looming shortages of food crops are causing an increase of food prices, which many poor countries cannot afford. Hundreds of thousands of children were recruited in these wars (from age 7 to 17). In South Sudan, there were more than 300,000 children under arms from age seven to seventeen. Similar figures were found in Angola, Zaire, Congo, etc. From 1986 to 1996 united Nations organization reported that killing of two million children, six millions were maimed and twelve millions were without homes. There are more than 100 million land mines over the globe. There are ten million in Afghanistan, another ten million in Angola, seven million each in Cambodia and Iraq, and so forth. Thousands are killed or maimed each year, mainly children. The United Nations called for moratorium in production of these land mines, but the largest producer USA objected, followed by Israel, Hungary and Romania. The manufacturing of a landmine costs $3 but to dismantle it costs up to $1000!!

Iraqi children suffered greatly since 1991 (2nd Gulf War) until 2003 (invasion of Iraq) when the suffering became worse. Millions died in these wars and its sequelae (being maimed, orphaned, malnourished, spread of malignancy due to the depleted uranium used in missiles during attacks in the war on Iraq, and to squash the mutiny and revolts in Ba'qooba. The war on Iraq was costing $4 billion a month (2003–2011).

Children in Labor

United Nations agencies report that 800 million children under 15 years of age are working daily to get sustenance allowance, losing their right to education and play. Many are involved in very serious hard jobs which expose them to physical and mental ailments. Between 50 and 60 million children aged 5–11 are exposed to such horrendous situations.

Street Children: United Nations agencies report 100 million children without homes living in the streets, and are used by gangs to distribute drugs, stealing (pick pocketing), begging and prostitution. About a million children are working in prostitution in Asia (Thailand, India, Cambodia, Philippines, etc.) and are used to attract tourist from Europe, Australia and USA. There are also another million in Latin America working in prostitution.

A BBC documentary film was broadcasted in June 2001, which exposed the horrifying situations in these countries. Millions of children suffer annually from sexually transmitted disease. Two million children between 10 and 14 get infected with HIV annually. About half a million are born with HIV from mothers already suffering from HIV. The brunt of the attack is in Subsaharan Africa. The total number of children suffering from HIV infection globally has reached ten million. The majority are in Subsaharan Africa, and are denied the new retrovirus drugs as they are very expensive. India and Brazil manufactured the generic drugs, but the big Pharma are fighting back and refusing to allow the distribution of these cheaper drugs.

Maldistribution of Wealth

The United Nations (UNDP) report of 1999 published in the media [8] included the following data:

(a) The three top wealthiest persons in the world possess the equivalent of Gross National Product (GNP) of 35 developing nations put together, whose population exceeds 600 million.
(b) The wealth of the richest 200 persons exceeds the income of 2400 million persons of world population.
(c) The developed nations constitute 15 % of the world population, but have 85 % of the world wealth.

Even in these wealthy countries there is a huge difference between the elite oligarchy controlling the wealth, and the masses; especially in USA, but not limited to it.

More recently, the Oxfam report to the last World Economic Forum held at Davos between 23 and 27 January 2013, declared that the wealthiest 85 persons in the world own half the wealth of the whole world, and their income exceeds the income of 3500 million of the world population.

Similarly in the developing or poor countries, there are few who are very rich while the rest of the populations are destitute.

Health services, when available in these countries, are located in the cities and mainly serve the rulers, the military, or their cronies. The rural areas are left with very little health services if any.

The Health Human Resources (health work force) is the number of people engaged in actions whose primary intent is to enhance health, according to WHO "World Health Report 2006" [9]. They include physicians, nurses, midwives, dentists, allied health professionals, community health workers, social health workers as well as health management and support personnel. Human resources for health are identified as one of the core building blocks of a health system [10].

Global Situation

The World Health Organization (WHO) estimates a shortage of 4.3 million personnel (physicians, nurses, midwives, and support workers) worldwide. The shortage is most severe in 57 of the poorest countries, especially in sub-Saharan Africa, reaching crises level as declared on World Health Day 2006 [11].

There is an estimated shortage of 1.18 million mental health professionals, including 55,000 Psychiatrists, 628,000 nurses in mental health and 493,000 Psychosocial Care providers [12]. There is also a severe shortage of Midwives and Obstetricians in many developing countries, which ends in higher maternal death and ailments, higher stillbirths and infant mortality rates.

The differences are staggering between developed and developing countries, and worse in rural and underserved areas. Unfortunately, when poor countries spend a large sum of money to bring forth physicians, nurses, and midwives, a substantial number of them migrate to wealthy countries to get better jobs and training. The brain drain is from the poor to the wealthy countries (from underdeveloped to developed countries of the West especially USA). The best of these physicians, nurses, and health professionals find lucrative jobs in these wealthy countries, including Arabian Gulf countries. The world map of health resources shows the worst shortages in Africa, India, and some parts of Latin America.

However, the availability of a sufficient number of health providers does not guarantee a high standard of health, as shown by the figures from Saudi Arabia. According to the report of Ministry of Health, Saudi Arabia published in 2008, there were 53,000 physicians and dentists (11,000 were Saudi) [1]. The population was reported at 25 millions which means one physician for 500 people; the number of hospital beds was also one for each 500 of the population. Saudi Arabia was spending 768 US dollars per capita. The number of health technicians including nurses was about 153,000, i.e., 2.9 health technicians and nurses for each Physicia [1].

These figures are fairly satisfactory (though there is a definite shortage of health technicians, including nurses) but the end result of infant mortality rate, 5-year-olds mortality rate, longevity, maternal death during delivery, and postpartum are not satisfactory. Malaysia, who spend less than Saudi Arabia has better health indices, viz, infant mortality rate, 5-years-old mortality rate, and so forth. Similarly, Cuba and Sri Lanka have performed well.

It is not only the money spent, the number of human power working in health services, or the number of beds available that determine the health and well being of a certain community or country. It is how the resources are spent and where they are spent. Inefficiency, waste, and spending more than 90 % of the resources on large fantastic hospitals, will not provide better health indices. The health services should be distributed in a fair way between rural areas and cities; and between tertiary hospitals and primary health care. Disease prevention, health education, and health promotion deserve its fair share; otherwise discrepancies will continue between the rich and the poor, the town and city dwellers and the rural, desert area and shanty town dwellers. The end result will be poor health indices.

There is no doubt that USA is the number one country in terms of spending on health, research and medical advancement, availability of hospitals, great physicians, surgeons, and health providers; nevertheless, it is no better than Malaysia in certain indices mentioned above set by the WHO. It is definitely far from the high standard of Singapore, Japan, Nordic countries, or Western Europe in these health indices.

Certainly, it is not only the number of physicians or nurses or beds that will improve the health standard of the nation. It needs equity in distribution of health resources and an efficient system of delivery.

Similarly on a global level, a better use of resources, equity in distribution, concentration on primary healthcare, provision of clean potable water, healthy food, healthy environment, good drainage system, changing lifestyle, no smoking, no prostitution or sodomy (sexually transmitted diseases and HIV), no famines, fair distribution of wealth and justice in all walks of life, will definitely improve the health of the world population. But nothing could be achieved if there is no world peace, if the machine of war goes on bringing havoc and misery to all except those who manufacture these wars and all types of weapons.

The world has to change to be more peaceful, more equitable, and more just, otherwise we will all suffer for many generations to come.

Although justice is a core value of USA, the actual facts of life show intolerance, injustice in different racial and ethnic groups of USA. The health disparities between the white Americans, especially the WASP (White Anglo Saxon Protestant) Americans and the Afro Americans and Latinos, are staggering.

In all diseases, e.g., diabetes, hypertension, malignancy, infant mortality, 5-year mortality, motality, and complication of parturition (delivery) and postpartum, sexually transmitted diseases including HIV, the Blacks and Latinos suffer to a much higher degree than the whites [13–16].

There is another factor discerned recently and dubbed Health Literacy. It is claimed that 90 million American adults lack the literacy skills needed to use the healthcare system [17–19]. The prevalence of limited literacy is high among those with lower levels of education, the elderly, the minorities, and those with chronic disease. An emerging literature has begun to describe the myriad of health consequences of limited literacy. Indeed, limited literacy has been shown to be an independent risk factor for worse health status, hospitalization, and mortality [18–20]. "Despite the clear injustice of health care system that is organized for the most literate and powerful members of our society, the medical ethics literature has neglected some of our most vulnerable patients by remaining largely quiet about the ethical implications of health literacy" [18].

Limited health literacy has been shown to be an independent risk factor of worse outcomes and health disparities independent of race and education [18]. There is no real autonomy if there is no health literacy, and there is no real justice for those who lack health literacy" [18].

Conclusion: What Should We Aim For?

The World Health Organization (WHO) defined health as "a state of complete physical, mental and social well-being and not merely the absence of disease." It decided in Alma Ata (1978) that the world should reach this Utopian level by the year of 2000.

By 2000, things got far worse than what they were in the 1970s of the twentieth century.

We do not think it is practical to assume reaching that Utopian level of health all over the world. Let us be more pragmatic and aspire to have:

(1) World peace
(2) Equity in distribution of wealth: It is shameful to find the wealthiest three have more than Gross National Product (GNP) of 35 developing nations whose populations exceed 600 million; and the 85 wealthiest persons own half the wealth of the whole world, and their income exceeds the income of 3500 millions of the world population.

It is a disgrace to find many millions dying from malnutrition, famines, diarrhea (6 million children die of diarrhea annually because of lack of clean potable water), malaria (more than 2 million die of malaria, mostly children in Africa), 2 million die of tuberculosis (mostly in Africa and many of them due to HIV).

These inequalities could be corrected if the wealthy people and wealthy countries donate 2.5 % of their wealth to the poor and needy both in their countries and outside their countries. The 2.5 % is the obligatory Zakat (alms-giving) in Islam required from all those who have more than their basic requirements for a decent life. If this corner of Islam is fulfilled, the problem of poverty, inequality, huge problems in health, and education will gradually be overcome.

Let us hope that at least the world population will get clean potable water, at least two nourishing healthy meals per day, good drainage system, child and maternal care which would reduce the infant mortality rate, the 5 years mortality, the stillbirths, the deaths and diseases occurring due to parturition and postpartum, and so forth. Health education for everybody, banning smoking all over the world, curbing diseases of obesity, diabetes, hypertension, and reducing the incidence of cancers by removing mutagens in food, water, air pollution, irradiation, and so forth.

The Utopian goal of WHO defining health as "a state of complete, physical, mental and social well-being and not merely the absence of disease and infirmity" will never be reached in this world. We must aim at preventing wars, preaching peace, and implementing the bare minimum of justice and equality. We cannot allow three persons to have more income than 600 million of the world population, and it is hazardous to world peace if the wealthiest 85 persons amass more income than 3500 million of the world population put together. Spending trillions on the war industry is not going to leave the world in peace; it has to make wars to continue usurping the wealth of the world.

Financial gimmicks and derivatives owned and played by a few experts in the financial field brought havoc to the world, the worst was the debacle of 2008, where trillions of dollars were lost, and the ordinary taxpayers were forced to pay the wealthy banks, otherwise the whole system would melt down. These inequalities and the abhorrent system behind them should be corrected; otherwise the whole world including the wealthy industrialized nations will suffer. There is a real need for a new world order, unlike that preached by President George W. Bush and his staff and advisers who waged wars and brought misery and havoc to different parts of the world.

The time for world peace and equity in distribution of wealth, education, and health has come. There is no other alternative. The people of the world should come together to fulfill these rightful ambitions for the future for the coming generations.

Notes and References

1. WHO statistics of 2010 (2011) Quoted in Zuhair AlSebayi: alRi'ya ass'hiyiah Nazra Mustaqbaliyiah (Healthcare: A Look to the Future). Saudi Publishing House, Jeddah, pp 14–37
2. Beauchamp T, Childress J (2001) Principles of biomedical ethics, 5th edn. Oxford University Press, New York, pp 240–282
3. Anderson G (1998) In search of virtue: an international comparison of cost, access and outcomes. Health Aff 16:163–171
4. The Kaiser Commission on Medicaid and the Uninsured in America. A Chart Book prepared by Catherine Hoffman (Kaiser Family Foundation), 1998, Sec. J, Fig. 10; Kenneth Thorpe: "Expanding Employment—Based Health Insurance: Is Small Group Reform, the Answer?" Inquiry 1992, 29:128–136 and Employee Benefit Research Institute; Issue Brief No. 104, July 1990
5. Veach R (2003) The basics of bioethics, 2nd edn. Prentice Hall, New Jersey, pp 125–126
6. The World Health Report (1996) Fighting disease, fostering development. World Health Organization, Geneva, pp 119–120
7. Mills RJ (2001) Health Insurance Coverage 2000. Consumer population reports, pp 60–215, Sept 2001
8. AlHayat Newspaper (Arabic-London) Issue No. 13275 on 13 July 1999

 9. World Health Organization (2006) The world health report 2006: working together for health, Geneva http://www.who.int/whr/2006
10. World Health Organization: Health System Topics http:/whoint/healthsystems/topics/en/index. html
11. http://en.wikipedia.og/wiki/health_human_resources
12. Scheffler RM et al (2011) Human resources for mental health-workforce shortage in low and middle income countries, Geneva–WHO 2011 http://whqlibdoc.who.int/publication2011eng. pdf/9789241501019
13. Manoach S, Goldfrank L (2002) Social bias and injustice in the current health care system. Acad Emerg Med 9(3):241–246
14. Gerrand M, Pai M (2008) Social determinants of black-white disparities in breast cancer mortality: a review. Cancer Epidemiol Biomark Prev 17(11):2913–2918
15. Norris K, Nissenson A (2008) Race, gender and socioeconomic disparities in Chronic Kidney Disease (CKD). US J Am Soc Nephrol 19:1261–1270
16. Donohoe M (2004) Luxury primary care academic medical centers and the erosion of science and professional ethics. J Gen Internal Medicine 19:90–94
17. Nielsen-Bohlman LT, Panzer AM et al (2004) Health literacy: a prescription to end confusion. National Academics Press, Washington DC
18. Volandes A, Paasche-Orlow M (2007) Health literacy, health inequality and just healthcare system. Am J Bioeth 7(11):5–10
19. Paasche-Orlow M et al (2005) The prevalance of limited health literacy. J Gen Intern Med 20 (2):175–184
20. Baker DW, Wolf MS, Feinglass J, Thompson JA, Gazmararian JA, Huang J (2007) Health literacy and mortality among elderly persons. Arch Intern Med 167(14):1503–1509

Part III
Selected Topics

Chapter 10
Abortion

Definition of Abortion

Abortion is the termination of a pregnancy before the infant can survive outside the uterus [1]. The age at which a fetus is considered viable has not been completely agreed upon. Many obstetricians use either 21 weeks or 400–500 g birth weight as the baseline between abortion and premature delivery. In one effort to resolve the matter, the American College of Obstetricians and Gynecologists has defined abortion as the expulsion or extraction of all (complete) or any part (incomplete) of the placenta or membranes, with or without an abortus, before the 20th week (before 134 days) of gestation. Early abortion is an abortion that occurs before the 12th completed week of gestation (84 days); late abortion is an abortion that occurs after the 12th completed week but before the beginning of the 20th week of gestation (85–134 days) [2]. Pregnancy is usually calculated from the beginning of the last normal menstrual period (LNMP).

An abortion may occur spontaneously, in which case it is also called a miscarriage, or it may be brought on purposefully, in which case it is often called an induced abortion.

Spontaneous abortions, or miscarriages, occur for many reasons, including disease, trauma, genetic defect, or biochemical incompatibility of mother and fetus. Occasionally a fetus dies in the uterus but fails to be expelled, and absorbed by the body of the mother's uterus; a condition termed a missed abortion [3]. It may also get calcified and has to be removed.

Moral Issues Connected with Induced Abortion

Induced abortion is still used in many countries as a means of family planning. The medical reasons for abortion are limited and constitute a small proportion of all abortion cases. A number of conflicting views on induced abortion from various

© The Author(s) 2015
M.A. Al-Bar and H. Chamsi-Pasha, *Contemporary Bioethics*,
DOI 10.1007/978-3-319-18428-9_10

religious groups, secular humanists, liberals, and feminists have created divisions and conflict, culminating in acts of violence and loss of life. Indeed, abortion is the most controversial area of family planning, and the least understood and socially accepted. However, it is, unfortunately, the most important method employed by the advocates of fertility regulation and family planning.

The moral, religious, and legal aspects of abortion are subject to intense debate in many parts of the world [4].

Abortion is highly stigmatized in the United States and elsewhere although it has been legalized since 1973. In many regions of the world, stigma is a recognized contributor to maternal morbidity and mortality from unsafe abortion, even when abortion is legal [5]. In USA, physicians who provide abortion care are targets of stigma, harassment, and violence [6].

Abortion Incidence

Approximately 44 million abortions are performed worldwide each year [7]. Of these, 26 million are said to occur in places where abortion is legal; the others happen where the procedure is illegal. The world ratio for induced abortions is 26 per 100 known pregnancies.

Among the 208 million women estimated to become pregnant each year worldwide, 59 % (or 123 million) experience a planned (or intended) pregnancy leading to a birth or miscarriage or a stillbirth. The remaining 41 % (or 85 million) of pregnancies are unintended [8].

According to Ms. Thoraya Obaid, the Executive director of United Nation Population Fund, in every minute in the world:

- 380 women become pregnant

  - 192 or half of them, did not plan or wish the pregnancy.
  - 100 women have an abortion.
  - 40 women have an unsafe abortion [9].

After declining substantially between 1995 and 2003, the worldwide abortion rate stalled between 2003 and 2008.

- Between 1995 and 2003, the abortion rate (the number of abortions per 1,000 women of childbearing age—i.e., those aged 15–44) for the world overall dropped from 35 to 29. It remained virtually unchanged, at 28, in 2008.
- Nearly half of all abortions worldwide are unsafe. In the developing world, 56 % of all abortions are unsafe, compared with just 6 % in the developed world.

Since 2003, the number of abortions fell by 600,000 in the developed world but increased by 2.8 million in the developing world. In 2008, 6 million abortions were performed in developed countries and 38 million in developing countries, a disparity that largely reflects population distribution [10].

Researchers estimate that about 2 million induced abortions occur each year in Indonesia and that deaths from unsafe abortion represent 14–16 % of all maternal deaths in Southeast Asia. It is generally accepted that the law allows abortion only if the woman provides confirmation from a doctor that her pregnancy is life-threatening, a letter of consent from her husband or a family member, a positive pregnancy test result and a statement guaranteeing that she will practice contraception afterwards [11].

Pakistan has an estimated abortion rate of 29 abortions per 1,000 women of reproductive age, and an estimated 890,000 abortions are performed annually in Pakistan [12]. The study found that pregnant women who wish to have an abortion in Pakistan often visit illegal clinics run by midwives. However, 23 % of women who go to an unskilled abortion provider are later hospitalized for complications. Abortion is considered illegal in Pakistan except on medical grounds.

The incidence of induced abortion is very high in Russia, China, and the former East European block countries, mainly because of the absence of the pill, and the use of abortion as a means of birth control [13].

Unsafe Abortion

The World Health Organization defines unsafe abortion as a procedure for terminating a pregnancy that is performed by an individual lacking the necessary skills, or in an environment that does not conform to minimal medical standards, or both [14]. Unsafe abortions result in approximately 70,000 maternal deaths and 5 million disabilities per year globally. Between 1995 and 2008, the rate of unsafe abortion worldwide remained essentially unchanged, at 14 abortions per 1,000 women aged 15–44 [15].

An estimated 21 million unsafe abortions occur each year, an annual rate of 16 for every 1,000 women in the developing world, where the vast majority of unsafe abortions take place [16].

In Africa, where abortion is restricted in most countries, almost all abortions are performed unsafely and the rates of unsafe abortion vary from 18 to 39, being highest in Eastern Africa and lowest in Southern and Northern Africa.

In Latin America and the Caribbean, the vast majority of abortions are, like in Africa, performed unsafely, and the estimated rates of unsafe abortion are 16–33. When focusing on Asia, the estimated rates of unsafe abortion are between 9 and 28 [17].

According to the Egyptian Ministry of Health database on maternal mortality rates, the number of deaths resulting from abortion for the years 1992, 2000, and 2006 were 4.6, 4, and 1.9 %, respectively [18].

Teenage Pregnancies

Pregnancy during adolescence is rarely planned and usually outside wedlock (Unmarried). Moreover, teenage pregnancies resulting in delivery have been associated with poorer health, increased social and economic burdens, and sexually transmitted infections [19].

Teenage pregnancy for married girls (in Saudi Arabia) is quite safe, and is no different from pregnancy at 20 years and over. Akinola et al. [20] concluded that there was no significant difference in the pregnancy outcome of the teenagers (13–19) with the control group (20 and over). In another study published by Johromi and Daneshvar the authors concluded that there was no difference in the obstetric and neonatal outcome of Parturients younger than 16 years compared to Parturients 24–28 years of age [21].

In a third study published on this subject the authors found out that "Teenage Pregnancy is not associated with bad obstetric outcome when adequate antenatal care is received" [22]. Similarly, Mahfouz et al. found that pregnant teenagers are not high risk group if good prenatal care is provided [23].

In a paper presented to Islamic Fiqh council of Islamic World League in December 2012, Dr. Adel Al Abid Al Jabar concluded that teenage marriage in Saudi Arabia is diminishing. Those married at the age 15 years or under constitute one marriage in 10,000 marriages. In other words, it is a disappearing phenomenon [24].

The real problem that will be faced in the near future is the pregnancy outside wedlock which will end in unsafe abortion or trying to get rid of the baby by putting him/her in front of a mosque or other places.

The proportion of teenage pregnancies ending in termination of pregnancy (TOP) varies by country. The incidence of teenage TOP is relatively low in Finland (13/1000 in 2009) [25] compared with Britain (24/1000) and Sweden (24/1000) [26]. In recent years, 61 % of all teenage pregnancies have resulted in termination of pregnancy in Finland, the figures being 80 % in Sweden and 23 % in the USA [27].

More than 60 % of all induced abortions in the USA, Canada, and Europe are carried out on young unmarried girls under the age of 20, one quarter of whom were under the age of 17.

It is evident that promiscuity and the sexual revolution constitute the major cause of unwanted pregnancies that result in induced legal and illegal abortions. The latter are fraught with serious and sometimes fatal complications. Despite the availability of contraceptive methods for young school girls in the USA, the rate of pregnancy there is very high indeed. By age 20, there are 2 million pregnancies outside wedlock, a million of which result in abortion annually.

In the last part of the twentieth century, abortions for teenage girls decreased in the USA, as girls became more adept at using contraceptive methods [28]. A new wave of female infanticide is now spreading in many countries, especially China and India, after the spread of ultrasonography. If ultrasound shows that the conceptus is a female, the parents resort to an abortion, which is unfortunately done in the second trimester and often results in serious complications, especially if done illegally [29].

The medical indications for an abortion are broadened to include not only physical ailments, but also supposed psychological disturbances that may result from the continuation of pregnancy. Similarly, if the continuation of pregnancy will somehow affect any member of the family, then abortion is resorted to (The British Law of 1967 regarding Abortion).

Abortion and in Vitro Fertilization

Another type of indication is called "reduction of pregnancy," in which the expectant mother treated for infertility with hormones or by in vitro fertilization (IVF) gets pregnant with multiple fetuses, when the treating physician had reintroduced more than three fertilized ova (pre embryos) into the uterus. This practice was deprecated by Islamic Jurists in their meeting in Kuwait in 1987 [30] and Amman 1986 (Jordan) [31]. Later, gynecologists all around the world passed a regulation limiting the reintroduction of fertilized ova to two in each cycle in the management of fertility by in vitro fertilization methods. Many papers were published claiming that even twin pregnancy increases the complications of pregnancy and are advising replacing one fertilized ova (morulla or blastula stage). Still many gynecologists reintroduce more than 3 fertilized ova, which ends in abortion or fetal reduction.

The Historical Aspect of the Legality of Induced Abortion

The medical profession took a stand many centuries ago against induced abortion. Imhotep of Egypt (3000 B.C; deified as the god of medicine) instituted an oath to be taken by all practicing physicians, which prohibited them from prescribing an abortifacient drug or pessary. Similarly, the well-known Hippocratic Oath enjoins doctors not to induce abortion by drugs, pessaries or any other means [32].

The Declaration of Geneva of 1968, as amended in Sydney, reiterated the Hippocratic Oath and pledged "to maintain the utmost respect for human life from the time of conception [33]." However, the Declaration of Oslo, while retaining this moral principle, recognized the different opposing opinions on the question of abortion: "The Diversity of opinion is the result of the varying attitudes towards the life of the unborn child. This is a matter of individual conviction and conscience [34]." This profound change in attitude is the result of cumulative change in the fabric of many societies, where mores and lifestyles have completely changed.

Although ancient civilizations prohibited and even harshly punished those who committed abortion, they were lax in some stages of their development and condoned clandestine acts of abortion. Potts and Diggory, in their Textbook of Contraceptive Practice, stated that abortion was practiced in the Middle Kingdom of Egypt (2133–1786 B.C), and the excavations at Pompeii revealed a vaginal speculum suitable for performance of abortion. The Roman Poet Ovid lamented, "There are few women nowadays who bear all the children they conceive [35]." The same seems equally true of the majority of women in many societies today, which have legalized abortion on demand, or for tenuous social or psychological reasons.

The Bible considers induced abortion a crime but not murder; the husband of the offending wife determined the punishment, which was a compensation to him. The judge could also punish the perpetrator by strapping or imprisonment [36].

The Catholic Church was more stringent, and in the seventh century instituted a canon for capital punishment of women who had abortions [37].

Laws were passed making abortion punishable by death, in England in 1524; in Germany in 1531; in France in 1562; and in Russia in 1649 [38].

With the advent of the industrial revolution and social upheavals in the eighteenth and nineteenth centuries, European countries gradually revoked the previous harsh laws and replaced them with less drastic penalties, e.g., imprisonment, fines, and withdrawal of the license to practice medicine.

By 1929, the law in Britain allowed abortion if continuation of pregnancy was expected to endanger the health of the expectant mother. The previous law had allowed abortion only if continuation of pregnancy endangered her life and not her health [39].

From 1929 to 1967, induced abortion without a clear medical indication was considered a criminal act and was punished by imprisonment, fine and withdrawal of the license to practice medicine. The 1967 amendment issued by the British Parliament authorized physicians to abort a fetus if there was likelihood of: (a) a threat to the life of the mother if pregnancy continued; (b) a threat to her physical or psychological health, or the health of children of the family (whether her own children, her husband's children or adopted children) if pregnancy continued; (c) the presence of congenital anomalies in the fetus.

The abortion should be performed in an institution recognized by The Ministry of Health, but not necessarily by a specialist [40].

The first country in the world to legalize abortion on demand was communist Russia, which passed a law on November 18, 1920, "permitting abortion to be performed freely without charge in Soviet hospitals" [41].

This resulted in the decline of the family and the population. Stalin saw the dangers clearly and hence passed a new law in 1935, which restricted abortion to medically indicated reasons. Pravda applauded the new law and wrote: "Our Soviet women have been given the bliss of motherhood. We must safeguard our families." In 1955 however, the 1920 law on abortion was reinstated [42]. The East European satellite countries soon followed suit, with minor changes. Several Scandinavian countries liberalized abortion laws in the 1930s. In 1935 Iceland did the same, and then Sweden and Denmark in 1938. Japan allowed abortion on demand and as a means of contraception in 1948, and China followed suit during the cultural revolution of the 1960s. Haiti and Great Britain passed their laws in 1967, India in 1971, and the USA in 1973. By 1980, about 60 % of the world's population lived in countries where abortion was allowed on demand or with minor restrictions.

The law in the United States varies from state to state, in general allowing abortion on demand in the first trimester of pregnancy, with more restrictions on certain medically indicated cases in the second trimester. The 1973 Roe v Wade decision removed many legal obstacles to abortion and was a public health watershed. The Roe v Wade decision in USA made safe abortion available but did not change the reality that more than 1 million women face an unwanted pregnancy every year. Forty years after Roe v Wade, the procedure is not accessible to many US women. The politics of abortion have led to a plethora of laws that create enormous barriers to abortion access, particularly for young, rural, and low-income women [43].

Forty percent of the world's women are living in countries with restrictive abortion laws, which prohibit abortion or only allow abortion to protect a woman's life or her physical or mental health. In countries where abortion is restricted, women have to resort to clandestine interventions to have an unwanted pregnancy terminated. As a consequence, high rates of unsafe abortion are seen, such as in sub-Saharan Africa where unsafe abortion occurs at rates of 18–39 per 1000 pregnant women [44].

The laws governing the practice of induced abortion in 197 countries were classified into five categories (to save a woman's life or prohibited altogether, to preserve physical health, to preserve mental health, socioeconomic grounds, and no restriction).

In 68 countries, abortion is not legally permitted on any grounds or only to save the woman's life, and 26 % of the world's population are living in countries with such restrictive laws [45] (most of them are Catholic countries). In 36 countries, around 10 % of the world's population, abortion is allowed only to protect a woman's physical health and in another 23 countries, around 4 % of the world's population, also to protect her mental health. Finally, 21 % of the world's population lives in the 14 countries that permit abortion on socioeconomic grounds and another 39 % are living in the remaining 56 countries, where abortion is available without restriction as to indication, albeit not gestational length [46].

Countries allowing abortion on demand include: Russia, China, Japan, the Scandinavian countries, Eastern Europe, Vietnam, North Korea, the USA, and Tunisia (the only Muslim country) [47]. This might change after the revolution and reintroduction of Islamic Laws.

Countries allowing abortion with some restrictions are: Great Britain, Canada, India, France, Germany, Holland, Italy, Switzerland, Turkey, and South Africa.

Countries allowing abortion only to save the life of the mother are: the Catholic countries such as those of Latin America; Ireland, Spain, Portugal, Malta, Belgium, the Philippines [48].

Almost all Muslim countries allow abortion only for strict medical reasons [49].

The Egyptian law criminalizes abortion in the Penal Code, according to articles 260, 261, 262, and 263. Abortions performed by doctors are regulated in article 29 of the physicians' Code of Ethics which states that physicians are allowed to perform the procedure to protect the pregnant woman's health if they obtain written approval from two other specialists. Egyptian law also finds a woman guilty if she willingly chooses an induced abortion, which carries a prison penalty (6 months to 3 years imprisonment) according to article 262 of the Penal Code [50].

Abortion and Birth Control

From 1970 to 1993, the cover of the "Contraception" journal featured a graph showing global population projections, reminding all readers that the development of new, more effective, acceptable and accessible contraceptives was urgently needed to assist women to voluntarily limit their family size [51].

It is unfortunate that induced abortion is used in many societies as a means of birth control. Many gynecologists, policy makers, Planned Parenthood organizations, and others related to the United Nations advocate the use of induced abortion as a means of birth control. They also indicate that the available methods, including sterilization of both males and females, be used for birth control.

The Encyclopedia Britannica mentions some contemporary views on birth control and the means of controlling populations, including strict government controls such as compulsory sterilization. This was enforced on 40 million people by the Mao Tse Tung regime in China and on 24 million in India by Indira Ghandhi [52]. As the law in China permitted couples to have only one child, millions in China were also forced to abort.

Potts and Diggory claim in their "Textbook of Contraceptive Practice" that "Both contraception and abortion are essential for controlling fertility. A society cannot meet its fertility goals purely by the use of contraception. Therefore, the combination of reversible methods of contraception (and sterilization), and induced abortion will remain necessary elements in fertility control. Throughout history, and with increasing force over the past 100 years, societies have used a combination of contraception and abortion to control fertility. The moral and political benefits of abortion services outweigh such factors as proven mortality rates or the evidence indicated in cost benefit studies. Abortion will occur in societies with low fertility, and is likely to be most common in those societies where the birth rate is falling in response to socioeconomic pressures" [53].

The paragraph quoted above contains many contradictory and illogical statements in support of abortion where it is employed despite dangers to the health and life of the expectant mother and in societies where fertility is low; where instead every effort should be made to improve fertility, prohibiting abortion, and encouraging the birth of as many children as possible.

American and European societies encouraged third world countries to curb fertility and population increase, even by resorting to methods unacceptable in their own societies. Governments of third world countries were encouraged to implement laws and take certain measures to enforce the policy of birth control, even if it involves compulsory sterilization, the use of unsafe contraceptives or even forced abortion [54].

The medical reasons for the therapeutic abortion constitute a very small proportion of the number of abortions carried out globally for social reasons. Potts and Diggory claim, "Few abortions are carried out because continuation of pregnancy threatens the woman's life, and a small proportion because of congenital anomalies of the fetus [55]." If a woman wishes to carry her pregnancy to term and delivery, almost all obstetricians will try their best to fulfill this desire. They will do this despite the fact that she may be suffering from a disease considered an indication for abortion, e.g., advanced renal, hepatic, cardiac problems, poorly controlled diabetes, hypertension, blood Dyscrasias, or the use of immunosuppressive drugs.

Hawkins and Elders, in their book "Human Fertility Control," emphasize that "Countries with a population problem have found it politically expedient, at least tacitly, to support increased facilities for abortion. The public in general is aware that abortion is either wrong or at least a medically and psychologically unsatisfactory solution to social problems. The church (Protestant) is faced with the difficulty that it cannot enforce its views without losing its adherents... Few doctors are happy with those aspects of society which produce the need for abortions; fewer still are satisfied with an environment which generates defects in motivation to employ effective contraceptive measures" [56].

The majority of medical practitioners and gynecologists agree that since criminal abortion is fraught with serious complications including loss of life, then for pragmatic reasons, if abortion is to be carried out, it should be done by a licensed professional in a safe environment. The complications of such procedure are much reduced and the mortality rate in first trimester abortions is very low indeed, especially after the introduction of regimens using the lower mifepristone dose, 200 mg, followed by misoprostol in early pregnancy which act successfully (90 %) if given to women less than 8 weeks pregnant. Treatment failure occurred in 4.8 %. Ongoing pregnancy was reported in 1.1 % [57].

The morality rate of illegal abortions is around 50 per 100,000, while that of legal abortions in the first trimester is approximately one or two per 100,000. In the second trimester, the mortality rate reaches 40 per 100,000 [58].

Abortions should not be used as a means of birth control. The social causes leading to unwanted pregnancy should be dealt with temporary means of contraception which should be made available to couples. Abortion should be strictly limited to medically indicated cases, which constitute a small proportion of all abortions carried out on demand and for social reasons.

Religious Aspects of Abortion

Islam, Christianity, and Judaism view procreation as an integral part of marriage. In the book of Genesis, God said to both Adam and Eve, "Be fruitful and increase in numbers, fill the earth and subdue it" [59].

In Islam, procreation is not only an integral part of matrimony; it is an act of worship. Even the sexual act with one's wife is considered to be an act of charity as proclaimed by Prophet Muhammad (PBUH) [60]. The Holy Qur'an proclaims: "Oh mankind, be conscious of your Sustainer, who has created you out of one living entity, and out of it created its mate, and of the two spread abroad a multitude of men and women" [61].

"And God has given you mates of your kind, and has given through your mates children and grand children" [62]. Prophet Muhammad said to all Muslims: "Get married, beget and multiply because I will be proud of you among nations" [63]. He also said: "Marry the kind and fertile, for I will be proud of your numbers among other nations" [64].

Though Islamic teachings encourage procreation within matrimony, it does not prohibit the temporary means of contraception. The Prophet himself (PBUH) allowed his companions to practice "aazel," i.e., coitus interruptus (Onanism) [65].

His teachings stand in stark contrast to what is found in the Old Testament, the Book of Genesis. Onan, the son of Judah and the grandson of Jacob, spilled his seed on the ground to avoid producing offspring for his deceased brother when he married his brother's widow Tamar. (The Jewish teaching then gave the offspring to the deceased husband if he left no children, rather than the actual father.) God was furious and caused the death of Onan [66].

The Catholic Church holds the most conservative and stringent position against any means of contraception except abstinence during and before ovulation, i.e., using the safe period. Similarly, it holds the most conservative point of view against abortion at any stage of pregnancy, since it views human life as beginning at the point of fertilization. The fertilized ovum is given the status of a human being, and hence killing it by any means is tantamount to the crime of manslaughter.

Abortion in Islam

Allah has made clear that killing people is forbidden, as their lives are made sacred by Allah's having created them. There are a lot of Qur'anic ayas and Hadiths on the sanctity of life. "We decreed upon the children of Israel that whosoever kills a soul for other than manslaughter or corruption in the land; it shall be as if he killed all mankind, and whosoever saves the life of one, it shall be as if he saved the life of all mankind" [67].

The Qur'an also says: "And do not kill anyone whom Allah has made sacred, except for a just cause…" [68]. This applies to killing anyone; and killing one's children is especially forbidden by Allah. "They are lost indeed who kill their children foolishly without knowledge, and forbid what Allah has given to them, forging a lie against Allah; they have indeed gone astray, and they are not the followers of the right course" [69].

The Qur'an deplores killing children for want, or fear of want, "Kill not your children on a plea of want. We provide sustenance for you and for them. Come not near to shameful deeds whether open or secret. Take not life, which God has made sacred, except by ways of justice and law. Thus does He command, that you may learn wisdom" [70].

"Kill not your children for fear of want. We shall provide sustenance for them as well as for you. Verily the killing of them is a great sin" [71].

Ibn Massoud (a companion of the Prophet) asked the Prophet: What is the gravest sin? The Prophet (PBUH) answered: "That you associate partners with God who created you." Ibn Massoud asked: What is next to this? And the Prophet answered "That you kill your offspring for fear of them sharing your food with you" [72].

Though Muslims generally consider the embryo from its earliest stages as "living," they do not give it the status of full human life except after ensoulment. Ibn Al Qaiyim, in his book "Attibian Fi Aksam Al Qur'an", brings up this question by asking: "Does the embryo before ensoulment (breathing of the spirit into it) have a life?" He answers that the embryo has the life of growth and nourishment like a growing plant, but once the spirit is breathed in he acquires perception and volition" [73].

Similarly, Ibn Hajar Al Asqalani, in his voluminous "Fatehul Bari", on the first organ to be formed in the embryo says, "The liver is the first organ formed as it is the site of nutrition and growth. Voluntary movement and perception are acquired only after ensoulment" [74].

Ensoulment only occurs after many stages through which the embryo passes. The Holy Qur'an says: "We created man from the quintessence of mud. Thereafter, we cause him to remain as a drop of fluid (Nutfa) in a firm lodging (the womb). Thereafter, we fashion the Nutfa into something that clings (Alakah), which we fashion into a chewed-like lump (Modgha). The chewed-like lump is fashioned into bones, which are then covered with flesh. Then we nurse him into another act of creation. Blessed is God, the best of artisans" [75].

All the ulama (jurists of the Islamic nation) and commentators of the Holy Qur'an agree that the "other act of creation" mentioned above is the time of ensoulment, where the spirit is inspired into the body of the fetus.

The Qur'an makes it clear that Allah creates humans in stages and that before the final stage they are not humans [76].

The Hadith (sayings) of the Prophet narrated by Ibn Massoud state: "The creation of each one of you is collected in the womb of his mother in forty days. And something that clings (Alakah) he becomes for forty days, and then he becomes Modgha (a chewed lump) for forty days. The angel is sent to him and the angel writes four things: his provision (sustenance), his life span, his deeds and whether he will be wretched or blessed. Then the spirit is breathed into him" [77].

This simply means that ensoulment occurs at 120 days computed from the beginning of conception. However, there is another Hadith narrated by Huzaifa Ibn Aseed which says: "When the Nutfa enters the womb and stays there for 42 nights, God sends an angel to give it a form and create its hearing, sight, skin, bone and flesh. Then the angel asks, "O God, is it a boy or a girl? And God determines whatever He decides. He then asks what his livelihood and God determines [78].

It is interesting to note that organogenesis (formation of organs in the embryo) takes place between the 4th and 8th week of conception (computed from fertilization) and reaches its zenith in 42 days. The embryo has an unidentified gonad until that period after which the gonad differentiates into either a testes or an ovary. Similarly, the brain stem forms and starts to function in an embryo after 42 days. However, the higher functions of the brain are still forming and the cerebral cortex does not have synapses with the lower centers before the beginning of the 20th week computed from the last menstrual period, which is equivalent to 120 days computed from fertilization (viz., beginning of conception). Dr. Koren J. presented a paper at the Conference on Ethics of Organ Transplantation in Ottawa, Canada August 20–24, 1989, in which he proved with dissection of many aborted fetuses that synapses between the higher centers of the cerebrum and the lower centers do not start to work before the beginning of the 20th week of pregnancy, computed from the LMP; which is equivalent to 120 days, computed from the moment of conception (fertilization) [79].

It is evident that both sayings of Prophet Muhammad (PBUH) speak of different times of development of the CNS of the fetus; the Hadith of 42 days refers to the development and functioning of the brain stem, while the Hadith of 120 days speaks about the higher centers and their control over the lower ones in the CNS. It clearly speaks of ensoulment; the spirit entering the body of the fetus.

There are a lot of Hadith which assign to the conceptus an important status that gradually increases with the time of pregnancy. If a lady commits a crime punishable by death, the execution of the penalty is postponed until after delivery and until after the baby has been nursed for 2 years. However, if a wet nurse is available for the mother's nursing period, it is much shorter. This applies even if the pregnancy is illegitimate [80].

In Islam, temporary means of contraception are allowed, provided they cause no harm, and are done with mutual consent of the spouses [81]. Sterilization is not allowed, except for clear medical indications, where pregnancy would seriously endanger the health or life of the expectant mother [82].

Similarly, abortion is allowed only if continuation of pregnancy would endanger the life or health of the expectant mother; or if there is proven serious congenital anomaly in the embryo or fetus. The performance of abortion should be done prior to elapse of 120 days from the start of conception, which is considered the time of ensoulment according to the Hadith (sayings) of the Prophet. However, if the life of the expectant mother is endangered, abortion or pre-term delivery can be performed at any time of pregnancy. The decision with clear medical indication for abortion should be agreed upon by three specialist physicians [83].

This was the Fatwa (decision) of the Islamic Fiqh council of Islamic World League held in Makkah from 10 to 17th February 1990. The decision was passed by the majority of votes, but with abstentions of the late president Shaikh Abdulaziz Bin Baz, and Shaikh Bakr Abu Zaid [84].

Many Islamic jurists are more stringent and would allow abortion only in the first 40 days of conception (computed from fertilization and not LMP). In fact, this was the official Fatwa in Saudi Arabia, until the Fatwa of the Islamic Fiqh council of Islamic World League; Makkah Al Mukaramah in 1990 extended it to 120 days from start of conception.

More conservative jurists like the Maliki School and Imam Al Gazali (from Shafii School of Jurisprudence) do not allow abortion at any time of pregnancy except to save the life of the expectant mother [85]. Nevertheless, there are some jurists who would allow abortion for social reasons, e.g., rape, or where continuation of pregnancy would affect a nursing child, or where a wet nurse was not available or the father was too poor to afford a wet nurse [86]. Prominent among those permitting abortion is the Zaidi School of jurisprudence which allows abortion for social and minor medical reasons in the first 120 days of conception. Some jurists of the Hanafi, Hanbali, and Shafii Schools also permit abortion with minor restrictions [87]. However, the majority of Islamic jurists throughout history, because of Islam's respect for life; do not allow abortion except for strong medical reasons.

Sheikh Yusuf Al-Qaradawi, states in his well-known book, "The Lawful and the Prohibited in Islam": "While Islam permits preventing pregnancy for valid reasons, it does not allow doing violence to the pregnancy once it occurs. Muslim jurists agree unanimously that after the fetus is completely formed and has been given a soul, aborting it is haram. It is also a crime, the commission of which is prohibited to the Muslim because it constitutes an offense against a complete, live human being" [88].

The fetus has the right of the lineage of his father, and if his father dies while he is in utero, his share of the inheritance will be kept for him/her until delivery. Sheikh Mohmoud Shaltout (Grand Imam of Al Azhar in the 1940s and early 1950s) wrote: "Old scholars have agreed that after quickening takes place (120 days from conception), abortion is prohibited to all Muslims, for it is a crime perpetrated against a living being. Therefore, blood ransom is due if the fetus is delivered alive and then dies immediately after delivery, and ghorra (1/20 of the diyah) if delivered dead" [89].

Imam AlGhazali (died 505 H = 1122 AD), in his well-known book "Ihyia Oloomaddin", considered abortion at all stages of conception as "Haram," with a gradation of the sin according to the length of pregnancy. It is tantamount to manslaughter if the child is delivered alive and then dies because of the abortifacient act or drug. However, the Imam recognized that the gravity of the crime is less if the abortion is of Nutfa (at 40 days) than the abortion of Alakah (40–80 days), which is less than the abortion of Modgha (80–120 days). It becomes a grave crime after ensoulment, i.e., after 120 days. In his opinion, abortion should be avoided at all stages of pregnancy except if the life of the expectant mother is endangered [90].

The Muslim physician Abubaker Al Rhazi (died 313 H/925 AD) mentioned in his book Al Mansouri and in his encyclopedic Al Hawi many abortifacient drugs and methods to be used if continuation of pregnancy would endanger the health or life of the expectant mother. Similarly, Ibn Sina (Avicenna) wrote in his well-known (Al Kanoon fi Tibb) a chapter on medical indications of abortion and how to perform them [91].

We think that their recognition of the need for abortion in certain cases where continuation of pregnancy would endanger the health or life of the expectant mother is more realistic and humane than the stance of the church in medieval Europe, and the Catholic Church at this moment.

Abortion and Population Control

Certainly, no school of Islamic jurisprudence intends to allow abortion as a method of population control. Muslim legal scholars have treated the subject of birth control in great detail, and a consensus has emerged regarding its permissibility if both spouses agree that it is not permanent and it is not harmful [92].

Other Indications

Many Fatwas have been given permitting abortion following rape, e.g., Islamic Fiqh council of Islamic World League, Makkah Al Mukaramah, The International Islamic Fiqh Academy of Organization of Islamic Conferences (OIC-IFA),and Sheikh Qaradawi, etc. [93]. It should be performed as early as possible and in the first 40 days of pregnancy. Abortions to avoid economic hardships are not condoned by Muslim jurists.

Abortion on Demand

Seeking abortion for no "good" reason at all, and indicating that the "mother" or "father" just do not want the baby—is considered to be inhumane and cruel.

Abortion on demand, as carried out in many countries, with liberal abortion laws, will never be condoned by Shari'ah (Islamic Law).

Unfortunately, Tunisia passed a law 65/24 dated July 1, 1965, which allowed abortion for tenuous reasons. The situation became worse when law no. 73–75 dated November 19, 1973 came into effect. It allowed abortion on demand in the first trimester of pregnancy, and on flimsy reasons in the second half of pregnancy [94]. After the toppling of the Secular regime in 2011, it is expected that these laws will be amended to conform to recognized Fatwas from Islamic jurists and Islamic conferences.

Turkey allows abortion with some restrictions based on some medical or social reasons. The remaining Islamic countries allow abortion to safeguard the expectant mother from serious problems in pregnancy that might put her health or life at risk. Many permit abortion when there is a seriously malformed embryo or fetus. The time limit for carrying out such abortions is 120 days computed from fertilization, which is equivalent to 134 days from the Last Normal Menstrual Period (LNMP) [95].

Punishment for Causing a Pregnant Woman to Miscarry

If someone causes a pregnant Muslim woman to have a miscarriage, that person must pay an indemnity to the woman's family but will not be submitted to the "hadd" punishment for taking life. The judge may order other punishment (Taazir).

Killing the fetus, intentionally or unintentionally, is penalized by the payment 1/20 of the diyha (blood fine), which is equivalent to 500 golden dinars. Another penalty is determined by the magistrate for intentionally induced abortion [96].

The question of indemnity for carrying abortion differs according to the time of abortion and according to different Islamic jurisprudence schools. If the abortion is carried out early and it is not possible to identify human features in the abortus, then there will be no indemnity according to Shafi, Hanbali, and Hanafi schools of jurisprudence.

The mother who intentionally tries to miscarry a fetus less than 120 days of gestation pays a penance, according to Ibn Hazm, as if she had broken a vow, but not an indemnity. If someone else causes a woman to abort before the fetus has reached 120 days gestation, this person would be liable for an indemnity [97].

References

1. The Encyclopedia Britannica (2013) http://global.britannica.com/EBchecked/topic/474704/pregnancy/76074/Abortion
2. Ibid
3. Ibid
4. Ilyas M, Alam M, Ahmad H, Sajid-ul-Ghafoor (2009) Abortion and protection of the human fetus: religious and legal problems in Pakistan. Hum Reprod Genet Ethics 15(2):55–59
5. Harris LH (2012) Stigma and abortion complications in the United States. Obstet Gynecol 120 (6):1472
6. Harris LH, Martin L, Debbink M, Hassinger J (2013) Physicians, abortion provision and the legitimacy paradox. Contraception 87(1):11–16
7. Shah I, Ahman E (2009) Unsafe abortion: global and regional incidence, trends, consequences, and challenges. J Obstet Gynaecol Can 31(12):1149–1158
8. World Health Organization (2012) Safe abortion: technical and policy guidance for health systems—2nd edn. www.who.int/reproductivehealth/.../unsafe_abortion/
9. Obaid TA (2005) Religion and reproductive health and rights. J Am Acad Relig 73(4):1155–1173
10. Sedgh G, Singh S, Shah IH, Ahman E, Henshaw SK, Bankole A (2012) Induced abortion: incidence and trends world wide from 1995 to 2008. Lancet 379(9816):625–632
11. Sedgh G, Ball H (2008) Abortion in Indonesia. Issues Brief (Alan Guttmacher Inst) 2:1–6
12. Ilyas M op. cit

13. Kovasc L (1997) Abortion and contraceptive practice in Eastern Europe. Int J Gynaecol Obstet 58(1):69–75
14. Sedgh G (2012) op. cit
15. Ibid
16. Singh S (2010) Global consequences of unsafe abortion. Womens Health (Lond Engl) 6 (6):849–860
17. Singh S, Wulf D, Hussain R, Bankole A, Sedgh G (2009) Abortion worldwide: a decade of uneven progress. Guttmacher Institute, New York
18. Necco E (2012) The Bioethics looks on abortion in Islam. A special case: Egypt. Published in: Berna A, Vardit R-C (eds) Islam and bioethics. A Publication of Ankara University, Turkey, pp 86–94
19. Paranjothy S, Broughton H, Adappa R, Fone D (2009) Teenage pregnancy: who suffers? Arch Dis Child 94:239–245
20. Akinola S, Manne N, Archiboug E, Sobandc AA (2001) Teenagers obstetric performance. Saudi Med J 7:580–584
21. Johromi B, Daneshvar A (2005) Pregnancy outcome of parturients below 16 years of age. Saudi Med J 26:1417–1419
22. Hammad S, Al-Enazi R (2008) Does Teenage Pregnancy affect obstetric outcome. Egypt J Community Med 20(3):25–35
23. Mahfouz A, El-Said M, Al-Erian RA, Homdi AM (1995) Teenage Pregnancy: are teenagers a high risk group. Euro J Obstet Gynecol Reprod Bid 59(1):17–20
24. Al Abid Al Jabar A (2012) A paper (Arabic) forwarded to Islamic Jurisprudence of Makkah, Islamic World League (21 Session), 8–12 Dec 2012
25. Induced abortions—reproduction—statistics by themes—stakes. http://www.tilastokeskus.fi/index_en.html
26. Gissler M, Fronteira I, Jahn A, Karro H, Moreau C, Oliveira da Silva M, Olsen J, Savona-Ventura C, Temmerman M, Hemminki E (2012) REPROSTAT group. Terminations of pregnancy in the European Union. Br J Obstet Gynaecol 119:324–332
27. Pazol K, Zane SB, Parker WY, Hall LR, Berg C, Cook DA (2011) Centers for disease control and prevention (CDC). Abortion surveillance—United States, 2008. Morb Mortal Wkly Rep Surveill Summ 60:1–41
28. Kaufman R, Spitz A, Moris L et al (1998) The decline in US teen pregnancy rates 1990–1995. Pediatrics 102(5):1141–7
29. Tifts (1988) Curse Heaven for little girls. Time Mag:46–47
30. Ibrahim MA (1987) What to do with excess fertilized ova? (Arabic) and discussions 3rd Symposium on some medical practices, April 18, 1987. Islamic Organization for Medical Sciences, Kuwait, pp 450–455
31. The complete works of the 3rd meeting of the International Islamic Jurists Council OIC. Amman, Jordan 1:425–515. Oct 11–16
32. Ahmed WD (1998) Oath of Muslim Physician. JIMA 20:11–14
33. Phillips M, Dawson J (1985) Appendix: the declaration of Geneva. Brighton (G. Britain). The Harvester Press, Doctors' Dilemma, p 211
34. Ibid
35. Potts M, Diggory P (1983) Abortion. Textbook of contraceptive practice. Cambridge University Press, Cambridge, pp 274–367
36. Ibid
37. Albar M (1991) Policy and methods of Birth control (Arabic: Siyasat wa wasayil Tahdid Annasl). Al Asr Al Hadith Publication, Beirut, pp 119–23
38. Ibid
39. Potts M op. cit
40. Hathout H (1984) Topics in Islamic Medicine. Islamic Medicine Organization, Kuwait, pp 93–135
41. Potts M op. cit
42. Albar M (1991) op. cit

43. Yanow S (2013) It is time to integrate abortion into primary care. Am J Public Health 103 (1):14–16
44. Rasch V (2011) Unsafe abortion and post abortion care—an overview Acta Obstetriciaet Gynecologica. Scandinavica 90:692–700
45. The World's Abortion Laws, Fact Sheet (2009). http://www.reproductiverights.org/document/world-abortion-laws-2009-fact-sheet
46. Ibid
47. Albar M (1991) op. cit
48. Ibid
49. Hessinil L (2007) Abortion and Islam: Policies and practice in the Middle East and North Africa. Reprod Health Matters 15(29):75–84
50. Necco E op. cit
51. Westhoff CL (2013) Contraception and the advances in family planning. Contraception 87 (1):1–2
52. Albar M (1991) op. cit
53. Potts M op. cit
54. Albar M (1991) op. cit
55. Potts M op. cit
56. Hawkins D, Elders M (1979) Human fertility control. Butterworths, London, pp 237–260
57. Raymond EG, Shannon C, Weaver MA, Winikoff B (2013) First-trimester medical abortion with mifepristone 200 mg and misoprostol: a systematic review. Contraception 87(1):26–37
58. Bennett M (1998) Abortion. In: Hacker N, Moore JG (eds) Essentials of obstetrics and Gynecology, 3rd edn. Saunders Co., Philadelphia, pp 477–486
59. Book of Genesis 1:27, 28. New International translation, Hodder and Stroughton, London; 1980. Holy Bible
60. Sahih Muslim Bishareh Al Nawawi (1972) Dar Al Fikr Beirut 7:92
61. The Holy Qur'an 4:4
62. The Holy Qur'an 16:72
63. Al-Souyoty (1976) Al-Jame Al-sageer: Hadith No. 3366, Dar Al Fikr, Beirut
64. Ibn Hanbal A, Musnad A (1999) Dar Al Maarif, Cairo 4:245
65. Al Bokhari M (1956) Sahih AlBoukhari, Maktabat Al Nahda, Cairo, Kitab Al Nikah, 96
66. Holy Bible. Book of genesis. 38:8–10
67. The Holy Qur'an 5:32
68. The Holy Qur'an 17:33
69. The Holy Qur'an 6:140
70. The Holy Qur'an 6:151
71. The Holy Qur'an 17:31
72. Al Bokhari M (1956) Sahih AlBoukhari, Maktabat Al Nahda, Cairo, 40:60
73. Ibn Al Qaiyim: Attibian fi Aksam Al Quran, Maktabat Al Kahira, Cairo (No date mentioned). p 255
74. Ibn Hajar Al Askalani: Fathu Al Bari Fi Shareh Sahihu Al Bokhari Al Malktabh Assalafiyah, Cairo Kitab Al Qadar. 11:481
75. The Holy Qur'an 23:12–14
76. Rogers T (1999) The Islamic Ethics of abortion. The Muslim World, vol LXXXIX, No. 2. (April)
77. Al Bokhari M (1956) Sahih Al Bokhari, Maktabat Al Nahda, Cairo
78. Sahih Muslim Bishareh Al Nawawi (1972) Dar Al Fikr, Beirut
79. Koren J (1989) Symposium on Ethics of Organ transplantation Ottawa (Canada) Aug 20–24; Abstracts
80. Albar M (1985) Mushkilat Al Ijhadh (The problem of abortion) Saudia Publishing House, Jeddah, pp 37–45
81. The council of Islamic Figh Academy, 5th session, held in Kuwait 10–15 December 1988, Islamic Figh Academy. Resolutions and Recommendations 1406-1409 H/1985-1989, 36. Organization of the Islamic conference; Resolution No 1 concerning Birth Control, Jeddah

82. Ibid
83. The 4th Resolution on Aborting a congenital malformed fetus, Islamic jurist council of Islamic World League, Makkah Al Mukaramah, 12th session 10–17th February 1990 and also quoted appendix No 1, in M. Albar: Al Ganin Al Mushawah (The congenitally malformed fetus), Dar Al Qalam Damascus and Dar Al Manara Jeddah. 1991:439
84. Ibid
85. Al Ghazali M. Ihyia Oloom Al Dein. Dar Al Maarif, Beirut 2:65
86. Albar M (1985) op. cit
87. Albar M (1991) op. cit
88. Al-Qaradawi Y (1994) The Lawful and the prohibited in Islam, Al Maktab Al Islami, Damscus
89. Shaltoot M (1966) Islam: Creed and Shari'ah. Dar al Qalam
90. Albar M (1991) op. cit
91. Ibid
92. Stephens M, Jordens CF, Kerridge IH, Ankeny RA (2010) Religious perspectives on abortion and a secular response. J Relig Health 49(4):513–535
93. Ilyas M op. cit
94. Albar M (1991) op. cit
95. Albar M (1985) op.cit
96. Albar M (1991) op. cit; Albar M (1985) op. cit
97. Rogers T op.cit

Chapter 11
Assisted Reproductive Technology: Islamic Perspective

Introduction

Infertility is defined as the inability of a couple to conceive after 1 year of regular, unprotected intercourse. Natural cycle fecundity, or the chance of a couple conceiving in a given month, is 20–25 % for a healthy couple. Approximately 10–15 % of couples experience infertility, and after 1 year of trying to conceive it is appropriate to evaluate a couple for infertility [1].

Recent research has shown that suffering from involuntary childlessness may be nearly equally distributed between women and men, but men have more difficulty in communicating this emotional crisis [2]. The psychological impact of infertility is a complex, integral part of the condition which must be taken into account by all treatment services associated with assisted reproduction [3].

Islamic View of Infertility

It is human nature to want to have children. The Qur'an says that "wealth and progeny are adornments for the life of this world," [4] which means that families seek two things: to have a secure financial future and children. Because one of the prayers of believers described in Qur'an is "O, Lord, grant us spouses and offspring who will be the comfort of our eyes," [5] seeking a cure for infertility is, thus, appropriate.

There are a few case scenarios depicted in the Holy Qur'an which helps us to gain a proper insight into the problem of infertility. The first illustrates the story of Ibrahim (May God give him His blessing) and his wife Sara as revealed in the Qur'an (surah 51: 28–30). "…And they (angels) gave him (Ibrahim) glad tidings of a son endowed with knowledge. But his wife came forward clamoring, she smote her forehead and said: A barren old woman! They said: Even so has thy Lord

© The Author(s) 2015   173
M.A. Al-Bar and H. Chamsi-Pasha, *Contemporary Bioethics*,
DOI 10.1007/978-3-319-18428-9_11

spoken and He is full of wisdom and knowledge." The aged Sara had willingly resigned to her destiny of being infertile but yet continued to be firm in her faith and true to her husband. She remained a complete, faithful woman in every other way. And she offered Hajar to Ibrahim in marriage, so as to enable him to have children. She was ultimately blessed with a child, Ishaq.

As with the example of Ibrahim, Zakaria remained faithful and supportive of his infertile wife. In surah 21: 89–90, Allah says: "And (remember) Zakaria, when he cried to his Lord: "O my Lord! Leave me not without offspring, though Thou are the best of inheritors." So We listened to him and granted him Yahya (John). We cured his wife (barrenness) for him. They were ever quick in emulation in good works; they used to call on us with love and reverence, and humble themselves before Us." Being infertile does not make one any lesser a man or woman. Like Zakaria, one should beseech Allah for the blessings of offspring [6].

The Prophet PBUH says: "Marry the kind and fertile women who will give birth to many children for I shall take pride in the great numbers of my ummah" (Nation) [7]. Islam gives strong and unequivocal emphasis to high fertility.

Artificial Reproduction

Dr. Edwards, an embryologist and Dr. Steptoe, a gynecologist in the United Kingdom first pioneered the fertility technique called In Vitro Fertilization Pre-Embryo Transfer (IVF–ET). In July 1978, they announced to the world the birth of the first test-tube baby, Louise Brown which was a landmark achievement in the science of reproductive medicine [8]. Since then, a myriad of assisted reproductive techniques have surfaced, further refining and superseding earlier technologies [9].

The use of medical techniques to enhance fertility is a topical issue that cannot be overemphasized, as recent studies show that Assisted Reproductive Technology (ART) is responsible for between 219,000 and 246,000 babies born each year worldwide [10].

ART today is being used for many different objectives. First, is the employment of ART as a succor to childless/infertile couples.

Second, it is also used to enable women without a male partner to have children by using sperm provided by a donor. Furthermore, assisted reproduction is equally being employed for baby gender selection and the quest for a particular sex (male or female) by fertile couples who resort to IVF just to be able to have a preferred gender. It is also used to avoid genetic and chromosomal diseases by pre-implantation diagnosis (PGD).

Islamic law frowns on any use of ART with no medical justification. Self-imposed single motherhood or fatherhood, as with lesbians or gays longing for children, is a sharp negation of Islamic law provisions.

In Vitro Fertilization (IVF)

IVF is a process by which a woman, through hormonal manipulation simultaneously produces several ova. These ova are needle aspirated at the proper time under ultrasonic guidance usually through the vagina or through the abdominal wall. In the lab, the husband's sperms fertilize these ova. Successfully fertilized ova (zygotes) reaching the four to eight cell stage are transferred into the uterus. At this point, the uterus has been prepared by hormones in order to begin implantation of the transferred zygotes (pre-embryos).

The current success rate, measured by fertilizations resulting in a live birth, is between 20 and 30 %. IVF, with its various modifications, i.e., GIFT (Gamete intra-fallopian transfer), ICSI (intracytoplasmic sperm injection) [11] etc., has been declared islamically permissible, only if the following conditions are satisfied. First, the IVF must involve a married couple. Second, the sperm must be from the husband, and the eggs from the wife. Third, this must occur within the context of a valid marriage. Fourth, the procedure must be conducted by a "competent team" in order to reduce the chances of failure or mixing of zygotes and pre-embryos of different couples when kept in liquid nitrogen. Fifth surrogacy is not accepted. Finally, no more than the appropriate number of fertilized eggs should be transferred to the uterus [12]. It is common to transfer only two to three fertilized eggs, although there are usually more fertilized eggs produced. Many centers transfer only one or two fertilized eggs.

Freezing the remaining fertilized ova is permissible by some Islamic Scholars as long as they are only used in subsequent cycles for the same couple, and the couple is still married. The fate of the unused eggs has not yet been decided upon. It is permissible to use them for medical research with the consent of the couple and within the appropriate guidelines. However, The International Islamic Fiqh Academy of Organization of Islamic Conferences (OIC-IFA) in 1990 refused the freezing of the pre-embryos as occurrences of mixing of gametes and pre-embryos happened.

Outcomes of ART

Pregnancy outcomes after ART treatment are not generally as favorable as for spontaneous conceptions. A substantial proportion of this excess risk is mediated through iatrogenic multiple pregnancy, as multiple embryos are routinely returned to increase the chance of pregnancy. Accordingly, early pregnancy loss, total miscarriage rates and stillbirth rates are elevated compared with the general population.

For the mother there is a low risk of hyperstimulation of the ovaries which is a serious complication. There are also elevated risks for preeclampsia, gestational diabetes, placenta previa, placental abruptia, and caesarean delivery. Gestations for ART pregnancies tend to be shorter and birth weights of singletons and twins are substantially reduced to a degree that can be comparable to smoking throughout pregnancy. The reasons for this are uncertain [13].

We are now developing a clearer view of the longer-term implications of ART. Cumulative evidence from a variety of sources including population registries, cohort studies, and meta-analyses indicate that ART is associated with an increased risk of major congenital malformation, and that this risk appears to vary by treatment modality in addition to patient's age and factors related to infertility.

The use of pre-embryo freezing appears to substantially reduce the risk, which suggests that the defects are in part intrinsic to the embryos, and that a freeze–thaw cycle adds a selection pressure against developmentally compromised pre-embryos [14].

Women undergoing IVF with multiple embryo transfer face an increased risk of twins and triplets. The social and economic consequences of multiple pregnancies are significant, as are risks to the mother and baby. Single Preembryo transfer can minimize the risk of multiples but the pregnancy and live birth rate was lower [15].

Multifetal pregnancy, particularly high-order multiple pregnancy, should be prevented in the first place because of its associated fetal and maternal complications and increased cost [16].

Islamic Views of ART

The teachings of the Qur'an and Hadiths have emphasized the vital role of the institution of marriage and the family structure, and inseparable from this is the act of procreation. To this effect Allah (God, Exalted be His Name) says in surah 16: 72; "And Allah has given you wives of your own kind, and has given you, from your wives, sons and grandsons, and has made provisions of good things for you. Is it then in vanity that they believe and in the grace of Allah that they disbelieve?"

Artificial reproduction is not mentioned in the primary sources of Shari'ah; however, when procreation fails, Islam encourages treatment, especially because adoption is not an acceptable solution. Thus, attempts to cure infertility are not only permissible, but also encouraged. The duty of the physician is to help a barren couple achieve successful fertilization, conception, and delivery of a baby [17].

All assisted reproductive technologies are permitted in Islam, if the semen source, ovum source, and the incubator (uterus) come from the legally married husband and wife during the span of their marriage [18]. According to Islam, a man's or woman's infertility should be accepted if it is beyond cure. Assisted reproduction was widely accepted after prestigious scientific and religious bodies and organizations issued guidelines, which were accepted by concerned authorities in different Muslim countries. These guidelines included a Fatwa from Dar El Iftaa, Cairo (1980) and a Fatwa from the Islamic Fiqh Council, Makkah (1984), the Islamic Organization for Medical Sciences (IOMS) in Kuwait (1983), the Fatwa of International Islamic Fiqh Academy in 1986, and the International Islamic Centre for Population Studies and Research, al. Azhar University. These guidelines are followed by most Muslims [19].

Third-Party Assistance

The dyad of the legal husband and wife must not be intruded by any third party. The involvement of a third person in the equation is totally unacceptable whether this take the form of a sperm, an ovum, an embryo or a uterus. Hence the widespread practice in ART facilities of sperm, ovum, and embryo donation and the "rental" of uterus is incompatible with the Islamic injunctions related to human reproduction [20]. Frozen pre-embryos are the property of the couple alone and may be transferred to the wife in a successive cycle provided the marital bondage is not absolved by death or divorce [21].

This ban on third-party assistance has been upheld in many fatwas and bioethical decrees Issued since 1980 in the Sunni Muslim countries [22]. For example, fatwas supporting assisted reproduction treatment but banning third-party assistance have been issued in Kuwait, Qatar, Saudi Arabia and the United Arab Emirates [23]. In 1997, at the ninth Islamic law and medicine conference, held under the auspices of the Kuwait-based IOMS in Casablanca, Morocco, a landmark five-point bioethical declaration included recommendations to prevent human cloning and to prohibit all situations in which a third party invades a marital relationship through donation of reproductive material [24]. Such a ban on third-party reproductive assistance of all kinds is now effectively in place in the Sunni world, which represents approximately 90 % of the world's 1.6 billion Muslims.

Surrogacy

Another form of ART is surrogacy. There are two types of surrogacy, partial and complete. In partial surrogacy, a couple will solicit or commission a woman to be artificially impregnated by the "husband" semen. The surrogate will then carry the pregnancy to term, and upon birth, give the baby away to the soliciting couple. In this case, the child will have the rearing father as the biological father, a rearing mother, and a biological birth mother.

In a complete surrogacy, the commissioning couple will undergo IVF. The embryo produced by IVF is transferred then to a surrogate woman. The surrogate gives the baby to the soliciting/rearing couple at birth. In this case, the biological parents are the rearing couple, and the surrogate is the birth mother [25].

Under Islamic law, surrogacy is prohibited [26]. Surrogacy between the wives of one husband is allowed by Ali Khamini of Iran.

The Fatwa of the Islamic Fiqh council of Makkah in 1984 allowed surrogacy by replacing the embryos inside the uterus of the second wife of the same husband who provided the spermatozoa. In 1985, the council withdrew its approval of surrogacy [27].

Linguistically and Islamically, the Arabic word for "to give birth" is Walad, and for "mother" it is Walidah, or the "one who gives birth." A verse from the Qur'an states that, "None can be their mothers except those who gave them birth" [28]. Even if there is an agreement between the parties, the confusion of lineage, which is inevitable in these surrogacy arrangements and which is of major importance in Islamic law, prohibits surrogacy. If surrogacy is still done despite the prohibition, it is the consensus of Islamic scholars that the birth mother is the "real" mother.

Shia's Views on ART

Major divergences in Islamic juridical opinion between Sunni and Shia religious authorities have led to striking differences in the practice of ARTs, particularly with regard to the use of donor gametes [29]. In the late 1990s, the Leader of the Islamic Republic of Iran, Ayatollah Ali Khamene'i issued a fatwa effectively permitting third-party donations including egg donation, sperm donation and surrogacy [30].

Iran is the only Muslim country in which ARTs using donor gametes and embryos have been legitimized by religious authorities and passed into law. This has placed Iran, a Shia-dominant country, in a unique position vis-à-vis the Sunni Islamic world, where all forms of gamete donation are strictly prohibited [31]. Most Shia scholars have also issued jurisprudential decrees (fatwas) that allow surrogate motherhood as a treatment for infertility, albeit only for legal couples [32].

In the Iranian clinics following Khamene'i's lead, all manner of egg, sperm, and embryo donation, as well as surrogacy, continue to take place, with his fatwa clearly displayed as moral justification. For over a decade, donor gametes are not only being donated and shared, but even purchased by infertile couples in IVF clinics in Iran and certain parts of Lebanon (Some Shia Lebanese) [33].

Many Shia religious authorities support the majority Sunni view: namely, they agree that third-party donation should be strictly prohibited. For example, Iraq's Ayatollah Sistani has opposed any form of third-party donation [34]. Several Shia jurists do not agree with Khamenei's position, nor his permissive fatwa on donor technologies. For example, Shaikh Muhammad Husayn Fadlallah, Lebanon's most prominent Shia religious authority, disagree with Khamenei's permission of sperm donation [35]. Besides, other sects of Shia: like Non-Iranian Jafari, Zaidi of Yemen and Ismaili disagree with Khamenei's fatwa.

Furthermore, Ayatollah Mohammad-Ali Taskhiri, the representative of Iran in OIC-IFA has also agreed to all decrees (fatwas) issued by this Academy on this subject.

Legal adoption does not exist in Islam. However, the Islamic scriptures emphasize on the kind guardianship of orphans. In Iran, an adoption law was sanctioned, giving Iranian couples the right to legally adopt orphaned children.. In some Sunni Islamic countries, abandoned child of unknown parents may be taken by a family who breastfeed him/her and therefore become a child of that family through Reezaa (breastfeeding) [36].

Cross Border Treatment for Infertility

Cross border treatment for infertility, commonly referred to as Cross-Border Reproductive Care (CBRC) is a relatively recent development in the history of assisted conception. CBRC is an international phenomenon and people travel overseas for a wide range of reasons [37]. These can include accessing treatment that is not available in their own country due to legal restrictions, shorter waiting lists, lower costs, higher success rates, better quality of care and availability of donor gametes [38]. Such an act is by no means restricted to one country or to followers of one religion. The pattern also exists in Europe among residents of different European countries with different regulatory mechanisms of the process of assisted reproduction [39].

Cryopreservation and the Use of Preserved Sperm

In medical terms, 'cryopreservation' is the freezing and storage of gametes, zygotes, or pre-embryos. Essentially, cryopreservation is used for two purposes. Patients who have been diagnosed as having a disease where treatment from the disease may result in infertility. The sperm is processed and is kept and thawed at a later date, and with the patient's consent, is used to fertilize the ovum from the wife. Similarly, ART procedures often result in the availability of numerous spare pre-embryos that are not transferred into the uterus of the mother. Cryopreservation or freezing techniques are able to store pre-embryo up to a few years which can be thawed and returned to the uterus of the same woman whenever she decides to have a child. The advantages of freezing embryos would be that the woman might not have to undergo the drug stimulation cycle again, and to save her the side effects of the stimulant drugs that are used [40].

Cryopreservation in itself entails no infringement of the Islamic law, but scholars have cautioned that the frozen embryos are the exclusive property of the couple who produced the gametes alone, and may be transferred only to the same wife in a successive cycle, restrictively during the duration of the marriage contract. In other words, storing the husband's sperm for the purpose of impregnating the wife in the event of his death is illegal. Under Islamic law, death terminates the marriage contract, and the widowed wife is free to remarry after the mandatory waiting period (al-'Iddah). The cryopreserved sperm or pre-embryo of an ex-husband in case of divorce should not be used either, as divorce equally renders the union void, legally [41].

Cryopreservation of gametes or gonads before exposure to radiotherapy or chemotherapy or for social reasons is allowed. These gametes or gonads can be used for conception later on by their owner. The cryopreserved gonads can be re-implanted after the end of chemotherapy or radiotherapy, based on the request of the owner of the gonads [42].

Another issue raised in this respect is state of a husband serving a prison term but still maintain the union with his wife. There is a ruling by some contemporary Muslim jurists that the stored sperm of the jailed husband can be used to impregnate his legitimate wife through artificial insemination. This is obviously premised on the presumed continuity of the marriage contract, until and unless the contrary is proven.

This could be pertinent succor to women who would like to bear legitimate children during long incarcerations of their spouses. Furthermore, it may provide in future a solid ground for the protection of conjugal rights of wives of prisoners, particularly in civil cases [43]. Actually, in Saudi Arabia the incarcerated husband is allowed to have conjugal contact with his wife in the prison itself on occassions, in civil cases.

Another topical issue concerning cryopreservation is the fate of frozen fertilized eggs if they are not used or are not needed by the owners. In Islam human life begins at ensoulment which is 120 days after conception. Therefore, doctors are not killing human beings when they leave these fertilized eggs to die.

In conclusion, the Islamic position on medically assisted conception is summarized as follows:

Artificial insemination with the husband's semen is allowed, and the resulting child is the legal offspring of the couple.

IVF of an egg from the wife with the sperm of her husband followed by the transfer of the fertilized embryo(s) back to the uterus of the wife is allowed, provided that the procedure is indicated for a medical reason and is carried out by an expert physician.

No third party should intrude into the marital functions of sex and procreation, because marriage is a contract between the wife and husband during the span of their marriage. This means that a third party donor is not allowed, whether he or she is providing sperm, eggs, embryos, or a uterus.

Adoption is not allowed. The child who results from a forbidden method belongs to the mother who delivered him/her.

If the marriage contract has come to an end because of divorce or death of the husband, medically assisted conception cannot be performed on the ex-wife even if the sperm comes from the former husband.

An excess number of fertilized embryos can be preserved by cryopreservation. The frozen embryos are the property of the couple alone and may be transferred to the same wife in a successive cycle, but only during the duration of the marriage contract.

Multifetal pregnancy reduction should not be intentionally performed as in ART, and therefore fetal reduction is only allowed if multiple pregnancies occurred spontaneously and is endangering the viability of the multiple embryos.

It is also allowed if the health or life of the mother is in jeopardy.

All forms of surrogacy are forbidden.

Establishment of sperm or egg banks is strictly forbidden, for such a practice threatens the existence of the family and should be prevented.

The qualified physician is the only person to practice medically assisted conception in all its permitted varieties. If he performs any of the forbidden techniques, he is guilty and he must be stopped from his morally illicit practice.

Regulations for ART should be laid down in all Muslim countries with clear adherence to the Islamic Fatwas on this important subject.

Gender Selection

"Are we having a boy or girl?" is one of the first things prospective parents wonder about the most. During pregnancy, couples wanting to know the sex of the future child may use ultrasound, chromosome analysis or testing of fetal DNA in maternal blood early in pregnancy, to find out the answer months before delivery. An estimated 50–70 % of parents want to learn the sex of their future child during pregnancy [44].

However, "More than 100 million women are missing." This was the title of an article written by social philosopher Amartya Sen and published in the New York Review of Books more than 20 years ago. Since then, the phenomenon of "missing" girls has been widely researched and publicized. It has been characterized by the feminist philosopher Mary Anne Warren as 'gendercide' and by The Economist (March 2010) as "the worldwide war on baby girls." About 40 million women were missing in China alone. Later and more sophisticated research by Western scholars indicates that, globally, the number of missing women has increased to over 100 million and that, in China, the figure is 40.9 million, with India having 39.1 million and Pakistan 4.9 million [45].

Due to strong cultural preferences for sons, marked sex ratio disparities have emerged in countries like China, Armenia, Azerbaijan, South Korea, and India. This lopsided preference for boys is often explained by gendered expectations that rely on sons to carry on the family name, support elderly parents, keep property within the family, perform specific religious rituals, or contribute more to the family's economic status [46]. In India, the girl has to pay a dower to the prospected husband and the father of the girl should bear that responsibility. If he has three or four girls, the expenses become unbearable (unless he is wealthy) and to avoid such situation he opts for abortion or infanticide.

The worst excesses are seen in parts of rural China where there are 140 male births for every 100 female. This leads to large numbers of unmarriageable men. Recent studies suggest that these men are marginalized, lonely, withdrawn, and prone to psychological problems [47].

The one child policy in China, enforced many parents especially in rural areas to abort a female fetus, whenever it was detected during pregnancy.

Gender Selection Methods

Modern reproductive medicine is able to offer reliable sex selection treatment.

Sex selection technologies may be broadly divided between post-pregnancy techniques and pre-pregnancy techniques and are conducted for medical or social ('nonmedical') reasons.

Post-pregnancy techniques, such as the use of prenatal screening through ultrasound, amniocentesis, or chorionic villi sampling, followed by selective abortion are generally condemned worldwide if undertaken for social reasons.

Pre-pregnancy techniques include microsorting or preimplantation genetic diagnosis (PGD).

Because they are not associated with abortion, pre-pregnancy techniques are argued by some to differ from post-pregnancy techniques and be more acceptable ethically.

Microsorting involves a patented process using a florescent dye to identify spermatozoa bearing the correct sex chromosome. Sperms can be sorted to produce an X or Y chromosome enriched sperm mixture, using flow cytometry. Sperm sorting, which is less effective but also less costly, can be used to increase the likelihood of producing a child of the desired sex [48].

PGD is used to determine the sex of embryos created by IVF and involves the removal of one or two cells (blastomeres) from an embryo at day 3 of development. This is followed by chromosomal analysis. Selected embryos are transferred to a woman's uterus on day 4 or 5. PGD is currently used to identify serious chromosomal or genetic disorders but may also be used for "nonmedical" sex selection in which only embryos of the desired sex are selected for transfer back to a uterus [49]. PGD is a technology that, when employed for sex selection, yields a near zero chance of a pregnancy with a fetus of the non-chosen sex [50].

The recent report of the International Federation of Fertility Societies notes that of 105 countries surveyed, sex selection by sperm-sorting techniques or PGD is allowed under legislation in 15 countries, not allowed in 43 countries and not mentioned in law in 15 countries. It is practiced in 26 countries [51].

Finally, sex can be determined by an ultrasound and embryos then selectively aborted. This remains the most common technique for sex selection in China and India today [52].

Gender selection is however permitted if a particular sex predisposes to a serious genetic condition. One of the first couple to use this technique of sex selection was hoping to escape a deadly disease known as x-linked hydrocephalus, which almost always affected boys. Embryonic sex selection would make possible the weeding out of other serious x-linked disorders including, Duchene muscular dystrophy, hemophilia, and fragile X syndrome [53]. Accordingly, decisions not to attempt replacement of embryos produced in vitro on the grounds that they show serious chromosomal or genetic anomalies, such as aneuploidy, cystic fibrosis, muscular dystrophy or hemophilia, are accepted [54].

The prophet Muhammad (PBUH) said: "Choose for your offspring the suitable woman for hereditary plays a role" [55]. The subject of Premarital examination to avoid genetic diseases will be discussed in another chapter (Genetics).

Ethics of Gender Selection

Although the successful development of sex selection technologies represents clear medical and scientific advancement, their use is a subject of intense ethical debate amongst clinicians, philosophers and bioethicists alike [56].

Although sex selection for medical purposes is generally accepted as ethically appropriate, concerns about endorsement of sexist practices, disruption of the sex ratio, or exacerbation of sexist discrimination has led the overwhelming majority of countries regulating PGD to prohibit its use for sex selection for social reasons [57]. Professional societies and international policy documents have also joined the opposition to this practice on similar grounds (ACOG 2007) [58], (FIGO 2006) [59].

Worldwide, sex selection for nonmedical reasons is generally defined as gender discriminatory (whether prior to pregnancy or post-pregnancy). A host of international human-rights laws, national laws and regulations, and ethical bodies of leading professional associations suggests that it infringes ethical practice and the shared responsibility of nations to protect and promote human-rights principles, particularly that of non-discrimination [60].

Islamic Views

Is it ever appropriate to select for gender? In Islam, gender selection is only up to God [61]. The Holy Qur'an unequivocally affirms that, "He (Allah) creates what He wills. He bestows female upon whom He wills, and bestows male upon whom He wills" [62]. Hence, it could be safely argued that gender selection on its own constitutes unacceptable interference in the divine demographic order and, ipso facto, a nullity under the law of Islam.

Abortion or infanticide has long been used as means of sex selection. Arabs more than 1400 years ago, before Islam, used to practice infanticide for gender selection. The Holy Qur'an described this act and condemned it. It states in one version: "On God's Judgment Day the entombed alive female infant is asked, for what guilt was she made to suffer infanticide?" [63]

Gender selection technologies have been condemned on the ground that their application will discriminate against female embryos and fetuses, so perpetuating prejudice against the girl child, and social devaluation of women. Such discrimination and devaluation are condemned in Islam [64]. Application of PGD or sperm sorting techniques for sex selection should be discouraged in principle. It should not be used for selection of the gender unless there is a clear medical indication.

Islamic Fiqh council of Islamic World League passed legal resolution (Fatwa) in its 19th meeting held in November 2007, and banned gender selection performed specifically for social reasons. It allowed gender selection for medical reasons only.

Sex ratio balancing in the family is considered acceptable by few scholars for very limited cases such as a wife who delivered five or six daughters and her husband has dire need for getting a boy! Centers performing the procedure should keep a record of all performed cases to ensure they are not choosing one sex only.

References

1. McLaren JF (2012) Infertility evaluation. Obstet Gynecol Clin North Am 39(4):453–463
2. Wischmann T (2013) 'Your count is zero'–counselling the infertile man. Hum Fertil (Camb) 16(1):35–39
3. Denton J, Monach J, Pacey A (2013) Infertility and assisted reproduction: counselling and psychosocial aspects. Hum Fertil (Camb) 16(1):1
4. The Holy Qur'an 18:46
5. The Holy Qur'an 25:74
6. Rodini M (2012) An investigation on Islamic perspective on the reproductive technologies. Webmed Cent Int J Med Mol Med 3(7):WMC003548
7. Sahih Abi Dawood Hadith No 2050, Maktibt Al Maaref, Riyadh
8. Steptoe PC, Edwards RG (1978) Birth after the reimplantation of a human embryo. Lancet 2:366
9. Rodini M. op.cit
10. Alaro AA (2012) Assisted reproductive technology (ART): the Islamic Law perspective. In: Berna A, Vardit R-C (eds) Islam and bioethics. Ankara University, Turkey, pp 95–108
11. Intracytoplasmic sperm injection as a process by which the doctor uses a tiny needle to manually insert a single sperminto an ova
12. Fadel HE (2002) The Islamic viewpoint on new assisted reproductive technologies. Fordham Urban Law J 30(1):147–157
13. Davies MJ (2013) Infertility treatment at the edge: discovery and risk converge at the limits ofknowledge. Arch Dis Child 98(2):89–90
14. Ibid
15. Pandian Z, Bhattacharya S, Ozturk O, Serour GI, Templeton A (2004) Number of embryos for transfer following in-vitro fertilisation or intra-cytoplasmic sperm injection. Cochrane Database Syst Rev 18(4):CD003416
16. Serour GI (2008) Islamic perspectives in human reproduction. Reprod BioMed Online 17 (Suppl. 3):34–38
17. Schenker JG (2005) Assisted reproductive practice: religious perspectives. Reprod Biomed Online 10(3):310–319
18. Fadel HE (2007) Prospects and ethics of stem cell research: an Islamic perspective. J Islamic Med Assoc 39(2):73–84
19. Serour GI (2008) op.cit
20. Fadel HE (2002) op.cit
21. Schenker JG. op.cit
22. Inhorn MC, Patrizio P, Serour G (2010) Third party reproductive assistance around the Mediterranean: comparing Sunni Egypt, Catholic Italy and multisectarian Lebanon. Reprod BioMed Online 21(7):848–853
23. Serour GI (2008) op.cit
24. Moosa E (2003) Human cloning in Muslim ethics. Voices Across Boundaries Fall, 23–26
25. Fadel HE (2002) op.cit
26. Hathout MM (1989) Surrogacy: an Islamic perspective. 21 J Islamic Med Assoc 105:105
27. Serour GI (2008) op.cit

28. Holy Qur'an 58:2
29. Inhorn MC (2011) Globalization and gametes: reproductive 'tourism', Islamic bioethics, and Middle Eastern modernity. Anthropol Med 18(1):87–103
30. Serour GI (2013) Ethical issues in human reproduction: Islamic perspectives. Gynecol Endocrinol 29(11):949–952
31. Abbasi-Shavazi MJ, Inhorn MC, Razeghi-Nasrabad HB, Toloo G (Spring 2008) The "Iranian ART Revolution": infertility assisted reproductive technology, and third-party donation in the Islamic republic of Iran. J Middle East Women's Stud 4(2):1–28
32. Aramesh K (2009) Iran's experience with surrogate motherhood: an Islamic view and ethical concerns. J Med Ethics 35(5):320–322
33. Inhorn (2011) op. cit
34. Clarke M (2009) Islam and new kinship: reproductive technology and the Shari'ah in Lebanon. Berghahn Books, New York
35. Abbasi-Shavazi. op. cit
36. Chamsi-Pasha H, Albar MA (2015) Assisted reproductive technology: Islamic Sunni perspective, Hum Fertil (Camb) 7:1–6
37. Hudson N, Culley L, Blyth B, Norton W, Rapport F, Pacey A (2011) Cross-border reproductive care: a review of the literature. Reprod BioMed Online 22:673–685
38. Hunt J (2013) Cross border treatment for infertility: the counseling perspective in the UK. Hum Fertil (Camb) 16(1):64–67
39. Serour GI (2008) op.cit
40. Ahmad NH (2003) Assisted reproduction- Islamic views on the science of procreation. Eubios J Asian Int Bioeth 13(2):59–61
41. Alaro AA. op.cit
42. Serour GI (2008) op.cit
43. Alaro AA. op.cit
44. Jesudason S, Baruch S (2012) Sex selection: what role for providers. Contraception 86 (6):597–599
45. Nie JB (2011) Non-medical sex-selective abortion in China: ethical and public policy issues in thecontext of 40 million missing females. Br Med Bull 98:7–20
46. Jesudason S. op.cit
47. Hesketh T (2011) Selecting sex: the effect of preferring sons. Early Hum Dev 87(11):759–61
48. Levy N (2007) Against sex selection. South Med J 100(1):107–109
49. Whittaker AM (2011) Reproduction opportunists in the new global sex trade: PGD and non-medical sex selection. Reprod BioMed Online 23(5):609–617
50. deMelo-Martín I (2013) Sex selection and the procreative liberty framework. Kennedy Inst Ethics J 23(1):1–18
51. Whittaker AM. op.cit
52. Levy N. op.cit
53. Rodini M. op.cit
54. Albar MA (2002) Ethical considerations in the prevention and management of genetic disorders with special emphasis on religious considerations. Saudi Med J 23(6):627–632
55. Al Dailamy SS (1987) Firdoos Al Hikmah, Dar Al Kitab Al Arabi, Beirut. Commented by Al-Zumerli FA and al-Baghdadi MM 2:76 Hadith No 2110
56. Strange H (2010) Cesagen, (ESRC centre for economic and social aspects of genomics). Non-medical sex selection: ethical issues. Br Med Bull 94:7–20
57. deMelo-Martín I. op.cit
58. American College of Obstetricians and Gynecologists, Committee on Ethics (2007) ACOG Committee opinion No. 360: sex selection. Obstet Gynecol 109:475–478

59. FIGO Committee for the Ethical Aspects of Human Reproduction and Women's Health (2006) Ethical guidelines on sex selection for non-medical purposes. FIGO committee for the ethical aspects of human reproduction and women's health. Int J Obstet Gynecol 92:329–330
60. Whittaker AM. op.cit
61. Athar S (2008) Enhancement technologies and the person: an Islamic view. J Law Med Ethics 36(1):59–64
62. Holy Qur'an 42: 49
63. Holy Qur'an 81:8–9
64. Serour GI (2008) op.cit

Chapter 12
Ethical Issues in Genetics (Premarital Counseling, Genetic Testing, Genetic Engineering, Cloning and Stem Cell Therapy, DNA Fingerprinting)

The Progeny—Islamic Views

The main relevant ethical aspects related to care for the family unit in Islam can be summarized as follows:

1. To ensure appropriate selection of the members of the "legal marriage" and to care for offspring throughout his or her life—preconception, prenatal, postnatal—and thereafter to ensure, as much as possible, a "stable marriage and healthy offspring."
2. Islam requires husband and wife to take necessary steps to protect themselves and their offspring, through the prevention of ill health and take appropriate steps to ensure their health as well as the health of their children at various stages of life.
3. To make use of "Advancement of Science" and seek means of protection from disease(s), including early diagnosis and intervention to ensure, as much as possible, freedom from ill health [1].

The Prophet (PBUH), more than fourteen centuries ago, had highlighted the importance of "selection of compatible couples" and indicated inheritance in children. The effect of genetic inheritance was also indicated by "Hadith" of the Prophet (PBUH) related to the "man" who came to the Prophet (PBUH) complaining that his wife gave birth to a black child. The Prophet asked him: "If he has camels?" The man answered: "Yes." The Prophet (PBUH) asked him: "What is their color?" The man said: "They are red." The Prophet (PBUH) asked him: "Is there any blackish (grey) among them?" The man answered: "Yes." The Prophet (PBUH) asked him: "Why do you think that is?" The man said: "This may be due to unseen 'Erg' (inheritance). The Prophet (PBUH) said: "your son has the same" [2].

© The Author(s) 2015
187
M.A. Al-Bar and H. Chamsi-Pasha, *Contemporary Bioethics*,
DOI 10.1007/978-3-319-18428-9_12

Genetic Disorders

A genetic disorder is an illness caused by abnormalities in genes or chromosomes, while some diseases, such as cancer, are due in part to a genetic disorders, they can also be caused by environmental factors. Except for genetic blood disorders like sickle cell anemia and thalassemia, and cystic fibrosis (in certain geographic location), most disorders are rare and affect one person in every several thousands. Chromosomal defects constitute a large number of early abortions. Both chromosomal and genetic defects are responsible for major part of late abortion, stillbirth and perinatal death. They also constitute an important part of early childhood diseases. Some cancers, e.g., polyposis coli are autosomal dominant.

In fact, nearly all diseases have a genetic component. Some, including many cancers, are caused by a mutation in a gene or group of genes in the cells of an individual. Such mutations can occur randomly or due to some environmental exposure (such as cigarette smoking).

Other genetic disorders are hereditary—such as Huntington disease or Marfan's disease—where a mutated gene is passed down through a family and each generation of children can inherit the gene that causes the disease.

But most genetic disorders are "multifactorial inheritance disorders," meaning they are caused by a combination of small variations in genes, often in concert with environmental factors.

Genetic disorders are classified into three categories

1. Single gene disorder: is the result of a single mutated gene and inherited as autosomal recessive, autosomal dominant, and x-linked. The mutation may be present on one or both chromosomes (one chromosome inherited from each parent). Sickle cell disease, and cystic fibrosis are examples of single gene disorders.
2. Chromosome disorders caused by an excess or deficiency of the genes that are located on chromosomes, or structural changes within chromosomes. Down syndrome, for example, is caused by an extra copy of chromosome 21.
3. Multifactorial inheritance disorders caused by a combination of small variations in genes, often in concert with environmental factors. Heart disease and most cancers are examples of these disorders.

Genetic and Congenital Disorders in Islamic World

Genetic and congenital disorders are more common in Arab countries than in industrialized countries. The incidence of congenital malformations and genetic disorders in Gulf countries amounts to 7.3 % of births, compared to the average of 4.4 % in Europe. In Saudi Arabia, the sickle cell gene and B-thalassemia occur at a rate of 1–20 % according to different regions, with 2000 affected newborns added to the pool annually [3].

Congenital and genetic disorders are responsible for a major proportion of infant mortality, morbidity, and handicap in Arab countries. The population of the region is characterized by large family size, high maternal and paternal age, and a high level of inbreeding with consanguinity rates in the range of 25–60 % [4].

Several factors may contribute to the high prevalence of genetically determined disorders:

- High consanguinity rates—25 to 60 % of all marriages are consanguineous, and the rate of first cousin marriages is high.
- The high prevalence of hamoglobinopathies, glucose-6-phosphate dehydrogenase deficiency, autosomal recessive syndromes, and several metabolic disorders.
- The rate of children with Down's syndrome in some Arab countries exceeds the 1.2–1.7 per 1000 typical for industrialized countries. This may be related to the relatively high proportion of births to older mothers in the region (up to 50 % of children with Down's syndrome in the region are estimated to be born to mothers aged 40 or over). In the west, prenatal diagnosis of Down syndrome ends in abortion in most cases.
- The lack of public health measures directed at the prevention of congenital and genetic disorders, with inadequate health care before and during pregnancy, particularly in low income countries.
- Services for the prevention and control of genetic disorders are restricted by certain cultural, legal, and religious limitations [5].

In the United Kingdom there are more than 250,000 people from the Middle East, among whom an estimated 3000 births occur each year [6]. Germany, Sweden, and the Netherlands have similar populations. Healthcare professionals in the West may assume that Muslim families will not consider termination of pregnancy, but this may not be the case. Families must be offered a full explanation of the risks they face and the range of interventions available to them [7]. People who have left their country of origin tend to preserve their original beliefs and cultural values [8].

Consanguinity

A consanguineous marriage is usually defined as marriage between people who are second cousins or closer. Incest is sexual intercourse between family members and very close relatives. Father-daughter marriage or sisters and brothers marriages are not allowed. All cultures and religions consider such a relation as a taboo. However it is well known that the Pharoes and the old Persians allowed marriage between brothers and sisters. In the old testament (book of Genesis) it is claimed that Abraham married his half sister Sarah [9], while "Lot" had sex with his two daughters and both of them became pregnant of that incest and delivered Moab and Benammi [10]. Islamic teachings refute such claims and consider the messengers of God as the purest persons on earth, and will never do such horrendous acts.

Consanguineous marriage is known to have many social and economic benefits, although Islamic teachings discourage it [11]. Omer Ibn Al-Khatab, the second khalifa, noticed that the progeny of the tribe of Bani Alsaa'b had become weak and unhealthy because of intermarriage of cousins. He advised the tribe to avoid close cousin intermarriage and to seek wives and husbands from tribes further afield, cautioning: "Marry from faraway tribes; otherwise you will be weak and unhealthy" [12].

It is estimated that 20 % of human population live in communities with preference for consanguineous marriage, and at least 8.5 % of children have consanguineous parents [13]. Consanguineous unions account for 20–70 % of all marriages in the Middle East, excluding Israel and Cyprus [14].

Studies of parental consanguinity in the general population in Egypt throughout the last 40 years showed an average consanguinity rate above 30 %. Parental consanguinity rates in groups of Egyptian patients with various birth defects are significantly higher than that of the general population according to the most recent estimate (33 %) [15].

This frequency of consanguinity leads to increased birth prevalence of infants with severe recessive disorders but has a relatively small effect on the prevalence of dominant and X-linked disorders, and its role in complex disorders is still uncertain.

Generally speaking, frequency of congenital and genetic diseases among newborns of first cousin unions is about 2 times the frequency among the general population. In other words instead of a rate of 2–3 % of birth defects in the general population, the risk to first cousin couples is around 4–6 %. Another estimate puts the offspring of first cousin unions at a 1.7–2.8 % increased risk above the population background risk [16]. The highest risks are from first degree marriage viz.: Parent child and sib to sib where they share half the genetic pool.

However, when the autosomal recessive gene in the community is very common namely Thalassemia, and sickle cell anemia, the carriers of the trait are one in 4, or one in 5 in the whole community, any marriage will have a high risk of marrying another carrier of the trait [17].

Genetic Disorders: A Community Hurdle in Islamic Communities

Genetic disorders occur at a high frequency in several Islamic communities.

The blood genetic disorders cause a variety of negative effects on health and psychosocial aspects due to the following: (1) Its wide spread in the community. (2) Chronicity and nonavailability of definitive treatment, and (3) Negative effect on the life style of the concerned individual, family, and the community at large.

Genetic diseases due to their chronic nature impose heavy medical, financial and emotional burdens. Therefore, the efforts to combat these problems are multifaceted and the effective control and prevention strategies gain a high priority beside care and rehabilitation of the affected in the community [18].

The whole family suffers from the daily strain of observing and caring for the affected individuals. It is notable that mothers with one affected child would be stressed; a mother with 2 or 3 affected children may become psychologically disturbed or depressed. Fathers are weary, visiting many hospitals, searching for someone who can offer treatment, or explain to them how to deal with the affected children better. In addition, financial difficulties often arise, especially in families with multiple affected children.

The responses from the concerned family to a genetic disease are associated with feelings of fear, misfortune, shame, guilt, anger, isolation, and blame and are accentuated by negative notions in the mass media, and unavailability of a definitive cure in most conditions. An increasing number of couples now seek premarital information on the risk of having genetically affected children [19]. Therefore, genetic services for patient care and control and prevention measures are necessary to:

- Help people with genetic disadvantage and their families,
- Live and reproduce as normally as possible,
- Make informed choices in reproductive and health matters,
- Assist people to obtain access to relevant medical services (diagnostic, therapeutic, rehabilitative, or preventive) and social support systems,
- Help affected people adapt to their unique situation, and
- Help affected people become informed on relevant new developments [20].

Premarital Examination Program

The main objectives of the premarital examination can be summarized as follows: (1) To limit the occurrence of genetic disorders. (2) To limit those marriages among those who are carriers or suffering from blood genetic disorders. (3) Explaining the pattern of inheritance of genetic disorders. (4) Save the families from having affected children suffering from a chronic disease and psychosocial problems. (5) Minimizing the economic burden on the family and on the government that results from seeking treatment for chronic and disabling genetic disorders [21].

Reassurance for carriers is important. The explanation should be given that to be a carrier is not an illness and not a God's punishment. Being a carrier is not shameful and is often associated with advantage for survival. In the case of sickle cell disease, carrier is selected by nature for survival against malaria. A carrier will have resistance to the illness later on. The advantage of knowing one is a carrier is to be able to plan a healthy family and avoid genetic disease. Any carrier can marry a non carrier of that gene.

Responses in the Arab World

Many Arab governments (Saudi Arabia, Egypt, Syria, Lebanon, Tunisia, Morocco, and Gulf countries) made a premarital medical examination mandatory. It resulted in some reduction of autosomal recessive blood disease (viz thalassemia and sickle cell anemia).

The premarital test for sickle cell, thalassemia and G6PD became compulsory. If both are carriers, they are counseled and advised against marriage, but the decision is theirs.

Genetic Testing

As currently practiced, genetic testing occurs at one of six stages in the life cycle: (1) Premarital Genetic Diagnosis (Vide Supra); (2) during the neonatal period; (3) prenatally, that is, between implantation and birth; (4) during the preimplantation stage of embryonic development, following in vitro fertilization; (5) when couples are considering whether to reproduce; or (6) when a person, often on the basis of family history, recognizes a higher-than-average risk of developing a particular disease later in life, for example, Huntington disease or breast cancer.

Genetic testing and screening raise some of the most difficult issues in the entire field of bioethics. On the one hand, it is clearly beneficial to reduce the incidence of severe disease, especially among children. In addition, individuals and couples can exercise their autonomy by deciding whether, when, and under what circumstances they will try to have children. And societies can focus their resources on people whose illnesses cannot be prevented and on people who are injured in accidents. On the other hand, deliberations about prenatal diagnosis and selective abortion are often agonizing for the people involved [22].

Genetic Counseling

Genetic counseling is the process whereby an individual or family obtains advice and information about a genetic condition that may affect the individual and family. The aim of such counseling is to enable appropriate decisions to be taken regarding marriage, reproduction, abortion, and health management. It is considered an important complementary approach to the screening procedure. As a service, it is offered to the members of the high risk groups, i.e., carriers of recessive genetic disease or those with an affected member of the family.

The principles and components of the "Informed Consent" that are generally acceptable in western countries are also applicable to Muslim community.

However, Muslims, in general, will often want to consult with family members and religious scholars, particularly in aspects of religious and social relevance [23].

Families with handicapped children should not be blamed, criticized, but should be supported in all ways possible. Health practitioners need to adopt a sensitive approach in providing health information paying attention to their vocabulary to ensure that unintended meanings are not communicated.

Every effort should be made to minimize diagnostic uncertainty [24].

Qualifications and Task of the Counselor

The counselor should be trustworthy, proficient, considerate, compassionate, and able to guard the confidentiality of the information he is given. The genetic counselor may not impose his views on his clients. Rather, he must let them reach their own decisions. The counselor's responsibility is to provide them with the necessary facts and information in plain language that they can understand easily and fully [25]. There are 3 main reasons why an appropriate counseling approach is essential: (1) Psychological, social, and ethical problems can arise as the result of genetic testing; (2) Genetic tests have high predictive values, thus can exclude or identify particular risks; (3) Currently, a large gap exists between the ability to diagnose, and the ability to treat genetic diseases.

Premarital carrier detection is important especially in communities where consanguinity is very high. If the fiancé and fiancée are found carrying the same autosomal recessive gene, then genetic counseling should be provided, and all the pertinent facts and risks to the progeny explained. If they insist on marriage, the decision is theirs, but reproductive alternatives should be discussed with them.

They should be counseled to choose a number of alternatives, should they still wish to marry.

Other Options

1. Contraception or sterilization to avoid pregnancy;
2. Adoption;
3. Donation of a sperm or ovum or pre-embryo;
4. Preimplantation diagnosis;
5. Diagnosis during pregnancy (e.g., chorion villus sampling, amniocentesis, blood tests from the expectant mother and the fetus, ultrasonography, etc.).

Each of these procedures needs to be scrutinized from an Islamic perspective:

1. Contraception and sterilization

Contraception is allowable under Islamic law as a temporary measure if the couple decide upon it and if there is no harm from the particular method used. Sterilization, however, is not acceptable unless there is danger to the mother's health from pregnancy. We may note that there is support for sterilization from at least some of our jurists in the situation where a couple have already had some congenitally affected children.

2. Adoption

Adoption was abrogated by the Qur'an, and in Islamic law adoptive parents are not recognized as parents in the way that natural parents are. The child must be attached in lineage to his or her natural parents, and legitimate pregnancy is, according to the law, only within wedlock. The Qur'an says: "He did not make your adopted ones your sons [26]. Bringing up orphans is a highly commended act of charity, encouraged by Islamic teachings, but even then the lineage of the child must remain to his or her natural parents."

3. Donation of a sperm, ovum or pre-embryo

In the West, a new technology of procreation is being made available to infertile couples. This technology, making use of semen banks and in vitro fertilization techniques, may involve donated sperm or ova; a donated pre-embryo (blastula or morulla). None of this technology is acceptable in the view of Islamic teachings which recognize procreation only within the bounds of wedlock excluding any third party from the process. Therefore, a Muslim couple who are carrying a lethal gene or serious disease gene cannot make use of either donated sperm or ova or pre-embryos. These methods are refuted by all Islamic jurists on the grounds that procreation must be limited to the spouses alone, without the intervention of third parties during the existence of matrimonial bondage. If divorce or death of a spouse occurs no procreation will be allowed.

4. Preimplantation genetic diagnosis (PGD)

Advances in medical technology over the last few decades have made it possible, at least in some specialist clinics, to remove one or more cells from the blastula (pre-embryo) prior to its implantation in the womb. A husband's semen is allowed to fertilize in vitro the ovum taken from his wife; when fertilization occurs, the zygote is allowed to grow to the blastula or morulla stage—this happens a few days after fertilization. If genetic disease or chromosomal abnormality (e.g., triosomy 13, 18 or 21) is suspected, one or more cells are taken from the blastula for appropriate testing. If the blastula is shown to have the defective gene or chromosome, it is discarded and another one tested. Only the unblemished blastula is reimplanted.

   PGD technology was made possible through the use of microinjection of an oocyte with a single spermatozoon as in intracytoplasmic sperm injection (ICSI) technique and the micromanipulation of the resulting embryo. Moreover, the technology involves removing 1–2 cells from each of the 6–8 cell stage embryos (usually 3 days after the ICSI procedure), studying each cell for chromosomal anomalies or screening for certain single-gene defects. Normal embryos are then transferred into the uterus while unwanted ones are discarded or used for research [27].

Although PGD screening has been available for nearly three decades in Western Europe currently, PGD is used mainly in two broad indication groups. The first group consists of individuals at high risk of having a child with a genetic disease, for example carriers of a monogenic disease or of chromosomal structural abnormalities such as translocations. The second group consists of those being treated with IVF, who might have a low genetic risk but whose embryos are screened for chromosome aneuploidies to enhance their chances of an ongoing pregnancy [28].

PGD is permissible in Islam provided the sperms and oocytes are from the husband and wife. PGD may be preferable to prenatal diagnosis for Muslim parents, because it is done when pre-embryos are only at the eight-cell stage and may avoid abortion. It is not an easy option, and couples must be selected and counselled appropriately [29].

PGD services in the Middle East is not available except in few centers. In summary, the procedure is still in its early stages, with many limitations.

5. Prenatal screening and diagnosis of genetic disorders

Better and more accurate diagnoses of congenital malformations, genetic diseases and chromosomal abnormalities are becoming available with the tremendous advances in medical technology. This will involve blood testing of the mother for alpha fetoproteins, gonadotrophins, and more recently for fetal cells.

Simple blood tests from the expectant mother can help the diagnosis of, for example, alpha fetoproteins in cases of neural tube defects, viz., anencephaly and spina bifida. Ultrasound can detect many dysmorphic abnormalities as well as congenital defects of the heart, brain anencephaly, and spina bifida and kidneys.

Chorion villous sampling (CVS) is carried out in the 9–10th week from last menstrual period of pregnancy and if the fetus is proved suffering from serious congenital anomaly then abortion is offered. If CVS was not available, then ultrasound study, amnniocentesis and blood sampling from the fetus will confirm the diagnosis. If the congenital anomaly is very serious, abortion could be carried, provided it is carried out prior to the 120 days from conception (134 days from last menstrual period).

Amniocentesis is done at a much later stage of pregnancy, between the 14 and 16th weeks. The advantage of early diagnosis by CVS is offset by higher percentage of abortions and complications (2–3 %), compared to amniocentesis which is safer albeit giving a much later diagnosis.

Prenatal screening and diagnosis of genetic disorders serves two purposes. First, it identifies fetuses that are affected with a disorder. Parents may then choose to terminate the pregnancy or, if they opt to continue the pregnancy be assisted with the management of a high risk pregnancy, be prepared for the birth with appropriate family and social support, and receive a modified delivery plan appropriate for the disorder. Second, for those with unaffected pregnancies, parents receive reassurance [30].

Screening tests have been primarily targeted towards the identification of two types of fetal disorders:

1. Chromosome abnormalities, notably Down syndrome, identified through the combination of maternal age, maternal serum biochemical tests, and fetal ultrasound; the definitive diagnosis is through CVS or amniocentesis.
2. Single gene disorders with Mendelian patterns of inheritance screened through carrier testing of parents (e.g., cystic fibrosis, hemoglobinopathies, neurodegenerative disorders, or other conditions that have a high prevalence in particular racial or ethnic groups).

Depending on the population screened and the test protocols, only a proportion of the affected pregnancies are identified as high risk. Screening protocols can be relatively expensive. Furthermore, women with positive-screening results require a definitive diagnosis through amniocentesis or chorionic villus samples (CVS). These "invasive tests" carry a small risk for miscarriage and maternal complications.

They are also expensive, anxiety provoking and likely to be completed relatively late in pregnancy [31].

Islamic Teachings and Prevention of Genetic Diseases

Islamic teachings concentrate on prevention of disease rather than cure. Islam encourages marriage and prohibits fornication and adultery.

The Prophet Muhammad (PBUH) advised Muslims to choose for their daughters, husbands with good character and free from physical and social illnesses. Similarly he warned not to marry a girl only for her beauty when her character is blemished [32]. He also said: "Choose for your offspring the suitable woman for hereditary plays a role" [33].

The premarital examination to avoid genetic diseases will be a welcome; especially in a community where the rate of consanguineous marriage is high [34]. These practices are carried out in a number of Islamic Countries and considered the method of choice in prevention of Single Gene Disorders. Congenital diseases such as Rubella are virtually eliminated in many countries by vaccinating school children girls at premarital age. Syphilis and other sexually transmitted diseases (STD) will not appear if all sexual desires are channeled through marriage as Islamic teachings implies. Fornication, adultery, and sodomy are all harshly punished in Islamic legal code, and religiously they are considered of the greatest sins, that each Muslim should avoid. Alcohol is the most frequent chemical teratogen substance causing mental retardation and congenital anomaly. Islam totally prohibits imbibing alcoholic beverages. Similarly smoking causes abortion, congenital anomalies and small for date babies. It is prohibited in Islamic teachings and many fatwas have reiterated its prohibition. Any substance that is going to be harmful to the baby (namely teratogen) should be avoided as the Prophet Muhammad (PBUH) him said: "Do no harm" [35].

Similarly, neonatal testing, avoiding of teratogens and provision of folate and iodine in the diet is encouraged as supportive measures. Simple tests for phenylketonuria, homocystinuria, galactosemia and many others for newborns can avert calamity in those affected.

Abortion for Genetic Diseases

The "Fatwa" number 4 of "Islamic Fiqh council of Islamic World League, Makkah Al Mukaramah," at its 12th session (Makkah, 10–17 February 1990) allows for the option of abortion under certain specific conditions. The fatwa determined that the abortion may take place only if a committee of specialized, competent physicians has decided the fetus is grossly malformed, and that its life would be a calamity for both the family and itself. The malformation must be untreatable, unmanageable and very serious, and the abortion may only be carried out prior to the 120th day of conception (computed from the date of fertilization, not the last menstrual cycle). Beyond 120 days, i.e., after the ensoulment, abortion only is allowed if there is a danger threatening the mothers' life and not only her health [36]. This Fatwa was a landmark, as previous Fatwas only allowed abortion in the first 40 days of conception. At such a period it was almost impossible to ascertain any of the congenital or hereditary diseases. By extending the time of permissible abortion to 120 days computed from the moment of conception (namely 134 days from LMP), gives ample time to ascertain the diagnosis of severely affected embryo's and fetuses. Abortion is one of the reproductive options offered to manage and prevent genetic diseases.

On the basis of this fatwa, abortions of fetuses with serious congenital diseases are carried out in the hospitals in Saudi Arabia.

Genetic Engineering

Genetic engineering is the direct manipulation of an organism's genome using biotechnology. Genetic engineering alters the genetic makeup of an organism using techniques that remove heritable material or that introduces DNA prepared outside the organism either directly into the host or into a cell that is then fused or hybridized with the host.

In medicine, genetic engineering has been used to mass-produce insulin, human growth hormones, other hormones for treating infertility, human albumin, monoclonal antibodies, antihemophilic factors, vaccines, and many other drugs.

Genetic engineering is used to create animal models of human diseases. Genetically modified mice are the most common genetically engineered animal model. They have been used to study and model cancer, obesity, heart disease, diabetes, arthritis, substance abuse, anxiety, aging, and Parkinson disease [37].

Potential cures can be tested against these mouse models. Also, genetically modified pigs have been bred with the aim of increasing the success of pig to human organ transplantation, but the occurrence of many porcine retroviruses hampered the whole project.

Gene Therapy

Gene therapy is the genetic engineering of humans by replacing defective human genes with functional copies. It derives its name from the idea that DNA can be used to supplement or alter genes within an individual's cells as a therapy to treat disease. The most common form of gene therapy involves using DNA that encodes a functional, therapeutic gene to replace a mutated gene. Other forms involve directly correcting a mutation, or using DNA that encodes a therapeutic protein drug (rather than a natural human gene) to provide treatment.

Gene therapy utilizes the delivery of DNA into cells, which can be accomplished by a number of methods. The two major classes of methods are those that use recombinant viruses (sometimes called biological nanoparticles or viral vectors) and those that use naked DNA or DNA complexes (nonviral methods).

Gene therapy has been used to treat patients suffering from immune deficiencies (notably Severe combined immunodeficiency) and trials have been carried out on other genetic disorders. The success of gene therapy so far has been limited and a patient (Jesse Gelsinger) has died during a clinical trial testing a new treatment [38]. There are also ethical concerns should the technology be used not just for treatment, but for enhancement, modification or alteration of a human being appearance, adaptability, intelligence, character, or behavior. The distinction between cure and enhancement can also be difficult to establish.

Gene therapy may be classified into the two following types:

- Somatic gene therapy
  In somatic gene therapy, the therapeutic genes are transferred into the somatic cell, or body, of a patient. Any modifications and effects will be restricted to the individual patient only, and will not be inherited by the patient's offspring or later generations. Somatic gene therapy represents the mainstream line of current basic and clinical research.
- Germ line gene therapy
  In germ line gene therapy, germ cells, i.e., sperm or eggs are modified by the introduction of functional genes, which are integrated into their genomes. This would allow the therapy to be heritable and passed on to later generations. Although this should, in theory, be highly effective in counteracting genetic disorders and hereditary diseases, many jurisdictions prohibit this for application in human beings, at least for the present, for a variety of technical and ethical reasons. In summary, the attention of researchers and bioethicists is now focused primarily on experimental approaches to the treatment of individual patients

suffering from either debilitating or lethal diseases. Unlike the situation in the late 1960s and early 1970s, germ-line intervention and the enhancement of human capabilities by genetic means are not the principal topics of debate. One hopes that in the future, gene transfer will join bone marrow transplantation, solid organ transplantation, and, perhaps, stem-cell transplantation as an effective therapeutic modality for an increasing number of human maladies [39].

Islamic Position on Genetic Engineering

The Islamic Fiqh council of Islamic World League, Makkah Al Mukaramah, in its 15th session (11th/07/1419Hijra/31 October 1998 Gregorian) gave the following guidance on the use of the genetic information and research technology:

1. Allow the use of genetic engineering for disease prevention, treatment, or amelioration on the condition that do not cause further damage;
2. Forbid the use of engineering in evil and criminal use or what is forbidden religiously;
3. Forbid using genetic engineering and its tool to change human personality and responsibility, or interfering with genes to improve the human race;
4. Forbid any research or therapy of human genes except in extreme need, after critical evaluation of its benefits and dangers and after an official consent of the concerned, respecting the extreme confidentiality of the information and human rights and dignity as dictated by Islamic Shari'ah;
5. Allow the use of bio-engineering in the field of agriculture and animals, on the condition that precautions are taken not to inflict harm (even in the long term) on humans, animals or vegetation;
6. Call on biotechnology companies and food and medical factories to reveal the structure of these bioengineered products so they can be dealt with and used with caution in light of potential harm or if any are forbidden religiously;
7. Recommend all doctors, factory and laboratory owners to fear Allah (God) and to watch out for Allah to avoid inflicting harm to humans, society or the environment [40].

Cloning and Stem Cell Research

Human cloning is the creation of a genetically identical copy of a human. The sheep Dolly (5 July 1996–14 February 2003), was the first mammal to have been successfully cloned from an adult cell.

To make Dolly, researchers isolated a somatic cell from an adult female sheep. Next, they transferred the nucleus from that cell to an egg cell from which the nucleus had been removed. After a couple of chemical tweaks, the egg cell, with its new nucleus, was behaving just like a freshly fertilized zygote. It developed into an embryo, which was implanted into a surrogate mother and carried to term.

The lamb, Dolly, was an exact genetic replica of the adult female sheep that donated the somatic cell nucleus to the egg. She was the first-ever mammal to be cloned from an adult somatic cell.

There are two commonly discussed types of human cloning: therapeutic cloning and reproductive cloning. Therapeutic cloning involves cloning cells from an adult for use in medicine and transplants, and is an active area of research. Reproductive cloning would involve making cloned humans, for couples wanting to have a child, but cannot naturally.

- Therapeutic cloning
  In this technique a somatic cell, e.g., a skin cell is fused with an enucleated ovum. The fused cell is then induced to divide and form a blastocyst. Stem cells are then harvested from the inner cell mass of this cloned embryo. It has the same DNA as the original somatic cell. This process termed Somatic Cell Nuclear Transfer (SCNT) holds great promise for regenerative medicine [41]. The applications of this technique are still in the realm of expectations.
  Muslim jurists have different views. SCNT raises many moral objections in addition to what will discussed in relation to hESC research. The cloned embryos will be produced exclusively for research, unlike other Human Embryonic Stem Cells (hESC) research that is utilizing 'spare' pre-embryos at IVF clinics [42].

Islamic Position on Cloning

Cloning is indeed a most serious issue as it is a reversion to the most primitive form, asexual reproduction. It conflicts with the Qur'anic verse: "God created consorts for you from amongst you and through them. He gave you children and grandchildren. Do they then believe in vain things and deny the blessing of God?" [43]. The bleak prospects of cloning are already manifested by the very high rate of fetal wastage before a clone is born [44].

In addition to the fact that a resulting embryo from reproductive cloning would be severely deformed with developmental abnormalities and early aging, the major problems of reproductive cloning are:

(1) the loss of kinship and lineage due to the unnaturalness of reproduction (mixing of kinship or the loss of it, would be considered haram) (unlawful in Isalm) and undermining the concept of reproduction and family (Holy Qur'an 4:1)
(2) the social harms, problems of personal identity and the psychological development of a clone and the disregard for human dignity
(3) the unjust eugenics (selecting genetic qualities by selective breeding) and trends towards "designer babies" (superior or inferior, depending upon the motives of the creator)
(4) the contradiction of the Islamic belief (God is the only and the best creator)

(5) the contradiction of the principle of creation of all beings (human, animal, plants) in pairs (male and female). However, as cloning produces the exact copy of the previously existent individual whether male or female, this leads to a disturbance of the natural existence of pairs, and finally

(6) the contradiction of the principle of diversity of creation of all beings, including human, animals, and plants in various colors and shapes [45].

Therefore, human cloning is forbidden in any method that leads to human reproduction.

The International Islamic Fiqh Academy of Organization of Islamic Conferences (OIC-IFA) in Jeddah in its 10th session (23–28. 2.1418H/28 June–3 July 1997 CE) explored all the research papers and recommendations of the 9th Medical & Fiqh Seminar held by the Islamic Medical Organization in Casablanca, Morocco, in collaboration with the Council and others (14–17 June 1997 CE), and declared Decree #100/2/D10:

1. Human Cloning is forbidden in any method that leads to human reproduction.
2. It is forbidden in all cases to introduce a third party into marriage, be it an egg donor, a surrogate womb, a sperm donor, or a cloned cell.
3. It is permissible to use genetic engineering and cloning in the fields of germs, microorganisms, plants, and animals, following legitimate rules which lead to benefits and prevent harm.
4. All Muslim countries are called upon to formulate the necessary legislation to prevent foreign research institutes, organizations and experts from directly or indirectly using Muslim countries for experimentation on human cloning or promoting it.
5. Specialized committees should be set up to look into the ethics of biological research and adopt protocols for study and research in Muslim countries.
6. Biological and bioengineering research institutions (other than cloning research) should be supported and established, according to the Islamic rulings, so that the Muslim World will not be dependent on others in this field.
7. The mass media are called upon to deal with recent scientific advances from an Islamic perspective in a faithful way and avoid employing their services against Islam, aiming to educate the public to be confident before any decision.

Stem cell research

Stem cell research is a very promising new field of medicine. It potentially holds the promise of a cure for many so far incurable diseases like Alzheimer's, genetic diseases, and malignancies.

The embryonic stem cells (ESCs) are the original cells from which all the 220 different types of cells that compose the human body develop.

Stem cells are also present in adult tissues in small numbers. Their ability to trans differentiate into cells of another lineage is very limited compared with that of ESCs. There is probably one exception, umbilical cord blood stem cells (UCB) SCs. Stem cells can be procured from fertilized eggs in storage following in vitro fertilization, but also are found in the placenta, umbilical cord and the blood in the normal human circulatory system. Up to now, the most readily available source seems to be the surplus fertilized ova left over after in vitro fertilization [46]. Cord blood is more readily available.

The ESC research is morally controversial because it involves sometimes the deliberate production, use and ultimate destruction of human pre-embryos.

To obtain hESCs one has to destroy a 5–7-day-old pre-embryo. The crux of this conflict is the question whether the 5–7-day-old pre-embryo is a human being entitled to protection against harm or destruction [47]. (The Catholic view and its supporters).

One side of the debate raises the dictum of the "sanctity of human life." From an Islamic point of view, we have already alluded to the inviolability of human life from the point of implantation onwards. A fertilized ovum in storage does not, however, possess the same rights as a fetus and it may be used if the purpose is to protect and save human life. Our argument rests on the following points:

- The Arabic word for embryo and fetus is "Janin" which means a conceptus hidden in the womb. If it is not in uterus, then it is not a "janin", i.e., not embryo nor fetus.
- If kept in storage, the fertilized ovum will acquire genetic anomalies and will, sooner or later, die.
- It is not part of the feto-maternal unit of a pregnancy.
- A somatic cell, such as a skin cell, can be made into an embryo through the process of cloning and yet, nobody ever claimed sanctity for skin cells.
- According to Islamic teaching, a fertilized egg, not yet residing in the mother's uterus, does not have the spirit instilled into it [48]. The ensoulement occurs at 120 days after fertilization.

On the basis of the concept that definitive human life does not start until ensoulment the great majority of Muslim scholars agree that research on the pre-embryo, especially the preimplantation pre-embryo—as it cannot grow independently outside the uterus—is permissible, provided that these pre-embryos were legitimately developed. The permissibility is also conditioned on the fact that these embryos are not produced specifically for research. Supernumerary embryos produced at infertility clinics are considered legitimate [49]. The surplus fertilized ova should be donated by the spouses who produced it.

Islamic Position on Stem Cells Research

In the opinion of most Muslim jurists, stem cell and cloning research, as scientific advancement, would have advantages and limitations.

While the majority of Islamic jurors permit Human Embryonic Stem Cells (hESC) research, all agree that that creating embryos for the sole purpose of research is prohibited.

Stem cell therapy is allowed if the source of the cells is legitimate including left over zygotes, and if the parents have consented to its use. Similarly spontaneous abortion or medically indicated abortion can be used as a source of Stem cells if the parents agree.

The practical application of the use of stem cells in therapy is the use of bone marrow transplant to treat blood disorders like thalassemia and leukemia and it is used to treat certain storage disorders. Umbilical cord blood banks are available in the Kingdom of Saudi Arabia and the UAE [50]. Because of the inevitable consequences of reproductive cloning; it is prohibited by the majority of Muslim reference decrees. However, stem cell research for therapeutic purposes is permissible with full consideration and all possible precautions in the pre-ensoulment stages of early fetus development.

The Islamic Fiqh council of Islamic World League, Makkah Al Mukaramah in its 17th session (19–23.10.1424 H/13–17 December 2003 CE) have declared Decree #3 on Stem Cell Therapy:

First: It is permissible to obtain stem cells, to be grown and used for therapy or for permissible scientific research, if its source is legitimate, as for example:

1. Adults if they give permission, without inflicting harm on them.
2. Children provided that their guardians allow it, for a legal benefit and without inflicting harm on the children.
3. The placenta or the umbilical cord, with the parents' permission.
4. A fetus if spontaneously aborted or when aborted for a therapeutic reason permitted by Shari'ah, with the parents' permission (Be reminded of Decree #7 of the Council in its 12th session about abortion).
5. Leftover zygotes remaining from in vitro fertilization, if donated by the parents, when it is ascertained that they will not be used in an illegal pregnancy.

Second: It is forbidden to use stem cells, if their source is illegal. As for example:

1. Intentionally aborted fetuses (that is, abortion without a legal medical reason).
2. Intentional fertilization between a donated ovum and sperm.
3. Therapeutic human cloning.

The Fiqh Council of North America in 2007 affirmed its earlier position of support for hESC research [51]. The Islamic Medical Association of North America (IMANA) Ethics Committee published a position paper on SC research and added its approval [52]. Both the Islamic Institute of Turkey and the Malaysian National Fatwa Council also supported hESC research [53].

DNA Fingerprinting

DNA fingerprinting, also called DNA typing, in genetics, method of isolating and making images of sequences of DNA (deoxyribonucleic acid). The technique was developed in 1984 by the British geneticist Alec Jeffreys, after he noticed the existence of certain sequences of DNA (called minisatellites) that do not contribute to the function of a gene but are repeated within the gene and in other genes of a DNA sample. Jeffreys also determined that each organism has a unique pattern of these minisatellites, the only exception being multiple individuals from a single zygote (e.g., identical twins) [54].

DNA profiling is employed by forensic scientists to assist in the identification of individuals by their respective DNA profiles. DNA profiles are encrypted sets of numbers that reflect a person's DNA makeup, which can also be used as the person's identifier. It is used in, for example, parental testing and criminal investigation.

A sample of blood, saliva, semen, or other appropriate fluid or tissue from personal items (e.g., toothbrush, razor, etc.) is required for the test. Although 99.8 % of human DNA sequences are the same in every person, enough of the DNA is different to distinguish one individual from another, unless they are monozygotic twins.

The technique was challenged, however, over concerns about sample contamination, faulty preparation procedures, and erroneous interpretation of the results. Efforts were made to improve its reliability, and today the technique has been refined through the use of more-specific techniques. DNA samples that are degraded or collected postmortem typically produce less-reliable results than do samples that are obtained from a living individual.

The procedure for creating a DNA fingerprint consists of first obtaining a sample of cells containing DNA (e.g., from skin, blood, or hair), extracting the DNA, and purifying it [55]. If only a small amount of DNA is available for fingerprinting, a polymerase chain reaction (PCR) may be used to create thousands of copies of a DNA segment.

DNA analysis is widely applied to determine genetic family relationships such as paternity, maternity, sibling ship, and other kinships.

On DNA fingerprinting, The Islamic Fiqh council of Islamic World League, Makkah Al Mukaramah, in its 16th session (21–26/10/1422 Hijra/5–10 January 2002 G) have issued the following guidance:

1. It is religiously allowed to use DNA fingerprinting in forensic interrogations to prove crime which has no definite penalty in Islamic law (Shari'ah) (Avoid punishment if there is any doubt, as doubt should always be used for the sake of the accused), this will lead to justice and to safety of the community, as the criminal will be punished and the innocent will be freed from guilt, which is one of the most important goals of Share'ah.
2. DNA fingerprinting may be used in lineage (genealogy) only with great caution and confidentiality as the Shari'ah rules take precedence over DNA fingerprinting.
3. It is forbidden to use DNA fingerprinting in paternity (lineage) disputes, which should not precede the oath of condemnation (the sworn allegation of adultery committed by one's spouse).
4. It is forbidden to use DNA fingerprinting to confirm or refute legally proven lineage; the state should forbid this and inflict punishment, in order to protect people's honor and to preserve their lineage.
5. It is allowed to use DNA fingerprinting in proving lineage on the following conditions;

   a. In case of a dispute about unknown lineage, as mentioned by the Islamic scholars because the evidence is either absent or equivocal, and to overcome (inundate) the vagueness (suspicion);

    b. in case of a dispute over babies in hospitals and nurseries or test tube babies;

    c. in case of children lost because of war, accidents or natural disasters, where their family could not be found;

    d. To identify babies or prisoners of war.

6. The human genome of an individual, nation, or race should not be sold for any reason; neither should it be given because of the harm it can cause. The counsel recommends that:

    a. The state to forbid DNA fingerprinting testing except on judge's orders and performed in the state laboratories; the private sector should be forbidden from doing such tests because of the great danger and harm.

    b. Each state should have a committee on DNA fingerprinting tests which should include legal scholars, physicians, and administrators to supervise and approve the result of such tests.

    c. There should be a precise mechanism to prevent deceit, cheating, contamination, or human error in such laboratories, so the results are compatible with reality. The accuracy of these laboratories needs to be confirmed.

    d. The number of genes [56] used for a test should be sufficient, in the opinion of specialists, to overcome any doubts about the accuracy of the results.

Unanswered Ethical Questions and Dilemmas

There are many dilemmas to be answered. Is it allowable to abort a fetus showing Downs syndrome although even with this condition it is possible to live a quiet, peaceful life? If the Huntington's disease gene is detected, is an abortion justified, although the disease will not appear until age 40 or even 60? Is it permissible to abort those who are homozygous for sickle cell disease or thalassemia or phenyl ketonuria or homocystinuria? For the last two diseases mentioned there is a treatment, namely to avoid foods that contain phenyl alanine or methionine.

It is hoped that, in the near future, advances in gene therapy will remove the need to consider abortion in such cases. In the meantime, the best policy is to encourage couples considering marriage to have premarital medical examinations for infectious and hereditary diseases common in their community. It is also important to educate people more effectively and actively about the sequel of consanguineous marriages which, as noted earlier, are very common in most Arab countries.

In conclusion, Islamic teachings offer a great deal in the prevention and control of genetic diseases to Islamic communities, which form the majority of the population in many Asian and African countries. It is important to educate people about the dangers of consanguinity, which is very common in several Islamic countries.

Premarital examination should be encouraged which may detect the trait in those intending to get married. Postnatal exam for newly born babies can detect many diseases (inborn errors of metabolism, hypothyroidism, etc.) which can be prevented by certain diets and drugs.

Proper counseling should be provided, the dangers explained, and the options discussed. Prenatal diagnosis and the option of abortion for serious devastating diseases (prior to 120 days from conception) will reduce the incidence of such diseases. Neonatal screening can avert havoc by simple measures namely specific diets, or certain operative measures. Avoiding teratogens and provision of folate and iodine in the diet will help in reducing congenital diseases.

References

1. El-Hazmi MAF (2009) Ethical issues on preventions and management of blood genetics disorders– Islamicviews. Hemoglobin 33(S1):S1–S6
2. Sahih AlBokhari, Sahih Muslim, Fathu AlBari, Sharieh Sahih AlBokhari, by Ibn HajarAlasqalani, Hadith No 5035, 6847 and No. 7314. He said one of the grandmothers of the child was black
3. Rajab AA, El-Hazmi MA (2007) The Gulf Cooperation Countries genetic services. Understanding individuals, families, and community needs. Saudi Med J 28(9):1321–1323
4. Al-Gazali L, Hamamy H, Al-Arrayad S (2006) Genetic disorders in the Arab world. BMJ 333 (7573):831–4
5. Ibid
6. Modell B, Darlison M, Birgens H, Cario H, Faustino P, Giordano PC, Gulbis B, Hopmeier P, Lena- Russo D, Romao L, Theodorsson E (2007) Epidemiology of haemoglobin disorders in Europe: an overview. Scand J Clin Lab Invest 67(1):39–69
7. Ibid
8. Bayoumi RA, Yardumian A (2006) Genetic disorders in the Arab world. BMJ 333:819
9. Good New Bible. The Bible societies, Collins/Fontana. Book Genesis 12:10–19
10. Good New Bible. Genesis 19:30–38
11. Albar MA (1999) Counseling about genetic disease: an Islamic perspective. Easter Med Health J 5:1129–1133
12. Al Aqeel AI (2007) Islamic ethical framework for research into and prevention of genetic diseases. Nat Genet 39(11):1293–1298
13. Modell B, Darr A (2002) Genetic counseling and customary consanguineous marriage. Nat Rev/Genet 3:225–229
14. Teebi AS, El-Shanti HI (2006) Consanguinity: implications for practice, research, and policy. Lancet 367:970–971
15. Temtamy S, Aglan M (2012) Consanguinity and genetic disorders in Egypt. Middle East J Med Genet 1(1):12–17
16. Hammay H (2012) Consanguineous marriages trends, impact on health and counseling. Geneva (Online)
17. Weatherall D (1998) Some aspects of the Hemoglobinopathies of particular relevance to Saudi Arabia and other parts of the Middle East. Saudi Med J 9:107–115
18. El-Hazmi MAF (2006) Pre-marital examination as a method of prevention from blood genetic disorders. Saudi Med J 27(9):1291–1295
19. Rajab AA. op.cit
20. El-Hazmi MAF (2009) op.cit
21. El-Hazmi MAF (2006) op.cit
22. Walters L (2012) Genetics and bioethics: How our thinking has changed since 1969. Theor Med Bioeth 33:83–95

23. El-Hazmi MAF Genehical Aspects of Research and Medical Services in Islamic Countries Mohsen A.F. El-Hazmi www.intechopen.com
24. Al-Odaib AN, Abu-Amero KK, Ozand PT, Al-Hellani AM (2003) A new era for preventive genetic programs in the Arabian Peninsula. Saudi Med J 24(11):1168–1175
25. Albar MA. op.cit
26. The Holy Qur'an 33:4
27. Eskandarani HA (2009) Pre-implantation genetic diagnosis in the Gulf Cooperative Council countries: utilization and ethical attitudes. Hum Reprod Genet Ethics 15(2):68–74
28. Alsulaiman A, Al-Odaib A, Al-Rejjal R, Hewison J (2010) Preimplantation genetic diagnosis in Saudi Arabia: parents' experience and attitudes. Prenat Diagn 30(8):753–757
29. Ibid
30. Benn PA, Chapman AR (2010) Ethical challenges in providing noninvasive prenatal diagnosis. Curr Opin Obstet Gynecol 22(2):128–134
31. Ibid
32. Al Darqutni AO (1966) Sunan Al Darqutni, Dar Al MahasinLittiba'a, Cairo, Commented by Abdullah Hashim Yamani, Kitab al Nikah (Book of Marriage) vol 3:299 (Hadith No 196, 197, 198) and vol 3:30 (Hadith No 212, 213)
33. Al Dailamy SS (1987) Firdoos Al Hikmah, Dar Al Kitab Al Arabi, Beirut, Commented by Al-Zumerli FA and al-Baghdadi MM, vol 2:76 Hadith No 2110
34. Albar MA. op.cit
35. AlBukhari M, Sahih AlBukhari (1958) Cairo: Matabi Asshab (1378H)
36. The Islamic Jurisprudence Council of the Islamic World League of the Organization of Islamic Countries, 12th session 1990
37. Knockout Mice (2009) Nation Human Genome Research Institute
38. Sheryl Gay (4 July 2010). Trials are halted on a gene therapy. The New York Times
39. Walters L. op.cit
40. The Islamic Jurisprudence Council of the Islamic World League of the Organization of Islamic Countries, in its 15th session, 1998
41. Fadel HE (2012) Developments in stem cell research and therapeutic cloning: Islamic ethical positions, a review. Bioethics 26(3):128–135
42. Al-Aqeel AI (2009) Human cloning, stem cell research. An Islamic perspective. Saudi Med J 30(12):1507–1514
43. The Holy Qur'an 16:72
44. Hathout H (2006) An Islamic perspective on human genetic and reproductive technologies. East Mediterr Health J Suppl 2:S22–8
45. Al-Aqeel AI (2009) op.cit
46. Hathout H. op.cit
47. Fadel HE. op.cit
48. Hathout H. op.cit
49. Al-Aqeel AI (2009) op.cit
50. Ibid
51. The Fiqh Council of North America. Embryonic Stem-Cell Research. http://www.fiqhcouncil. org/Articles/GeneralFiqhIssues/
52. IMANA Ethics Committee (2007) Stem cell research: the IMANA perspective. Islamic Medical Association of North America, Lombard
53. Fadel HE. op.cit
54. Encyclopedia Britannica (2013). http://global.britannica.com/EBchecked/topic/167155/DNA-fingerprinting
55. Ibid
56. Genes are composed of exons and introns. Exons are templates for proteins, introns are filler, and critical for DNA fingerprinting. The genes are not used for DNA fingerprinting (Exons). Introns are used

Chapter 13
Organ Transplantation

Organ transplantation is one of the major medical achievements of the twentieth century. Nowadays, many diseased organs are being replaced by healthy organs from living donors, cadavers, and from animal source. Successful bone marrow, kidney, liver, cornea, pancreas, heart, and nerve cell transplantations have taken place. The incidence is limited only by cost and availability of the organs. The discovery of effective immunosuppressive drugs in the late 1970s was an important step toward increasing the success rate of organ transplants and thus paved the way for organ transplantation to become a medical routine affair in the twenty-first century [1].

Definition

Organ donation is the donation of biological tissue or an organ of the human body, from a living or dead person to a living recipient in need of a transplantation.

The Encyclopedia Britannica (2013) defines organ donation, as the act of giving one or more organs (or parts thereof), without compensation, for transplantation into someone else. Organ donation is a very personal yet complex decision, intertwined with medical, legal, religious, cultural, and ethical issues. Today organ donation, strictly defined, encompasses the donation and transplantation of the heart, intestines, kidneys, liver, lungs, and pancreas (e.g., the islets of Langerhans) [2]. It also involves corneas, bones, skin, joint, blood, etc.

Types of Transplant

Autograft: Autotransplantation is the transplantation of organs, tissues from one part of the body to another in the same individual. Tissue transplanted by such "autologous" procedure is referred to as an autograft or autotransplant.

Allograft: An allograft is a transplant of an organ or tissue between two genetically non-identical members of the same species. Most human tissue and organ transplants are allografts.

© The Author(s) 2015
M.A. Al-Bar and H. Chamsi-Pasha, *Contemporary Bioethics*,
DOI 10.1007/978-3-319-18428-9_13

Xenograft: A transplant of organs or tissue from one species to another. An example is porcine heart valve transplant, which is quite common and successful.

Historical Background

Organ transplantation is not a twentieth century novelty. Indeed, it was known in one form or another even in prehistoric times. Ancient Hindu surgeons described methods for repairing defects of the nose and ears using auto grafts from the neighboring skin, a technique that remains to the present day. Susruta Sanhita, an old Indian medical document written in 700 BC, described the procedure, later emulated by the Italian Tagliacozzi in the sixteenth century, and by British surgeons working in India in the seventeenth and eighteenth centuries [3]. Tooth transplantation was practiced in ancient Egypt, Greece, Rome, and pre-Colombian North and South America. Arab surgeons were adept at this technique one thousand year's ago [4].

At the time of Prophet Muhammad (PBUH)—AD 570–632—one of his companions, Qatada ibn Nu'man, lost his eye during the battle of Uhud. The Prophet replanted it and it became the better of his two eyes [5]. In the battle of Badr, the Prophet (PBUH) replaced the arm of Muawath bin Afra and the hand of Habib bin Yasaf [6]. Muslim jurists sanctioned transplantation of teeth and bones, which had been practiced by Muslim surgeons for over a thousand years. Imam Nawawi (631-671H/AD1233-1272) fully discussed the subject of bone and teeth transplantation in his voluminous reference textbook AL Majmu, [7] and his concise text book Minhaj Attalibin [8]. Al Imam Asshirbini commented on the same subject in his book Muqhni Al Muhtaj [9]. The bone to be implanted could be from the same person (autograft) or from the corpse of another person (allograft) or from an animal (xenograft). The latter could be from a slaughtered (Halal) animal or from a Najas, i.e., a dead corpse (Carcass) or of porcine origin, both of which will not be allowed unless there is no other alternative and is deemed necessary. However, Zakaria Al Qazwini, a grand Qhadi (judge) in Iraq (600-682H/1203-1283AD), noticed that porcine bone grafts function more efficiently than other xenografts, and reported this fact in his book "Wonders of Creatures" [10].

Ibn Sina (Avicenna (607-687H/1210-1288AD) (the greatest Muslim physician), in his voluminous textbook "Canon" [11] regarded bone transplantation as a hazardous operation that he would never attempt to perform.

Timeline of Successful Transplants

- 1905 First successful cornea transplant by Eduard Zirm [Czech Republic]
- 1954 First successful kidney transplant by J. Hartwell Harrison and Joseph Murray (Boston, U.S.A.)

- 1966 First successful pancreas transplant by Richard Lillehei and William Kelly (Minnesota, U.S.A.)
- 1967 First successful liver transplant by Thomas Starzl (Denver, U.S.A.)
- 1967 First successful heart transplant by Christian Barnard (Cape Town, South Africa)
- 1981 First successful heart/lung transplant by Bruce Reitz (Stanford, U.S.A.)
- 1983 First successful lung lobe transplant by Joel Cooper (Toronto, Canada)
- 1984 First successful double organ transplant by Thomas Starzl and Henry T. Bahnson (Pittsburgh, U.S.A.)
- 1986 First successful double-lung transplant (Ann Harrison) by Joel Cooper (Toronto, Canada)
- 1995 First successful laparoscopic live-donor nephrectomy by Lloyd Ratner and Louis Kavoussi (Baltimore, U.S.A.)
- 1997 First successful allogeneic vascularized transplantation of a fresh and perfused human knee joint by Gunther O. Hofmann
- 1998 First successful live-donor partial pancreas transplant by David Sutherland (Minnesota, U.S.A.)
- 1998 First successful hand transplant by Dr. Jean-Michel Dubernard (Lyon, France)
- 1999 First successful Tissue Engineered Bladder transplanted by Anthony Atala (Boston Children's Hospital, U.S.A.)
- 2005 First successful ovarian transplant by Dr P N Mhatre (wadia hospital Mumbai, India)
- 2005 First successful partial face transplant (France)
- 2006 First jaw transplant to combine donor jaw with bone marrow from the patient, by Eric M. Genden Mount Sinai Hospital, New York
- 2006 First successful human penis transplant [reversed after 15 days due to 44 year old recipient's wife's physiological rejection] (Guangzhou, China)
- 2008 First successful complete full double arm transplant by Edgar Biemer, ChristophHöhnke and Manfred Stangl (Technical University of Munich, Germany)
- 2008 First baby born from transplanted ovary by James Randerson
- 2008 First transplant of a Vertebrate trachea|human windpipe using a patient's own stem cells, by Paolo Macchiarini (Barcelona, Spain)
- 2008 First successful transplantation of near total area (80 %) of face, (including palate, nose, cheeks, and eyelid) by Maria Siemionow (Cleveland, USA)
- 2010 First full facial transplant, by Dr Joan Pere Barret and team (Hospital Universitari Valld'Hebron on July 26, 2010 in Barcelona, Spain.)
- 2011 First double leg transplant, by Dr Cavadas and team (Valencia's Hospital La Fe, Spain)
- 2013 First successful entire face transplantation as an urgent life-saving surgery at Maria Skłodowska-Curie Institute of Oncology branch in Gliwice, Poland.
  2014: First successful uterine transplant resulting in live birth (Sweden)
  2014: First successful penis transplant (South Africa)
  2014: First neonatal organ transplant (U.K) [12]

World Activity in Transplantation

The greatest numbers of living donor kidney transplants, on a yearly basis, were performed in the United States (6435), Brazil (1768), Iran (1615), Mexico (1459), and Japan (939). In the Arab world, Saudi Arabia had the highest reported living kidney donor transplant rate [13].

The scarcity of organs has dire consequences. An average of 19 people dies each day waiting for a transplant that never comes. The World Health Organization WHO global observatory showed that in 2009 about 100,900 people received a lifesaving organ transplant, representing only less than 10 % of the global needs. The entire issue has raised serious ethical concerns and the debate over them rages unabated.

The increasing incidence of vital organ failure and the inadequate supply of organs, especially from cadavers, have created a wide gap between organ supply and organ demand, which has resulted in very long waiting times to receive an organ as well as an increasing number of deaths while waiting [14]. These events have raised many ethical, moral and societal issues regarding supply, the methods of organ allocation, and the use of living donors including minors. It has also led to the practice of organ sale by entrepreneurs for financial gains in some parts of the world through exploitation of the poor, for the benefit of the wealthy.

Renal Transplantation in the Arab World

The first successful renal transplantation in the Arab world took place in Jordan in 1972. Surprisingly, the kidney transplanted was from a non-heart beating deceased donor. Many Arab countries followed suit, starting their transplantation programs in the 1970s and 1980s, but all were from living related donors. Very few Arab countries managed to start deceased donor programs, notable among which is the Kingdom of Saudi Arabia [15]. Religion has an important part in personal life and government legislation in the Arab world; thus, organ procurement and transplantation had to wait for religious edicts (fatwas) to be passed about the permissibility of organ donation and brain death diagnosis before starting transplantation activities. In Saudi Arabia, the renal transplantation service went through several developmental phases, culminating in the establishment of the Saudi Center for Organ Transplantation, which has become the prototype of a successful multiorgan procurement center. Many patients from the Arab countries, especially from the Gulf countries, traveled abroad to get "commercial" transplants. These were usually done in poor countries where there was much abuse of the donors and poor results for the recipients [16].

All Arab countries that have deceased organ programs follow the opt-in (required consent) system. The only exception is Tunisia, which has had an opt-out (presumed consent) system since 1991 [16].

Types of Organ Donors

The sources of organs for transplantation, i.e., living donor (related and nonrelated), cadaveric donor, and brain-dead patients. In countries where transplantation is well established, organs are sourced from living and deceased (cadaveric) donors using different strategies, i.e., an opt-in (explicit consent), opt-out (presumed consent), and donation after brain death

What Is "Opt-in" and "Opt-Out" Systems?

The United States and many other countries all use what is commonly referred to as the "opt-in" organ donation system, in which individuals have to sign up to become a donor before their death, and then the final decision to use the organs from a given individual's body rests with the potential donor's family after their death.

Some European countries (including France Belgium, Finland, Denmark, Italy, Spain, Norway, and Sweden) have shed the restrictions of the opt-in system in favor of an opt-out system. The opt-out system presumes that all individuals would presumably consent to have their organs used for transplant. In Belgium, for example, only 3–4 % opt out, leaving 96–97 % of the population still in the pool of potential donors, as compared with the roughly 30 % of Americans who are organ donors in the opt-in system. The opt-in systems give a higher respect for the requirement of consent than the opt-out systems [17].

In practice many countries, have legislation allowing for implied consent [18] which pays little regard for informed consent and autonomy.

Islamic Principles and Rules Related to Organ Transplantation

Islam differs from many other religions in providing a complete code of life. It encompasses the secular with the spiritual and the mundane with the celestial. Man is the viceregent of god (Allah) on earth. "Behold the lord said to Angels: I will create viceregent on earth" [19]. He fashioned man in due proportion and breathed into him something of his spirit [20] and not only Adam was honored by Allah, but his progeny also, provided they followed the right path. "We honored the progeny of Adam, provided them with transport on land and sea; given them for sustenance things good and pure; and conferred on them special favors above a great part of our creation" [21]. Human life begins at the time of ensoulment, which is stated in the sayings of the prophet (PBUH) to be the 120th day from the time of conception [21]. Prior to that moment, the embryo has sanctity, but not reaching that of a full human being. Life ends with departure of the soul (or spirit); a process that cannot be identified by mortals except by the accompanying signs—the most important of which is the cessation of respiration and circulation. Some jurists described weakening of vision, limpness of the feet, bending of the nose, whitening of the temples and the stretching of the face and loss of the ability to wrinkle as the signs of death [23].

The sanctity of the human body is not lessened by the departure of the soul and declaration of death. The human body, whether living or dead, should be venerated likewise. The prophet Muhammad (PBUH) rebuked a man who broke a bone of a corpse that he found in a cemetery. The prophet said, "the sin of breaking the bones of a dead man is equal to the sin of breaking the bones of a living man" [24].

The dead body should be prepared for burial as soon as possible in order to avoid putre-faction (which occurs rapidly in hot climates). Cremation is not allowed. Due respect and reverence should be given to the funeral, as exemplified by the prophet Muhammad (PBUH) who stood in veneration for the passing funeral of a Jew, at a time when Jews were waging war against him. One of his companions exclaimed: "It is the funeral of a Jew"—the prophet answered, "Is it not a human soul"? [25] Islam considers disease as a natural phenomenon. It is not caused by demons, stars or evil spirit. Indeed, disease is not even caused by the wrath of God or any other celestial creature. Diseases and ailments are a type of tribulation by God and expiate sin. Those stoics who forbear and endure in dignity are rewarded in this world and on the Day of Judgment. However, man should seek remedy for his ailments. The Prophet Muhammad (PBUH) told Muslims to seek remedy and treatment [26]. He ordered his cousin Saad ibn AbiWaqqas to seek the medical advice of Al Harith ibn Kaledah, a renowned physician of the time [27]. He also declared that there is a cure for every illness, although we may not know it at the time [28]. New methods of treatment should be searched for and applied if proven successful.

The prophet ordered Muslims to be compassionate to every human being. He also said, "All mankind is the family of Allah. Those who best serve his family are best loved by God" [29].

The human being should always maintain his dignity even in disease and misfortune. The human body, living or dead, should be venerated likewise. Mutilation of humans or animals is not allowed [30]. However, performing post-mortems or donating organs from a cadaver are not tantamount to mutilation of the corpse or an act of disrespect [31]. The harm done, if any, by removing any organ from a corpse should be weighed against the benefit obtained, and the new life given to the recipient. The principle of saving human life takes precedence over whatever assumed harm would befall the corpse [32]. Nevertheless, Sheikh Shaarawi, a renowned commentator on the Holy Qur'an, but not a Mufti (Jurisconsult), rejected all types of organ donation.

In the case of living donor, the principle of doing no harm—premium non nocere —is invoked. The donor cannot give one of his vital organs, which would end his life. It is an act of homicide or suicide, both of which are considered among the most detestable crimes in Islam. The donation of an organ whose loss would usually cause no harm, or a minimal increased risk to the health or life of the donor, is acceptable if the benefit to the recipient is greater than the harm. It invokes the principle of accepting the lesser harm when faced with two evils. The harm done by the disease, which can kill a human life, is not to be compared with the harm incurred by donation [33].

Organ transplantation is a new method of treatment that can save many human lives and improve the quality of life for many others. Islam encourages a search for a cure and in-vokes Muslims not to despair, for there is certainly a cure for every ailment, although we may not know of it at the present time. The donation of organs is an act of charity, benevolence, altruism and love for mankind. God loves those who love fellow humans and try to mitigate the agony and sorrow of others and relieve their misfortunes. Any action carried out with good intentions and which aims at helping others is respected and indeed encouraged, provided no harm is inflicted. The human body is the property of God; however, man is entrusted with the body as well as other things. He should use it in the way prescribed by God as revealed by His messengers. Any misuse will be judged by God on the Day of Judgment, and transgressors will be punished. Suicide is equated, in Islam, with homicide. Even cremation of the corpse is not allowed. The only accepted and dignified way is burial of the corpse—which should be performed as soon as possible, but not immediately for medical certainty. Donation of organs should not be considered as acts of transgression against the body. On the contrary, they are acts of charity and benevolence to other fellow humans, which God loves and encourages. Human organs are not a commodity. They should be donated freely in response to an altruistic feeling of brotherhood and love for one's fellow beings [34]. Encouraging donation by the government (by any means) is allowed by Islamic Jurists, and is practiced in Saudi Arabia, Gulf Countries, and Iran.

Islamic Jurists Fatwas (Juridical Resolutions) Regarding Organ Transplantation

Muslim surgeons practiced autograft transplantation, which they learned from other nations, especially the Indians. They also practiced teeth and bone grafting from both animal and human sources (i.e., xenograft and homografts) as far back as a thousand years ago, having first obtained the consent of the jurists. Table 1 illustrates some of the recent Fatwas on organ transplantation. In the 20th century, Muslim jurists sanctioned blood transfusion, although blood is considered as Najas—i.e., unclean. The Fatwa of the Grand Mufti of Egypt, No. 1065 dated June 9, 1959, is an example of Islamic jurists' attitude toward new methods of treatment [35].

A Fatwa by Grand Mufti is almost a decree and not a mere juridical opinion; so is a Fatwa by a Conference of Jurists. However, each country legislative parliament should endorse it to become a law.

The majority of the Muslim scholars and jurists belonging to various schools of Islamic law invoked the principle of priority of saving human life and hence gave it precedence over any other argument. Sheikh Hassan Mamoon (the Grand Mufti of

Table 1 Fatwas relating to organ transplantation

Source	Date	Fatwa
Sheikh Maamoon (Grand Mufti, Egypt)	1959	Sanctioned blood transfusion
Sheikh Maamoon (Grand Mufti, Egypt)	1959	Sanctioned corneal transplants
Sheikh Hureidi (Grand Mufti, Egypt)	1966	Sanctioned organ transplants
Islamic Int. Conference (Malaysia)	1969	Sanctioned organ transplants
Algiers Supreme Islamic Council	1972	Sanctioned organ transplants
Sheikh Khater (Grand Mufti, Egypt)	1973	Allowed harvesting skin from unidentified corpses
Saudi Grand Ulema	1978	Sanctioned corneal transplants
Sheikh Gad Al Haq (Grand Mufti, Egypt)	1979	Sanctioned live and cadaveric donation
Kuwaiti Fatwa of Ministry of Endowment	1980	Sanctioned organ transplants
Saudi Grand Ulema	1982	Sanctioned organ transplants
3rd Int. Conference Islamic Jurists (OIC)	1986	Equated brain death with cardiac death
4th Int. Conference Islamic Jurists (OIC)	1988	Sanctioned organ transplants and trafficking
6th Conference Islamic Jurists (OIC)	1990	Discussed transplantation from embryos, IVF projects, CNS and auencephalics

Egypt) also sanctioned corneal transplants from cadavers of unidentified persons and from those who agree to donate upon their death (Fatwa No. 1084 dated 14 April 1959) [36]. His successor, Sheikh Hureidi, extended the Fatwa to other organs in 1966 (Fatwa No. 993) [37]. In 1973, the Grand Mufti, Sheikh Khater, issued a Fatwa allowing harvesting of skin from an unidentified corpse [38].

Grand Mufti Gad Al Haq sanctioned donation of organs from the living provided no harm was done and provided it was donated freely in good faith and for the love of God and the human fraternity. He also sanctioned cadaveric donors provided there was a will, testament or the consent of the relatives of the deceased. In the case of unidentified corpses, an order from the magistrate should be obtained prior to harvesting organs (Fatwa No. 1323 dated 3 December 1979) [39]. The Saudi Department of Research Fatwa studied corneal transplantation in H1376 (1976) and H1397 (1977). The Saudi Grand Ulama sanctioned corneal transplant the following year (Decree No. 66 H1398/1978) [40].

In Algiers, the supreme Islamic Council sanctioned organ transplantation in 1972, while in Malaysia, the International Islamic Conference sanctioned organ transplantation in April 1969 [41].

The Saudi Grand Ulama Fatwa No. 99, 1982, addressed the subject of auto-grafts, which was unanimously sanctioned. It also sanctioned (by a majority) the donation of organs both by the living and by the dead, who made a will or testament, or by the consent of the relatives (who constitute the Islamic next of kin) [42]. The Kuwaiti Fatwa of the Ministry of Charitable Endowments No. 132/79, 1980 sanctioned live and cadaveric organ donation [43]. The Kuwaiti law No. 7, 1983, reiterated the previous Fatwa and pointed out that living donors should be over the age of 21 years in order to give their own consent.

The subject of the brain death was not addressed in any of these Fatwas. It was discussed for the first time in the Second International Conference of Islamic Jurists held in Jeddah in 1985. No decree was passed at that time, until further studies and consultations were obtained. In the Third International Conference of Islamic Jurists (Amman 1986), the historic resolution (No. 5) was passed with a majority of votes, which equated brain death to cardiac and respiratory death [44]. Death in the true Islamic teaching is the departure of the soul, but, as this cannot be identified, the signs of death are accepted. This decree paved the way for an extension of organ transplantation projects, which were limited to living donors. Campaigns for organ donation from brain-dead persons were launched both in Saudi Arabia and in Kuwait.

The unfortunate high incidence of road accidents in the Gulf area provides many cases of brain death. The tragedy should be averted by issuing and pursuing stricter traffic laws, and by other means. Meanwhile, it is a pity to waste such candidate cadavers without trying to save the life of many others who need their organs.

The Islamic Fiqh council of Islamic World League held in Makkah Al Mukaramah (December 1987), which passed Decree No. 2 (10th session), did not equate cardiac death with brain death. Although it did not recognize brain death as death, it did sanction all the previous Fatwas on organ transplantation. This decree received little publicity in the media, and cardiac and kidney transplants from brain dead individuals continued without any hindrance from the jurists.

The most detailed Fatwa on organ transplantation was that of the Fourth International Conference of Islamic Jurists, held in Jeddah in February 1988 (Resolution No. 1). It endorsed all previous Fatwas on organ transplantation, clearly rejected any trading or trafficking of organs and stressed the principle of altruism [45].

Later, the Islamic jurists started to discuss new subjects related to organ transplantation, viz. (A) Transplantation of the nerve tissue as a method for treating Parkinsonism or other ailments

- Transplantation from anencephalics;
- Transplantation of tissues from embryos aborted spontaneously, medically or electively;
- Leftover pre-embryos in vitro fertilization (IVF) projects [46].

The Sixth International Conference of Islamic Jurists, held in Jeddah in March 1990, addressed all these issues fully [47]. It sanctioned transplantation of nerve tissues to treat ailments such as Parkinsonism, if this method of treatment proved superior to other well-established methods of treatment. The source of the nerve tissues could be:

1. The suprarenal medulla of the patient himself (autograft);
2. The nerve tissues from an animal embryo (xenograft);
3. Cultured human nerve cells obtained from spontaneous abortion or medically indicated abortions.

However, the conference deplored the performance of abortion for the sake of procuring organs. It reiterated the Islamic views against elective abortion, which is only allowed to save the life or health of the expectant mother. If, however, the fetus is not viable, organs can be procured if the parents donate and only when the fetus is declared dead. The aborted fetus is not a commodity and commercialism is not allowed.

Anencephalics cannot be used as organ donors until declared brain or cardiac dead. The fully informed consent of the parents should be obtained in every case.

Regarding leftover pre-embryos from IVF projects, the jurists recommended that only the needed ova should be fertilized by the husband's sperms. However, if excess fertilized ova were found, they should be left to die spontaneously. Cryopreservation or donation of these fertilized ova was not allowed.

The jurists also discussed transplantation of genital organs. They did not allow the transplantation of gonads, as they carry all the genetics inheritance from the donor. However, they sanctioned the transplantation of the other internal sex organs.

In 2003, the Islamic Fiqh council of Islamic World League, Makkah Al Mukaramah in its 17th session passed a Fatwa No. 3, which allowed using leftover pre-embryos for stem cell research and treatment of serious ailments.

Organ Donation Among Muslims in Europe

In his article, "Religio-ethical discussions on organ donation among Muslims in Europe," Dr Ghaly sheds light on the discussions among Muslim religious scholars on organ donation particularly related to Muslims living in Europe. The article examines three main religious guidelines (fatwas) issued respectively by the UK Muslim Law (Shari'ah) Council in 1995 in the UK, the European Council for Fatwa and Research (ECFR) in 2000 in Ireland and the Moroccan religious scholar Mustafa Ben Hamza during a conference on "Islam and Organ Donation" held in March 2006 in the Netherlands.

The three fatwas studied in this article show that by the end of the twentieth century Muslim religious scholars started to specifically address Muslims in Europe.

The three fatwas examined in this article shared one main purport; organ donation is in principle permitted in Islam [48].

The fatwa issued by the ECFR in 2000 quoted the pro-organ donation fatwas issued earlier in the Muslim world but further added some points of specific relevance to Muslims in Europe. For instance, the fatwa stated that there are no ethical objections to directed organ donation and that donor's wishes should be respected in this regard as much as possible. As for the role of the deceased's family, the fatwa opined that if the deceased did not make up his/her mind before death about organ donation, then the deceased's family has the right to decide. The ECFR went even further by giving the same right to "the authority concerned with the Muslims' interests in non-Muslim countries" if the deceased's family was missing. The ECFR fatwa also indicated that there are no objections, from an Islamic perspective, to the opt-out system [49].

The second fatwa analyzed in this article was issued by the UK Muslim Law (Shari'ah) Council in 1995. Different to the ECFR fatwa, this fatwa was much less dependent on the religio-ethical discourse in the Muslim world. The UK fatwa also dedicated much more space to the concept of brain death and argued that this death-criterion is accepted from an Islamic perspective. The fatwa also clearly stated that Muslims may carry donor cards. Like the ECFR fatwa, the UK fatwa expressed no objection to the idea that the deceased's family can decide if the deceased did not have a donor card nor expressed his/her wish before death. Finally, the fatwa stressed that organ donation should be done freely without reward and that trading in organs is prohibited [50].

The third fatwa studied in this article was issued by a Moroccan scholar, Mustafa Ben Hamza, during a conference on "Islam and organ donation" held in 2006 in the Netherlands. This fatwa approved for a Muslim to donate his/her organs to a non-Muslim. A similar Fatwa was issued by Mufti of Singapore Sheikh Bin Sumait in early 1990s.

Contemporary English Sunni E-Fatwas on Organ Donation

Van den Branden and Broeckaert analyzed 70 English Sunni e-fatwas and subjected them to an in-depth text analysis in order to reveal the key concepts in the Islamic ethical framework regarding organ donation and blood transfusion [51].

They found all 70 fatwas allow for organ donation and blood transfusion. Autotransplantation is no problem at all if done for medical reasons. Allotransplantation, both from a living and a dead donor, appears to be possible though only in quite restricted ways. Xenotransplantation is less often mentioned but can be allowed in case of necessity. Transplantation in general is seen as an ongoing form of charity.

They state that their findings are very much in line with the international literature on the subject. They also found two new elements: debates on the definition of the moment of death are hardly mentioned in the English Sunni fatwas and organ donation and blood transfusion are presented as an ongoing form of charity.

The impact of globalization and migration on Muslim minorities living in non-Islamic countries during the past 20 years has been very strong [52].

In view of the positive evaluation these fatwas give; and in view of the worldwide shortage of organs for donation, the importance of these English Sunni e-fatwas must not be underestimated [53].

Fatwas in Malaysia

The issue of organ transplantation has been discussed since the 1960s. As a result, a fatwa regarding organ transplantation was issued in 1970 by the National Fatwa Council. The fatwa is used as reference for matters pertaining to organ transplantation and donation in Malaysia, and is adopted by states which do not have a specific fatwa regarding the issue.

The latest one is the Penang Fatwa Committee which sat on December 30, 2009 issued a comprehensive fatwa regarding organ transplantation and donation. The fatwa was gazetted on 9th December 2010, stating that the organ and tissue transplantations are permissible under certain conditions [54].

For Living Donor, the Conditions Are as Follows

a. Careful and professional medical examinations must be conducted by medical specialists to guarantee the safety of the donor to continue his or her life, the benefits, the advantages and disadvantages, as well as the success and failure of the transplantation.
b. The transplantation is performed with the willingness and consent from the donor without any kind of coercion from any parties [55].
c. Organ transplantation is the final resort in a critical and crucial situation, and there is an urgent need to save the life of other people especially those with family relationship.
d. Written consent is obtained from the donor, and the donor is free to withdraw the consent at any time.
e. The organ and tissue taken are from paired organs or a small part of an organ that can be taken without endangering the life of the donor.
f. Medical practitioners should observe medical ethics.
g. The transplanted organ and tissue are not for the purpose of trade.

For Cadaveric Donor, the Conditions Are as Follows

1. The death is not part of a pact or a plan to gain profit.
2. The death of the donor should be carefully ascertained.
3. It is performed under the donor's consent through a will or through his/her guardian and it must be witnessed by two witnesses.
4. There should not be any humiliation to the deceased.
5. Medical experts have verified that the organ and tissue from the donor can be used for donation.
6. The transplantation has a high degree of success.

7. The transplantation is performed with full discipline, knowledge, faith and piety, and respect should be accorded to the deceased following Islamic law, and humiliation should not take place.
8. The cadaver should be managed for burial.
9. If the donor is under aged or mentally-incompetent, consent from his or her legal guardian should be obtained [56].
10. Organ transplantation is the final resort in a critical and crucial situation, and there is an urgent need to save the life of other people especially those with family relationship.
11. Prayers (du'a) should be offered to the deceased (for Muslims).
12. The transplanted organ and tissue are not for the purpose of trade.

Penang's fatwa also stresses the following matters:

- The recipient of the organ and tissue must use the organ and tissue responsibly.
- It is permissible to transplant organs and tissues from a Muslim donor to a non-Muslim recipient, and vice versa.
- It is not permissible to donate organs and tissues from a Muslim donor to a kafirharbi (non-Muslim who wages war on Muslims) [57].

Organ Sale

Paying people to donate their kidneys is one of the most contentious ethical issues being debated at the moment. The most common arguments against this practice include:

- Donor safety;
- Unfair appeal of financial incentives to the economically disadvantaged;
- Turning the body into a money-making tool "commodity";
- Wealthy people would be able to access more readily.

The idea of nonfinancial incentives may be rising in popularity as a way to entice people to donate their organs. Financial incentives aimed at encouraging living donation have received much attention from bioethicists lately. Most experts argue that buying and selling human organs is an immoral and disrespectful practice [58]. The moral objection raised most, is that selling organs will appeal to the socio-economically disadvantaged (poor, uneducated people) and these groups will be unfairly pressured to sell their organs by the promise of money. International trade in human organs, occur particularly in the developing countries of the world where cadaveric organs are not easily available and where there is marked disparity in wealth. As a consequence, a deplorable type of medical practice has emerged, where human kidneys are bought from the poor for transplantation into the wealthy clientele with soaring profits for brokers, private hospitals and physician [59]. It is estimated that since 1980, over 2,000 kidneys are sold annually in India, Iraq, Philippines, Iran and elsewhere, to wealthy recipients from the Middle East, the Far

East and Europe. Human organ ("Kidneys") trade has shifted from India to Pakistan [60]. Media had gone to the extent of labeling it as shifting of "Kidney Bazar," "Bombay Bazar" from India to Karachi, Lahore and Islamabad [61].

In Saudi Arabia, the government controls the organ transplantation through SCOT (Saudi Center for Organ Transplantation). It gives incentives to the living donors and the families of the deceased donors.

In Iran, the government control and distributes the incentives for the living donors.

The World Health Organization argues that transplantation promote health, but the notion of "transplantation tourism" has the potential to violate human rights or exploit the poor, to have unintended health consequences, and to provide unequal access to services, all of which ultimately may cause harm. Thus WHO called to ban compensated organ transplanting and asked member states to protect the most vulnerable from transplant tourism and organ trade [62]. However, as disincentives becomes a must, adding incentives back, such as improving life condition for organ donors after donation, becomes difficult [63].

The Role of the Relatives in Postmortal Organ Procurement

Respecting the decision of the deceased person, whether in favor of or against organ donation, is a common starting point for the different legal systems which regulate the procurement of postmortal organs for transplantation.

However, opt-in systems claim a higher respect for the requirement of consent than the opt-out systems. When no legally valid decision of the deceased was registered, the family of the deceased can donate the organs of their deceased relative.

The opt-out systems allow harvesting the organs because of the absence of actual rejection from the side of the deceased [64]. The family cannot reject the donation of the organs of their loved one.

Public Media Campaigns

Public media campaigns should "demand the highest standard of transparency and accuracy of information related to healthcare issues so as to enable the general public to make informed decisions about health and lifestyles." In order to overcome these ethical concerns and rehabilitate the ethical image of these media campaigns, Rady et al. propose five practical guidelines: "(1) media campaigns should communicate accurate information to the general public and disclose factual materials with the least amount of bias; (2) conflicting interests in media campaigns should be managed with full public transparency; (3) media campaigns should disclose the practical implications of procurement as well as acknowledge the medical, legal, and religious controversies of determining death in organ donation; (4) organ donor registration must satisfy the criteria of informed consent; (5) media campaigns should serve as a means of public education about organ donation and should not be a form of propaganda" [65].

In conclusion, Organ transplantation is a highly complicated issue from an ethical perspective and thus cannot be reduced to one single ethical value. The noble desire to help patients who are in need of organ transplantation by making more donated organs available does not justify overlooking other ethical values such as objectivity in communicating information, the requirement of informed consent, providing psychological care whenever needed and doing justice to the religious aspects of the issue. Overlooking such ethical values can be counterproductive on the long run because potential donors might lose their trust in the whole system and thus decline to donate their organs in the future [66, 67].

New frontiers have been opened and Islamic jurists are keeping pace with the tremendous advances in medicine and technology. This chapter has discussed the pragmatism that prevails in interpreting the Islamic heritage as applied to present-day science.

References

1. Schmidt VH (2003) Transplant medicine as borderline medicine. Med Health Care Philos 6:319–321
2. Encyclopedia Britanica (2013). http://escola.britannica.com.br/article/476842/organ-donation
3. Bollinger R, Stickel D (1986) Historical aspects of transplantation. In: Sabiston D (ed) Textbook of surgery, 13th ed, Philadelphia. W.B. Sunders, London, pp 370–380
4. Peer LA (1955) Transplantation of tissues. William & Wilkins, Baltimore
5. Hawa S (1971) Arrasul (The messenger), 2nd edn, vol 2. Assharikah AlMutahida, Beirut, p 97
6. Asshibani AR (Ibn Adaiba) Hadaiq AlAnwar Wa Matali Aasrar Fi Sirat Annabi AlMokhtar, vol. 1. Ministry of Endowment (nd), Qatar, p 244
7. AlNawawi MS, Almajmooh Shareh AlMohzab. In: AlMutteei M (ed) vol 1. AlFajalah press, Cairo, p 293
8. AlNawawi MS (1978) Minhaj Attalibin. Dar AlFikir, Beirut, vol 1, p 190
9. Asshirbini M, Mughni, Al muhtaj Limarifat Alfaz AlMinjah. Dar AlFikir (nd), Beirut, pp 190–191
10. AlQawzini Z (1978) Ajayib AlMakhlohat (Wonder of creatures). Dar AlAfaaq AlJadidah, Beirut, p 422
11. Ibn Sina, AlHusein ibn Ali, AlKanoon fi Tibb commented by Edward AlQush, Ezzuldin (1987) Publishing House, Beirut 3:2075–2076
12. Wikipedia online en.wikipedia.org/wiki/Organ_transplantation. Accessed 3 May 2015
13. Horvat L, Shariff S, Garg A (2009) Global trends in the rates of living kidney donation. Kidney Int 75:1088–1098
14. Ehtuish E (2011) Ethical controversies in organ transplantation. In understanding the complexities of kidney transplantation. Jorge Ortiz and Jason Andre (ed). InTech Publisher

15. Al Sayyari AA (2008) The history of renal transplantation in the Arab world: a view from Saudi Arabia. Am J Kidney Dis 51(6):1033–1046
16. Al-Meshari K, Al-Shaibani K, Hamawi K et al (2005) The kidney transplant program at king faisal specialist hospital and research center. Clin Transpl 19:119–129
17. Ghaly M (2012) The ethics of organ transplantation: how comprehensive the ethical framework should be? Med Health Care Philos 15:175–179
18. Implied consent is a consent which is not expressly granted by a person, but rather inferred from a person's actions and the facts and circumstances of a particular situation
19. Holy Qur'an 2: 30
20. Holy Qur'an 3:9
21. Holy Qur'an 17: 70
22. AlBukhari M, Sahih AlBukhari C (1958) Matabi Asshab (1378H) 4:135
23. Rispler-Chain V (1989) Islamic medical ethics in the twentith century. J Med Ethics 5: 203–208
24. Abu Dawud, Sunan AbiDaw'ud. Beirut: Dar AlFikir (nd); Kitab AlGanayiz, 3: Hadith No. 3207
25. AlBukhari M, Sahih AlBukhai, Kitab Al Ganayiz; Cairo (1958) MatabiAsshab (1378H) 2:107
26. Ibn AlQayim M. Zad Al ma'ad Fi Hadiy Khir Allbad, Cairo: Mustafa AlBadi Alhalabi
27. AlBukhari M, Sahih AlBukhari, KitabAttib (1958) Cairo: MatabiAsshab (1378H) 7:148–182
28. AlQushairi M. Sahih Muslim Bishareh AlNawawi (1972) Dar AlFikir. Beirut 14:191–200
29. AlBukhari M. Sahih AlBukhari, KitabAzzabayeh, Cairo (1958) MatabiAsshab (1378H) 7:121–122
30. AlQushairi M. Kitab Sahihmuslim Bihsreh A. Nawawi, Kitab AlJihad (1972) Beirut Dar AlFikir 12:37
31. Ahmed ibn Hanbal, Musnad Ahmend, Cairo: Dar Almaarif Publishing Co. (nd) 1;338; 2:13, 5:168, 173
32. Sharafuddin A. AlAhkam Asriyah Lil-Amal Attibiyah (1983) National council for culture, Arts and literature. Kuwait, pp 89–160
33. Ibid
34. Dar Allfta Almisryah, Al-Fatwa Allslamiyah (1982) Cairo: The Supreme Islamic Council, Ministry od Endowment, Fatwa of Sheikh Hassan Maamoon (No. 1065, 9 June 1959), 2278–2282, and Fiqh Academy Book of Decrees. Decree No. 1:55-58
35. Dar Allfta Almisryah, Al-Fatwa Allslamiyah (1982) Cairo: The Supreme Islamic Council, Ministry of Endowment, 7:2495
36. Dar Allfta Almisryah, Al-Fatwa Allslamiyah (1982) Cairo: The Supreme Islamic Council, Ministry of Endowment, 7:2552
37. Dar Allfta Almisryah, Al-Fatwa Allslamiyah (1982) Cairo: The Supreme Islamic Council, Ministry od Endowment, 6:2278–2282
38. Dar AllftaAlmisryah, Al-Fatwa Allslamiyah (1982) Cairo: The Supreme Islamic Council, Ministry od Endowment, 7:2505–2507
39. Ibid (1983) 10:3702–3715
40. Abu Ziad B (1988) Attashrith AlGothmani Wanagel Watta'weed Allnsani. Majalat Majmah AlFiqh Allslami, Jeddah: organization of Islamic Conference, vol 1, pp 145–146
41. Ibid
42. Saudi Grand Ulema (1987) Fatwa No. 99 dated 6/11/1402H (25 August 1982). Majalat AlMajma AlFiqhi: J Fiqh Acad 1:37
43. Ibid
44. Fiqh Academy Book of Decrees (1988) Decree No. 5, 3rd Conference of Islamic Jurists (Amman: 11-6 October 1986). Jeddah: Figh Academy and Islamic Organization of Medicine Sciences p. 34
45. Ibid
46. Seminar on new issues in organ transplantation (Kuwait: October 1989). Jeddah: Fiqh Academy and Islamic Organization of Medical Sciences (not yet published); & Fiqh Academy

Decree and Recommendations for the 6 th Conference of Islam Jurists (Jeddah, 14-20 March 1990). Decrees No. 56/5/6; 58/8/6

47. Fiqh Academy Decree and Recommendations for the 6th Conference of Islam Jurists (Jeddah, 14–20 March 1990). Decrees No. 56/5/6; 58/8/6; and Islamic Jurisprudence Council, Islamic World League, Makkah- Saudi Arabia, session 17, 2003, Fatwa No. 3, Book of Resolutions 17th session, 13-17 December 2003, Makkah: Islamic World League; 2003. pp 33–35

48. Ghaly M. op.cit

49. Majlis al-Urubbıli al-Ifta' waal-Buḥuth, al- (2002) Qararat wafatawa [Resolutions and fatwas]. Cairo: Daral-Tawzai wa al-Nashral-Islamiyya; and Ghaly, M op.cit

50. Ghaly M. op.cit

51. Van den Branden S, Broeckaert B (2011) The ongoing charity of organ donation. Contemporary English Sunni fatwas on organdonation and blood transfusion. Bioethics 25 (3):167–175

52. Buskens L (2009) An Islamic Triangle. Changing Relationships Between Shari'a, State Law, and Local Customs. ISIM Newsletter 2000; 5: 8; A. Cairo

53. Van den Branden S. op.cit

54. Warta Kerajaan Negeri Pulau Pinang—HukumTransplan Organ danTisu. (2010). Ref. no.: JMNPP/ (S)/19/1101/001(16); PUNPP 152.100.1/2/2 Jld. 2. Enakmen No. 864

55. The living donor should be competent adult over the age of 18 years as, other Fatwas have delineated. The guardian of a minor or incompetent person, cannot donate the organs of the person under his guardianship

56. The Fatwas from Saudi Arabia (Senior Ulema), Kuwait, Islamic jurist council of Islamic World League, Makkah Al Mukaramah and Organization of Islamic Conferences' Islamic Fiqh Academy (OIC-IFA) stipulated that a living donor should be adult and the donation of the guardian of the minor is invalid

57. Organ Transplantation from the Islamic perspective. Ministry of Health Malaysia in collaboration with Malaysia department of Islamic development (JAKIM) (2011)

58. Daar AS (1998) Paid organ donation-the grey basket concept. J Med Ethics 24:365–368

59. Danovitch GM, Delmonico FL (2008) The prohibition of kidney sales and organ markets should remain. Curr Opin Organ Transplant

60. Noorani MA (2008) Commercial transplantation in Pakistan. BMJ 336:1378

61. Sajjad I, Baines LS, Patel P et al (2008) Commercialization of kidney transplants: a systematic review of outcomes in recipients and donors. Am J Nephrol 28:744–754

62. Bulletin of the World Health Organization (2007) by World Health Organization, 85(1):1–84

63. Organ trafficking and transplantation pose new challenges (2004) Bull World Health Organ 82 (9):639–718

64. Ghaly M. op.cit

65. Rady M, McGregor J, Verheijde J (2012) Mass media campaigns and organ donation: managing conflicting messages and interests. Med Health Care Philos 15(2):229–241

66. Ghaly M. op.cit

67. Chamsi-Pasha H, Albar MA (2014) Kidney transplantation: ethical challenges in the Arab world. Saudi J Kidney Dis Transpl 25(3):489–495

Chapter 14
Brain Death

Introduction

The diagnosis of death is, in most countries, the legal responsibility of a medical practitioner. It marks a point in time after which consequences occur including no medical or legal requirement to provide resuscitation or life-sustaining technologies, loss of personhood, and most individual rights, the opportunity for organ donation and autopsy proceedings, execution of the decedent's legal will, estate and property transfer, payment of life insurance, final disposition of the body and, of course, religious, or social ceremonies to mark the end of a life [1].

A definition of death, just like a definition of life, continues to elude philosophers. Death can be considered in terms of medical, legal, ethical, philosophical, societal, cultural, and religious rationales. The medical definition of death is primarily a scientific issue based on the best available evidence [2].

Definition of Death

Death is defined by almost all cultures and religions as the departure of the soul out of the body. The old Egyptians, Chinese, Hindus, Judiasm, Christianity, and Islam agreed to this definition, but they differed on the concept of soul and whether it will depart into another body or remain in limbo until resurrection when it will go back to its old body with new formulation that will give it the ability for life forever.

Both the Hellenic and Judeo Christian cultures identified death with the departure of soul from the body. In 1957, Pope Pius XII speaking to an International Congress of Anesthetists, raised the question of whether one should continue the resuscitation process despite the fact that the soul may already have left the body [3].

In Islam death is the departure of the soul out of the body. The soul is created by Allah (God) but remains afterwards eternal and will not die, but will either be

© The Author(s) 2015
M.A. Al-Bar and H. Chamsi-Pasha, *Contemporary Bioethics*,
DOI 10.1007/978-3-319-18428-9_14

chastised or eulogized until the day of resurrection when it will be reunited with the body for a new eternal life either in Hell or Paradise.

The embryo and fetus has a vegetative and then animated life but will not have a human life except after ensoulment which only occurs at 120 days from the moment of conception (fertilization) as narrated by Prophet Muhammad (PBUH) [4]. Ibn AlQaiym said: If it is asked "Does the embryo before breathing of the soul unto it, has a life? It is answered that it has a vegetative life like a growing plant. Its movements and perception are not voluntary. When the soul is breathed in it acquires sentience and volition" [5].

It is clear that the embryo and fetus has a pumping heart and circulation long before ensoulment occurs. The circulation and pumping heart denote a lower level of life (vegetative or even animated but not a human life which only occur after ensoulment and which is directly connected to the higher functions of the brain). As death is defined as departure of the soul out of the body, and as the soul cannot be identified by mortal human beings, the signs accompanying this departure are looked for, the most important of which is the irreversible loss of respiration. The word "nafs" in Arabic means Soul, and the word "nafas" means Respiration and if respiration (nafas) ceases irreversibly then the "nafs" (the soul) has left the body.

There are other signs described by the Islamic Jurists like glaring of eyeballs (the vision following the soul as it departs), limpness of the feet, bending of the nose, whitening of the temple, etc. [6]. These signs are not definite of death. The important sign is the irreversible loss of respiration plus the irreversible loss of consciousness.

Christopher Pallis conceived human death as a state in which there is irreversible loss of the capacity of consciousness combined with the irreversible loss of the capacity to breath [7]. The concept is a hybrid one, expressing both Philosophical and Physiological attributes.

It also agrees with the old observation of linking "nafs" (soul) with "nafas" (respiration) as already explained. The irreversible loss of consciousness and responsiveness to external or internal stimulation is of paramount importance.

Clinical examination should provide evidence of the irreversible damage of the brain especially the brain stem. (These will be discussed later in more detail).

Death is a result of the irreversible loss of these functions in the brain; either from an intracranial cause such as trauma or hemorrhage, or from an extracranial cause such as cardiorespiratory arrest, where impaired cerebral perfusion will culminate in cerebral and brainstem damage.

There is growing consensus that there is a unifying medical concept of death; all human death is anatomically located to the brain. That is, human death involves the irreversible loss of the capacity for consciousness, combined with the irreversible loss of the capacity to breathe. These two essential capacities are found in the brain, particularly the brainstem, and represent the most basic manner in which the human organism can sense and interact with its environment [8].

The most appropriate set of criteria to use is determined by the circumstances in which the medical practitioner is called upon to diagnose death. The three criteria sets are somatic (features visible on external inspection of the corpse), circulatory (after cardiorespiratory arrest), and neurological (in patients in coma on mechanical ventilation); and represent a diagnostic standard in which the medical profession and the public can have complete confidence [9].

Brain Death: Medical Background

Although it is more than 40 years since the concept of brain death was first introduced to clinical practice, many of the controversies that surround it have not been settled. These include the relationship between brain death and death of the whole person, the international differences in the nomenclature and criteria for the determination of brain death, and the inextricable links between brain death and organ donation [10].

The development of organ transplantation and the associated need to determine death before organ retrieval led to the publication of the first widely accepted standard for the confirmation of brain death by an ad hoc Committee of the Harvard Medical School in 1968 [11]. Although this early link with organ donation might give the impression that brain death was a construct designed only to facilitate donation, this is incorrect. Most importantly, the confirmation of brain death allows the withdrawal of therapies that can no longer conceivably benefit an individual who has died.

In the UK, a Conference of the Medical Royal Colleges and their faculties produced guidance for the diagnosis of brain (stem) death in 1976 [12] and, in a subsequent memorandum 3 year later, equated brain death with death of the whole person for the first time [13]. In the USA, the 1981 Uniform Determination of Death Act (UDDA) gave equivalence to death determined by neurological and cardio-vascular criteria, although it did not mandate a standard by which brain death should be determined, confirming only that this should be in accordance with accepted medical standards [14].

The UDDA relies on the whole-brain formulation and states that "an individual, who has sustained irreversible cessation of all functions of the entire brain, including the brain-stem, is dead."

This forms the standard for the determination of death by neurological criteria in the USA and most European countries and is based, in theory at least, on confirmation of the loss of all brain function including, but not limited to, the brainstem [15].

Unlike whole-brain death, the diagnosis of brainstem death, such as that used in the UK, does not require confirmation that all brain functions have ceased, rather that none of those functions that might persist should indicate any form of consciousness [16].

The determination of brainstem death requires confirmation of the "irreversible loss of the capacity for consciousness combined with the irreversible loss of the capacity to breathe" and relies on the fact that key components of consciousness and respiratory control, the reticular activating system and nuclei for cardiorespiratory regulation, reside in the brainstem [17].

Death is not a single event but a process that leads progressively to the failure of all functions that constitute the life of the human organism. There have always been individuals that do not accept that brain death equates to the death of the individual.

Initially, it was argued that brain death equates to the death of the individual because, after brain death, the body ceases to be an integrated organism and rapidly becomes a disintegrating collection of organs which have permanently lost the capacity to work as a coordinated whole [18]. However, it is now clear that brain-dead patients can show levels of somatic integration that may persist for some time [19, 20].

The US President's Council on Bioethics proposed a new unifying concept of death in 2008. The Council reiterated its support for a whole brain formulation and rejected a reliance on brainstem death, arguing that the inner state of a person with residual cortical activity in the complete absence of brainstem activity is unknown.

Preconditions for the Diagnosis of Brain Death

Before proceeding to make the diagnosis of Brain Death, the following conditions should be present:

- Patient in deep coma, and the cause of the coma firmly established.
- The patient has no spontaneous respiration and is on the ventilator.
- The event causing brain death occurred at least 6 h previously and the cause of death has been established.
- Complete areflexia (spinal reflexes excepted).

<u>Exclusions</u>

- Core body temperature above 35.5 C.
- Toxicology testing for drug overdose, narcotics, alcohol and hypnotics should be done in unexplained cases of coma or in road traffic accidents. If no toxicology lab is available and there is suspicion of drug overdose, an interval of 5 days should lapse before testing for brain death.
- The patient should not be receiving any sedatives, muscle relaxants, hypnotics, narcotics, or antidepressants.
- Patients with metabolic and endocrine causes of coma should be excluded until the metabolic and endocrine derangements corrected.
- Patients shall not have any signs of cerebral activity like decerebrate or decorticate posture and seizure activities.
- Patient is not in cardiovascular shock.
- No physician should determine brain death in patients with a (possible reversible) septic shock or rapidly proceed with testing in patients seen soon after arrival in the emergency department [21].

Clinical Assessment

1. Lack of response to stimulation (spinal reflexes excepted).
2. Absence of brain stem reflexes:

    a. Fixed pupils to light
    b. Corneal reflexes
    c. Occulocephalic reflexes
    d. Occulovestibular reflexes (50 ml of ice cold water)
    e. Gag reflex
    f. Cough reflex
    g. Apnea test: absence of spontaneous breathing when the patient is disconnected from the ventilator for 10 min so that the arterial CO_2 pressure is more than 50 mm of Hg (Pa CO_2 54 mmHg) i.e. hypocapnia is excluded. At the same time O_2 is administered through a catheter into the trachea. This test is only done at the end of the second examination and confirmatory tests performed. It is mandatory to repeat the clinical tests by two consultant Physicians and done separately.

Confirmatory Tests (Required in Saudi-Arabia and some other countries)

- EEG of 30 min duration should be silent or
- Absence of blood flow to the brain proved by Doppler or cerebral angiograms or CT Angiography or MRI Angiography, etc.

The period between the two tests depends on the age of the patient:

1. Infants: (7 days to 2 months) : 48 hours confirmed by two flat EEGs
2. Infants: (2 months to 1 year) : 24 h confirmed by 2 flat EEGs
3. 1 year-Puberty: 12 h confirmed by one flat EEG
4. Adults: 6 h confirmed by one flat EEG

As the EEG denotes cerebral activity, it is imperative to confirm the absence of blood flow to the brain by cerebral angiography or CT Angio or MRI angio or Doppler.

Both clinical examinations should be completed and signed by the two consultants Physicians conducting the tests (Neurologist, Neurosurgeon, Anesthetist, or Intensivist).

The Executive Medical Officer (CMO) or designee should countersign, before any supportive means are disconnected. The relatives of the brain dead person should be approached tactfully to either donate organs of their beloved one or to disconnect the deceased from the ventilator. The Fatwas of the ulema and Islamic Jurisprudence Councils which allow disconnections of the machines help the relatives to accept the diagnosis. However, many relatives ask for continuation of ventilation and management until asystole occurs. This is a big burden on the staff, expense to the community and deprivation of the machines when the sources are limited.

Differences in Establishing the Diagnosis

Despite general consensus on the concept of brain death, there are major international differences in its diagnosis. The majority of countries have followed the lead of the USA and the UK in specifying that the clinical diagnosis of brain death is sufficient for the determination of death in adults [21].

While there is unanimity that confirmation of the absence of brainstem reflexes is fundamental to the clinical determination of brain death, there are wide variations in the requirements for the conduct of the apnea test. This is concerning because the confirmation of apnea is fundamental to the determination of brain death (either whole brain or brainstem) and this can only be assured if the degree of acute hypercarbia is sufficient to stimulate the respiratory centre.

A second clinical examination is required in many countries and this was presumably introduced to minimize the likelihood of errors in diagnosis.

However, while there is no convincing evidence that a second test is necessary, there is evidence that it delays the determination of brain death [22]. A second apnea test is not required in some countries that mandate two clinical examinations, but omission of this crucial component from one of the examinations is illogical. The mandated time interval between the two examinations also varies. While a 24 h period is usual after hypoxic–ischemic brain injury, the time frame is already mentioned depending on the age of the individual.

Some brain death guidelines specify the qualification and level of experience of those determining death, and most explicitly exclude anyone involved in organ transplantation.

The number of doctors required to determine brain death also varies widely, although most commonly a single doctor is sufficient. Two doctors (the UK standard) are required in only around one-third of countries. Some jurisdictions mandate that two different doctors must determine brain death only when organ transplantation is being considered. There is variability in the diagnostic criteria for brain death reported between hospitals and different countries.

Confirmatory Tests

It is widely accepted that brain death is a clinical diagnosis and that confirmatory laboratory tests are recommended when specific components of the clinical testing cannot be evaluated. An ideal confirmatory test should be safe, accurate, and inexpensive [23]. Confirmatory investigations generally fall into two general categories. These either demonstrate the loss of electrical activity of the brain or confirm the absence of intracerebral blood flow [24].

Confirmatory tests are optional in most countries and reserved for circumstances where some doubt exists about the clinical diagnosis of brain death (e.g. after infusion of long-acting sedative drugs such as thiopental) or because the patient might be too unstable to undergo an apnea test [25].

In clinical practice, EEG, cerebral angiography, nuclear scan, transcranial Doppler (TCD), CT Angiography (CTA), and magnetic resonance angiography (MRI/MRA) are currently used ancillary tests in adults. Most hospitals will have the logistics in place to perform and interpret an EEG, transcranial Doppler, nuclear scan, or cerebral angiogram, and these tests may be considered the preferred tests. Transcranial Doppler is the easiest and cheapest.

CT-A is easily accessible in almost every hospital, offers a high spatiotemporal resolution, is operator independent and inexpensive. The results of CT-A are comparable to other established brain perfusion techniques in brain death [26].

Ancillary tests can be used when uncertainty exists about the reliability of parts of the neurologic examination or when the apnea test cannot be performed. The interpretation of each of these tests requires expertise. In adults, ancillary tests are needed to confirm the clinical diagnosis of brain death. Physicians ordering ancillary tests should appreciate the disparities between tests and the potential for false-positives (i.e., the test suggests brain death, but the patient does not meet clinical criteria).

Rather than ordering ancillary tests, physicians may decide not to proceed with the declaration of brain death if clinical findings are unreliable [27]. Ancillary tests may play an important role in shortening periods of observation, but the Subcommittee of the American Academy of Neurology concluded that there are not enough data to show that newer tests confirm the termination of whole brain functioning.

Confirmatory tests are not specifically recommended in current UK guidance and it is time for a broad debate on the role, type, and application of ancillary tests and publication of consensus guidance that has professional support [28]. The High Committee on brain death in Saudia Arabia insists on performing an EEG before establishing the diagnosis of brain death. Other ancillary tests are optional.

We think that confirming the absence of intracerebral brain flow e.g. by transcranial Doppler is feasible, inexpensive and will reduce the resistance against accepting brain death as death.

Islamic Views of Brain Death

Death etymologically means departure of the soul out of the body, and cessation of the signs of life. Al-Ghazzali (d 505 AH/1111 CE), an influential Islamic scholar, says that separation of the soul from the body is the end of its dominance over the body [29].

According to Al-Ghazzâlî and all Muslim Scholars, the event of death occurs when the soul is separated from the body [30]. Thus, the event of death is just a 'change of state'. The fact pointed out by certain Qur'anic verses and hadiths (prophetic traditions) pertaining to this subject that death is not simply a type of change; but the soul separated from the body is either in a state of punishment, or in a mode of blessing [31].

The Islamic faith values human life. It values any means to save a human life, and condemns the termination of a human life without just cause: "And kill not anyone whom God has forbidden, except for a just cause (according to Islamic law)" [32]. Muslim scholars who advocate organ donation commonly cite the verse:

"if anyone killed a person—not in retaliation of murder, or (and) to spread mischief in the land—it would be as if he killed all mankind, and if anyone saved a life, it would be as if he saved the life of all mankind" [33] and emphasizing the latter, i.e., the saving of a human life being of a paramount value with such actions to be rewarded as if they involved the saving of the whole of mankind [34].

Is brain death equal to cardiopulmonary (traditional) death or is brain death just an intermediate state between life and death?. Which formulation, whole-brain or brain-stem death, is consonant with Islamic bioethics?. Finally what are the clinical responsibilities of physicians to patients in these states? [35]

An Islamic consensus on brain death is lacking. Some equate brain death with cardiopulmonary collapse, both being death proper in Islamic law. Others hold brain death to be an in-between state between life and death, where life support need not be continued, while some have rejected the concept in toto [36].

The Fatwa of Khomeni and Mufti of Egypt in early sixties allowed procurement of organs from "dead" persons with the classical definition of death with irreversible cardiac and respiratory failure and followed by death of the whole body. Iran officially accepted "Brain Death" in 2003.

In their Fatwa of 1982, The Senior Religious Scholars of Saudi-Arabia mentioned only obtaining organs from living and dead donors. They never recognized "Brain Death" as "Death" up till now. However, they allowed stopping the ventilators and resuscitative measures. When the heart and circulation stops, then organs could be retrieved if the family agrees.

Two of the most influential bodies of Islamic bioethicolegal deliberation are the Organization of Islamic Conferences' Islamic Fiqh Academy (OIC-IFA) and the Islamic Organization of Medical Sciences (IOMS). Both organizations bring together scholars of Islam and medicine for Islamic ethico-legal deliberation around bioethical challenges faced in the Muslim and non-Muslim world.

The first discussion of Brain Death started by Islamic Organization for Medical Sciences (IOMS) in Kuwait in 1985 and both the The Islamic Fiqh Academy of the Organization of Islamic Conference (OIC-IFA) and The Islamic jurist council of Islamic World League, Makkah started then to discuss the issue of Brain Death.

During a 1985 meeting of the Islamic Organization for Medical Sciences (IOMS) Islamic scholars and medical scientists equated brain stem death, and allowed for removal of life support [37].

The Fatwa of the The Islamic Fiqh Academy of the Organization of Islamic Conference on resuscitation apparatus (October 1986) incorporated the concept of brain death into the legal definition of death in Islam:

[A] Person is pronounced legally dead and consequently, all dispositions of the Islamic law in case of death apply if one of the two following conditions has been established: (1) there is total cessation of cardiac and respiratory functions, and doctors have ruled that such cessation is irreversible; (2) there is total cessation of all cerebral functions and experienced specialized doctors have ruled that such cessation is irreversible and the brain has started to disintegrate [38].

Some Muslim countries adopted this definition of death after the enactment of the Uniform Determination of Death Act (UDDA) in the United States, which stated that: An individual who has sustained either (1) irreversible cessation of circulatory and respiratory functions, or (2) irreversible cessation of all functions of the entire brain, including the brain stem, is dead. A determination of death must be made in accordance with accepted medical standards. (National Conference of Commissioners on Uniform State Laws 1981).

The Islamic jurist council of Islamic World League allowed in 1987 stopping the ventilators in brain dead persons. It resisted taking organs from brain dead patients. The Pulmonary Circulatory death should be announced first; then organs could be taken if the relatives agree.

This Fatwa concurs with the Fatwa of High Scholars of Saudi Arabia (including the grand Mufti Sheikh Bin Baz) which was passed in 1983, and allowed stopping the ventilators from brain dead persons, as it was considered futile to continue hooking such persons to machines; but death will not be announced until after the stoppage of circulation and respiration [39].

The IOMS revisited the issue in 1996 after they sent three members to participate in an international bioethics conference. These members reported back to the IOMS, this time with some eminent Islamic Scholars attending the meeting including Sheikh Yousef Al-Qardawy, Sheikh Khaled Al-Mathkoor, Professor of Islamic Law in Kuwait University, Dr. Ibrahim Ali Hasan, the Vice President of the High Government Council in Egypt, and Dr. Abdullah Al Isa, Vice President of the High Court of Kuwait. (Dr. Mohammed Albar had the privilege of presenting a paper in that meeting as well).

The meeting was called for because an Egyptian professor of Anesthesia (Dr. Safwat H Lutfi) campaigned against brain death both in the medical circles and media (newspaper, television and public meetings) in Egypt, and stirred antagonism against the physicians who wanted to take organs from poor people and give them to wealthy persons for money!! It was then discussed by Al-Azhar and the parliament which was about to accept brain death. He succeeded in stopping this approval. He was called to Kuwait to attend this meeting and IOM sent a delegation of three people to attend an international conference on brain death held in San Francisco, 21–25 November 1996 to obtain an update on the subject.

Utilitarian reasoning would be invoked to facilitate end-of-life organ procurement because "…it is a pity to waste such candidate cadavers without trying to save the life of many others who need their organs" [40].

The Islamic Medical Association of North America (IMANA) also contributes to the discussions of brain death through an Islamic lens. IMANA's support of brain death is as follows: A person is considered dead when the conditions given below are met… A specialist physician (or physicians) has determined that after standard examination, the function of the brain, including the brain stem, has come to a permanent stop, even if some other organs may continue to show spontaneous activity [41].

In summary, the literature most accessible to practicing clinicians uses the OIC-IFA and IOMS assessments as support for brain death within Islamic law [42]. It is important to note that no mention of brain death was available in Islamic countries before 1985. All the discussions since the time of Ibn Sina (Avicenna) and Nawawi were on death of the whole person.

Controversies in Brain Death

Despite its name, the Universal Determination of Death Act has not been universally accepted. Ethicists and physician experts have taken issue with the concept of brain death and the medical standards by which it is diagnosed. Some feel that the clinical examination alone is insufficiently sensitive to detect loss of all brain function and that ancillary tests of cerebral blood flow or electroencephalographic activity should be mandatory [43]. Others feel that we are too lax in our definition of "all functions of the brain" and that we inappropriately declare dead patients in whom neuroendocrine function persists. Still others feel that brain death is an artificial construct created expressly for the purpose of generating more organ donors and creating the illusion of moral soundness [44].

The public must believe that the priority of the medical system is to save lives rather than to obtain organs to feel confident that they would become organ donors only after all reasonable attempts to save their lives have failed.

Strict adherence to published guidelines and medical standards for determining brain death is the minimum requirement for maintaining public trust [45].

A person should be declared (brain) dead because he or she is in fact dead, rather than because of any potential for organ donation. In this way, the professional and legal acceptability of withdrawal of treatment (including mechanical ventilation) which is merely prolonging somatic function can be assured. The recently updated Code of Practice in the UK has separated completely the diagnosis and confirmation of death from issues surrounding organ donation and this is helpful.

Opponents of Brain Death concept

The Muslim opponents of Brain Death concept criticize it in several points:

I. They claim that the 2010 update of the American Academy of Neurology guidelines for determining brain death fail to meet the three essential requirements stated in the Islamic definition of death: (1) total cessation of all brain functions, (2) irreversibility of cessation, and (3) the onset of disintegration of the brain [46].

The opponents argue that there are two consequences of using a medically faulty criterion of death in organ donation. First, organ procurement is performed in the operating room with no general anesthesia because donors are presumed dead [47]. To avoid Lazarus Phenomenon, most surgeons require general anesthesia to procure organs from brain dead individuals.

Second, donors are not legally dead if they do not fulfill the criterion of death stipulated in the Resolution of the Council of Islamic Jurisprudence on Resuscitation Apparatus (1986).

Padela et al. [48] have pointed out the serious gaps in contemporary medical understanding and clinical diagnosis of brain death and its endorsement as human death in the Islamic faith. These gaps pertained to: (1) the retention of residual brain functions; (2) the recovery of some previously ceased brain functions; (3) the absence of whole brain degeneration and necrosis; and (4) the uncertainty of medical tests and bedside examination in determining this condition with reasonable accuracy [49].

Bedir and Aksoy [50] concluded that brain-dead patients should be cared for as living humans who could still suffer from surgical procedures performed on them. Prof. Sachedina has acknowledged that the Western concept of death that equated brain death with human death was incompatible with Islamic teachings because: .... the Qur'anic view of human person, the nafs [soul], that rejects the dichotomization of human personality into a body and mind, is at the root of theological debate on the relationship between life and death. As a nafs who dies through the divine decree any definition of this nafs's death must focus on the criteria that determines the death of the whole human rather than just a part of his biological existence. In other words, no definition of death that fails to take a living person, as seen in the Qur'an, can have a valid ground for acceptance in Islamic jurisprudence [51].

II. The opponents say that: the guidelines should reliably establish the irreversible cessation of all functions of the entire brain including the brainstem, yet neither "irreversibility" nor "function of the brain" (or "of the entire brain") is defined. Both of these terms have engendered unresolved controversies. The American Academy of Neurology Subcommittee does not identify the gold standard by which sensitivity, specificity, and predictive accuracy of the guidelines as a diagnostic tool are measured, with respect to either the irreversibility or the totality aspects. This gold standard does not and will never exist in the opinion of some authorities. Therefore, diagnostic guidelines for brain death are inherently unable to be validated through an evidence-based methodology [52].

III. Some state that there is mounting scientific evidence that neither the Neurological Standard (namely, whole brain or brain stem death) nor the circulatory criteria (namely absent arterial pulse and circulatory arrest for 2–5 min), specifically developed to declare death for procuring transplantable organs, is consistent with human death [53, 54].

In medical practice, there are two types of end-of-life organ donation.

The first is called "heart beating organ donation" and is performed on a person with spontaneously beating heart and circulation after declaring death using a Neurological Standard of whole brain (in USA) or brain stem death (in Europe).

The second is called "non-heart beating organ donation" and is performed on a person who has controlled or non-controlled cessation of spontaneously beating heart and absent arterial pulse of 2–5 min. However, there are scientific flaws with this criterion: (1) the heart is capable of recovering its mechanical function and spontaneous regular beating, and (2) the whole brain, including the brainstem, can remain viable after 2–5 min of absent arterial pulse [55, 56]. Therefore, the ceased physiological functions of the cardiovascular, respiratory, and neurological systems are reversible at the time of procuring organs from non-heart-beating donors.

This criterion was opposed by The High Committee on brain death in Saudi-Arabia.

IV. The opponents state that the concern regarding the validity of the clinical criteria has been reinforced by a recent report of 2 cases of well-documented clinical brain death with return of spontaneous respiration during the period of preparation for organ harvesting [57].

Rebuttal

I. The authors of the updated American guidelines state that: The gold standard for the diagnosis of brain death is a neurologic examination and irreversible loss of all brainstem function. They never claimed that the clinical examination of brain death implies loss of all neuronal function [58].

II. The American Evidence-based guideline update published in 2010 stated that "in adults, there are no published reports of recovery of neurologic function after a diagnosis of brain death using the criteria reviewed in the 1995 American Academy of Neurology practice parameter." All "recovered" adult cases reported in the literature and those in the media are suspect due to presence of confounders, no detailed description of testing, or no mention of the apnea test [59, 60].

Dr. Martin Smith from Queen Square, London confirms that: "The criteria for the determination of brain death are robust" [61]. He also states that the recent reports describing the apparent "reversibility" of brain death have been refuted because of failure to adhere to such standard guidelines [62].

The authors of the updated American guidelines also states that rare cases of brain death claimed to being reversible have been reported [63–66]. These cases report transient return of some neurological function after a diagnosis of death using neurological criteria [67]. In some cases, the details are unclear regarding whether an acceptable apnea test was performed. In two infants aged 3 months, apnea testing was adequately described, and brain death confirmed for >24 h, with later return of some brainstem function [68]. Together with the other report in an infant aged 10 months, these three cases illustrate that brain death as currently diagnosed can be reversible [69]. The author of one of these reports clearly says that "It should be noted that in most cases of children pronounced brain dead these guidelines are not followed" [70].

The outcome in these three cases with a confirmed apnea test and reversal of brain death was dismal, with profound brain injury, and ultimate death [71].

Recommendations for brain death determination may require revision for infants, to more clearly define a time interval between examinations and to incorporate consideration of confounding sedative drug effects.

III. The preservation of spinal and autonomic (cardiovascular) function and reflexes after the diagnosis of death using neurological criteria has led to concern by some clinicians that this residual function represents evidence for continued or potential consciousness. There is overwhelming evidence that continued spinal cord activity, including complex withdrawal movements (Lazarus sign), is possible and indeed expected after a diagnosis of death using neurological criteria [72, 73].

IV. The continued secretion of pituitary hormones observed in some cases of confirmed "brain death" is not a surprise, since anatomically the posterior pituitary and, to a lesser degree the anterior pituitary (indirect partial supply via short portal vessels), is supplied by the inferior hypophysial artery, which is extra-dural in origin [74, 75].

Conclusion

Although guidelines are available in many countries to standardize national processes for the diagnosis of brain death, the current variation and inconsistency in practice make it imperative that an international consensus is developed. This should clarify the criteria for the determination of brain death and provide specific instructions about the clinical examination necessary and the conduct of the apnea test. It should also stipulate the role and type of confirmatory investigations, and detail the required level of documentation. An international consensus on the determination of brain death is desirable, essential, and long overdue [76].

Following established guidelines scrupulously can maintain the foundation of a transplantation system that saves thousands of lives a year [77]. Confirmatory test is mandatory to establish the absence of blood flow to the brain by cerebral angiography or CT Angio or MRI angio or Doppler. Infants diagnosed as Brain Dead should have a longer period (48 h) for the second test, prior to declaration of Brain Death.

On the issue of equating brain death with human death, the Islamic jurist council of Islamic World League held in Makkah Al Mukaramah (December 1987), which passed Decree No. 2, did not equate cardiac death with brain death. Although it did not recognize brain death as death, it did sanction all the previous Fatwas on organ transplantation. It allowed harvesting organs if the circulation stops irreversibly [78].

Islamic juridical deliberations around brain death largely took place over 25 years ago in response to medical developments and ethical controversies in the Western world. As these developments have been transplanted into Muslim contexts, the debates within Muslim bioethics need both updating and deepening with regard to the early rulings on brain death [79].

References

1. Shemie SD (2007) Clarifying the paradigm for the ethics of donation and transplantation: was 'dead' really so clear before organ donation? Philos Ethics Humanit Med 2:18
2. Gardiner D, Shemie S, Manara A, Opdam H (2012) International perspective on the diagnosis of death. Br J Anaesth 108(Suppl 1):i14–i28
3. Pope Pius XII (1957) Prolongation of Life. Pope Speaks 4:393–398
4. AlBokhari M:(Sahih AlBokhari) Kitab Al Qadar, Kitab Al Anbiya, Kitab Al Tawhid and Sahih Muslim, Kitab Al Qadar
5. Ibn AlQaiym: AlTibyan fi Aksam Al Qur'an. Dar Alkitab Alarabi, Beirut, 1989
6. Albar M (1995) Organ transplantation: an Islamic perspective. In: Albar M (ed) Contemporary topics in Islamic medicine. Saudi Publishing House, Jeddah, pp 3–11

7. Pallis C (1983) ABC of brain stem death. BMJ Publication, London, p 2
8. Gardiner D. op.cit
9. Ibid
10. Smith M (2012) Brain death: time for an international consensus. Br J Anaesth 108(Suppl 1): i6–i9
11. A definition of irreversible coma (1968) Report of the Ad Hoc Committee of the Harvard Medical School to examine the definition of brain death. J Am Med Assoc 205:337–340
12. Diagnosis of brain death (1976) Statement issued by the honorary secretary of the Conference of Medical Royal Colleges and their faculties in the United Kingdom on 11 October 1976. Br Med J 2:1187–1188
13. Ibid
14. Uniform Determination of Death Act. http://www.law.upenn.edu/bll/archives/ulc/fnact99/1980s/udda80.pdf
15. Smith M. op.cit
16. A code of practice for the diagnosis and confirmation of death (2008) Academy of the Medical Royal Colleges, London. http://www.aomrc.org.uk/reports-guidance.html
17. Smith M. op.cit
18. Pallis C (1983) Whole-brain death reconsidered—physiological facts and philosophy. J Med Ethics 9:32–37
19. Shewmon DA (1998) Chronic 'brain death': meta-analysis and conceptual consequences. Neurology 51:1538–1545
20. Wijdicks EF, Varelas PN, Gronseth GS, Greer DM (2011) Evidence-based guideline update: determining brain death in adults: report of the Quality Standards Subcommittee of the American Academy of Neurology. Neurology 76(3):308 (author reply 308–9)
21. Smith M. op.cit
22. Lustbader D, O'Hara D, Wijdicks EF et al (2011) Second brain death examination may negatively affect organ donation. Neurology 76:119–124
23. Wijdicks EF (2006) The clinical criteria of brain death throughout the world: why has it come to this? Can J Anaesth 53:540–543
24. Young GB, Shemie SD, Doig CJ, Teitelbaum J (2006) Brief review: the role of ancillary tests in the neurological determination of death. Can J Anaesth 53:620–627
25. Smith M. op.cit
26. Welschehold S, Kerz T, Boor S, Reuland K, Thömke F, Reuland A, Beyer C, Wagner W, Müller-Forell W, Giese A (2013) Detection of intracranial circulatory arrest in brain death using cranial CT-angiography. Eur J Neurol 20(1):173–179
27. Wijdicks EF (2011). op.cit
28. Smith M. op.cit
29. Al-Ghazzalı, AbuHamıd Muhammad B. Muhammad: Ihya' Ulumal-Dın, vol 4 Beirut: Dar al-Ma'rifah: 493–495. No publication date
30. Ibid
31. Al-Tabarı, Muhammad B. Jarır Jami' al Bayan 'anTawilAyial-Qur'an, vol 1. Beirut: Dar al-Fikr, 1405. AH: 189
32. The Holy Qur'an 6:151
33. The Holy Qur'an 5:32
34. Rady MY, Verheijde JL, Ali MS (2009) Islam and end-of life practices in organ donation for transplantation: new questionsand serious sociocultural consequences. HEC Forum 21 (2):175–205
35. Padela AI, Arozullah A, Moosa E (2013) Brain death in Islamic ethicolegal deliberation: challenges for applied Islamic bioethics. Bioethics 27(3):132–139
36. Ibid
37. Ebrahim AF (1998) Islamic jurisprudence and the end of human life. Med Law 17:189–196
38. Albar MA (1996) Islamic ethics of organ transplantation and brain death. Saudi J Kidney Dis Transplant 7(2):109–114

39. Albar MA (2007) Seeking remedy, abstaining from therapy and resuscitation: an Islamic perspective. Saudi J Kidney Dis Transplant 18(4):629–637

40. Albar MA (2012) Organ transplantation: a Sunni Islamic perspective. Saudi J Kidney Dis Transplant. 23(4):817–822

41. Islamic Medical Association of North America. Mission and Vision. Lombard, IL. http://www.imana.org/mission.html

42. Padela AI (2013). op.cit

43. Tibballs J (2010) A critique of the apneic oxygenation test for the diagnosis of brain death. Pediatr Crit Care Med 11:475–478

44. Joffe AR (2007) The ethics of donation and transplantation: are definitions of death being distorted for organ transplantation? Philos Ethics Humanit Med 2:28

45. Shore PM (2013) Following guidelines for brain death examinations: a matter of trust. Pediatr Crit Care Med 14(1):98–99

46. Rady MY (2009). op.cit

47. Rodriguez-Arias D, Smith MJ, Lazar NM (2011) Donation after circulatory death: burying the dead donor rule. Am J Bioeth 11(8):36–43

48. Padela AI, Shanawani H, Arozullah A (2011) Medical experts and Islamic scholars deliberating over brain death: gaps in the applied Islamic bioethics discourse. Muslim World 101(1):53–72

49. Padela AI (2013). op.cit

50. Bedir A, Aksoy S (2011) Brain death revisited: It is not 'complete death' according to Islamic sources. J Med Ethics 37(5):290–294

51. Sachedina A (2000) Brain death in Islamic jurisprudence. http://people.virginia.edu/*aas/article/article6.htm

52. Shewmon DA, Sylmar CA, Verheijde JL, Rady MY (2011) Evidence base guideline update: Determining brain death in adults: report of the Quality Standards Subcommittee of the American Academy of Neurology. Neurology 76(3):308 (author reply 308–309)

53. Rady MY, Verheijde JL (2009) Islam and end-of-life organ donation. Asking the right questions. Saudi Med J 30(7):882–886

54. Bernat JL, Capron AM, Bleck TP, Blosser S, Bratton SL, Childress JF et al (2010) The circulatory-respiratory determination of death in organ donation. Crit Care Med 38(3):963–970

55. Joffe A, Carcillo J, Anton N, deCaen A, Han Y, Bell M et al (2011) Donation after cardiocirculatory death: a call for a moratorium pending full public disclosure and fully informed consent. Philos Ethics Humanit Med 6(1):17

56. Rady MY, Verheijde JL (2010) General anesthesia for surgical procurement in non-heart-beating organ donation: why we should care. Anesth Analg 111(6):1562

57. Roberts DJ, MacCulloch KAM, Versnick EJ, Hall RI (2010) Should ancillary brain blood flow analyses play a larger role, in the neurological determination of death? Can J Anaesth 57 (10):927–935

58. Smith M. op.cit

59. Joffe AR, Kolski H, Duff J, deCaen AR (2009) A 10-month-old infant with reversible findings of brain death. Pediatric Neurol 41:378–382

60. Wijdicks EF, Varelas PN, Gronseth GS, Greer DM (2011) Evidence base guideline update: Determining brain death in adults: report of the Quality Standards Subcommittee of the American Academy of Neurology. Neurology 76(3):308 (author reply 308–309)

61. Wijdicks EF, Varelas PN, Gronseth GS, Greer DM (2010) Evidence-based guideline update: determining brain death in adults: report of the Quality Standards Subcommittee of the American Academy of Neurology. Neurology 74:1911–1918

62. Wijdicks EF, Varelas PN, Gronseth GS, Greer DM (2011) There is no reversible brain death. Crit Care Med 39:2204–2205

63. Okamoto K, Sugimoto T (1995) Return of spontaneous respiration in an infant who fulfilled current criteria to determine brain death. Pediatrics 96:518–520

64. Joffe AR. op.cit

65. Webb AC, Samuels OB (2011) Reversible brain death after cardiopulmonary arrest and induced hypothermia. Crit Care Med 39:1538–1542

66. Streat S (2011) 'Reversible brain death'—is it true, confounded, or 'not proven'? Crit Care Med 39:1601–1603

67. Gardiner D. op.cit

68. Okamoto K. op.cit

69. Joffe AR. op.cit

70. Mathur M, Petersen L, Stadtler M et al (2008) Variability in pediatric brain death determination and documentation in southern California. Pediatrics 121:988–993

71. Joffe AR. op.cit

72. Jain S, De Georgia M (2005) Brain death-associated reflexes and automatisms. Neurocrit Care 3:122–126

73. Gardiner D. op.cit

74. Lechan RM, Toni R (2008) Functional anatomy of the hypothalamus and pituitary. www.endotext.org, http://www.endotext.org/neuroendo/neuroendo3b/neuroendo3b_2.htm

75. The adenohypophysis receives the majority of its blood supply from the paired superior hypophyseal arteries, which arise from the medial aspect of the internal carotid artery, within the ophthalmic segment. The neurohypophysis is supplied by the inferior hypophyseal arteries. These vessels are terminal branches of the meningohypophyseal trunk, which arises from the cavernous portion of the internal carotid artery. The hypophyseal portal veins drain the primary capillary plexus formed by the superior hypophyseal arteries, which deliver blood to the pars distalis. The pars distalis in turn houses the secondary capillary plexus. Thus, a portal venous system allows delivery of hypothalamic prohormones to the adenohypophysis, and the neurohypophysis secretes hormones directly into the venous draining system of the pituitary

76. Smith M. op.cit

77. Shore PM. op.cit

78. Albar M. op.cit

79. Padela AI (2013). op.cit

Chapter 15
End-of-Life Care

Introduction

Muslims believe that death is the departure of the soul from the body by divine decree. Death marks the transition from one state of existence to the next and the beginning of the journey in the life hereafter, which is perpetual and infinite.

> It is He Who gives life and death; and when he decides upon an affair, He says to it, "Be", and it is [1].

The earth is described as a resting place for the purpose of worshipping God and doing good deeds [2]. Death is inevitable and occurs only with a command from God: "Every soul shall have a taste of death: in the end to Us shall you be brought back" [3]. It also states "Wherever you are, death will find you out, even if you are in towers built up strong and high" [4].

Death is unpredictable and can happen at any time and as such Muslims should always be prepared for the inevitable and for what is about to occur.

The time of death is predetermined by God. "When their time comes they cannot delay it for a single hour, nor can they bring it forward by a single hour" [5].

It is but a gateway from this short but mortal existence to a life of immortality in the afterlife [6].

The Prophet (PBUH) quoted saying "None of you should wish for death because of a calamity befalling him; but if he has to wish for death he should say: O Allah! Keep me alive as long as life is better for me and let me die if death is better for me" [7].

Muslims view illness as trial or a test of faith from Allah and is intended as a cleansing by Him, not as a punishment. At the same time, Allah and His Prophet clearly command that Muslims are obligated to seek treatment, and may not terminate life [8].

The purpose of medicine is to search for a cure through the application of human knowledge and scientific Endeavor, and to provide the necessary care to those afflicted with diseases. The primary obligation of a Muslim doctor is to provide care

© The Author(s) 2015
M.A. Al-Bar and H. Chamsi-Pasha, *Contemporary Bioethics*,
DOI 10.1007/978-3-319-18428-9_15

and alleviate pain. However, resorting to extraordinary means to sustain life does not in any way "prolong" life. The Qura'n states: "And for all people a term has been set. And when the end of the term approaches, they can neither delay it by a single moment, nor can they hasten it" [9].

Medical advances make it possible to restore health and sustain the life in circumstances previously regarded as hopeless. This capability brings with it considerable clinical, moral, socio-cultural, legal, and economic issues that challenge the values and goals of patients' care.

End-of-life treatment choices are increasing in intensive care units (ICUs) around the world. Many dying patients suffer prolonged and painful deaths, receiving unwarranted, expensive, and invasive care threatening their physical, psychosocial, and spiritual integrity.

The Intensive Care Unit or Critical Care Unit (CCU) is the special hospital ward within which the highest levels of continuous care and treatment are provided to patients after major surgery, with severe head injuries, life-threatening illnesses, respiratory insufficiency, coma, hemodynamic insufficiency, severe fluid imbalance, or with failure of one or more of the major organ systems.

Highly skilled specialized nursing staff mans the ICU, which is undoubtedly the most expensive and the most highly technological area of medical care [10].

Generally, patients whose conditions are expected to improve with intensive care aid are admitted to the ICU. In other words, patients are not admitted to the ICU to die. However, families of patients in the ICU are plagued with a host of dilemmas. Some of these dilemmas pertain to: (a) the justification for "prolonging" the suffering of their loved ones; (b) what extent they must outlay their financial resources in order to keep their loved ones in the ICU; (c) whether or not to give their consent to disconnect the ventilator once their loved ones are diagnosed to be brainstem dead; and (d) the validity of seeking extraordinary treatment measures for their loved ones when the prognosis is poor [11].

Although ICUs present many challenges to providing excellent end-of-life care, they also have special resources available, including a low patient-to-nurse ratio that allows better care for the dying patient. Terminally ill patients consume significant resources, including nursing care, transportation, and medications. Almost half of those who die in the hospital have been cared for in an intensive care unit (ICU) within 3 days prior to their death.

The Prophet Muhammad PBUH said: Seventy Thousands would enter paradise without being questioned. When asked who are they? He said "those who refused Ruqia (Incantation) and treatment" [12]. In another hadith he lauded the black lady who agreed not to be treated for epilepsy and said she would go directly to paradise. Many of the Sahaba (companions of the Prophet) refused to be treated in their final illness. Among them was Abubaker Al Sadiq, Abu Dardaa, Muath Ibn Jabal, etc.

Islam acknowledges that death is an inevitable phase of the life of a human being; medical management should not be given if it only prolongs the final stage of a terminal illness as opposed to treating a superimposed, life-threatening condition.

Terminally ill patients usually question the meaning of life, and the approach of death may stimulate serious spiritual questions that contribute to psychological symptoms such as anxiety, depression, hopelessness, and despair. Spiritual care is not necessarily religious, but religious care, at its best, should always be spiritual [13].

Persistent Vegetative State

The persistent vegetative state (PVS), a chronic neurological disorder of consciousness characterized by wakefulness without awareness, is a tragic and ironic artifact of modern medical technology. Patients reach a PVS after suffering a pathological process that has produced widespread damage to cerebral cortical neurons, thalamic neurons, or the white matter connections between the cortex and thalamus, but that largely spares the brain stem and hypothalamic neurons. Common etiologies of acute PVS are traumatic brain injury, stroke, and neuronal hypoxia and ischemia suffered during cardiopulmonary arrest [14].

The diagnosis and prognosis of PVS have reached public attention through several landmark high court rulings involving termination of life-sustaining treatment, most notably the cases of Karen Ann Quinlan in the 1970s, Nancy Beth Cruzan in the late 1980s, and the case of Terri Schiavo in 2005.

Karen Ann-Quinlane was the first case of PVS brought to courts in 1975. The ventilator was stopped in 1976, but she lived for 9 years and finally died of pneumonia. She was kept alive with artificial nutrition and hydration.

Thousands of cases have been recognized all over the world annually. Nancy Cruzan (1990) was another PVS whose family requested to stop hydration and nutrition after 4 years of loss of her cognitive functions, as she expressed her wishes previously.

The Case of Terri Schiavo

On March 31, 2005, a 41-year-old patient, Terri Schiavo died 2 weeks after her feeding tube was removed in a Florida, USA nursing home.

The saga of Mrs. Schiavo started in 1990 when she developed cardiac arrest of undetermined etiology; she was resuscitated, but never regained consciousness. A percutaneous endoscopic gastrostomy (PEG) tube was introduced for feeding and hydration.

Neurological evaluation established the diagnosis of PVS.

In August 1992 Michael Schiavo, her husband, received $250,000 in an out-of-court settlement with a physician and he later received $300,000 for loss of consortium.

In May 1998 Michael Schiavo filed a petition in Court to have the PEG tube removed, because she had no chance of improvement.

On April 24, 2001 the PEG tube was removed. From that point on, a major conflict started, and became the focus of heated and prolonged medical, legal, religious, ethical, social, and political controversy. Several contradicting court or administrative orders were issued to remove or maintain the tube, or to reinstate it after its removal! During that period, there were active movements by ethical and human rights groups to defend Terri's right to live, and others to defend her right to withdraw Life-Sustaining Treatment (LST) and die.

After prolonged trials, litigations, and accusations the High Court agreed to remove the PEG tube of Terri Schiavo on March 18, 2005. She died on March 30, 2005 by starving to death. It would have been less traumatic if she had an injection that put her agony to end in a few minutes.

On January 26, 2006 Michael Schiavo married his girlfriend with whom he has two children.

The practical questions that must be answered in Terri's case, as well as many other similar cases, could be summarized in the following points:

- Is it ethically and legally permissible to withdraw or withhold life-sustaining treatment?
- Who speaks for the patient when he/she cannot speak?
- What are the duties of a surrogate decision maker or proxy?
- Surrogate or proxy decision makers are persons appointed to speak and make decisions for the unconscious patient.
- What should be done when it is suspected that a surrogate may not be acting in the best interests of the patient?
- Is artificially supplied fluid and nutrition considered a medical treatment or a mandatory comfort care? [15]. People rarely execute living wills or advance directives, to help in delineation of their wishes regarding medical interventions when they face end-of-life stages, or when they become unconscious. Physicians rarely discuss such issues with patients and families when they face terminal illnesses. And if they do so they do not usually document patients' and families' opinions and wishes in the medical records.

Concepts Involving End-of-Life Care

Full Resuscitation: Aggressive ICU management up to and including full resuscitative attempts.

Withholding Resuscitation: Aggressive ICU management up to, but not including Cardio-Pulmonary Resuscitation (CPR).

Withholding Life Support: Decision not to institute a medically appropriate and potentially beneficial therapy, with the understanding that the patient will probably die without the therapy in question.

Withdrawing Life Support: Cessation and removal of an ongoing therapy with the explicit intent not to substitute an equivalent alternative treatment.

Palliative Care: Prevention or treatment of suffering, including the administration of drugs such as narcotics and sedatives.

Do Not Resuscitate (DNR) order: An order stating that in case of cardiac arrest or respiratory arrest, cardiopulmonary resuscitation will not be undertaken by any means.

Withdrawal of Life-Sustaining Treatments

Withholding or withdrawing life support, however, is still an area of controversy. Its applicability is weighed with benefits and risks and how futile the treatment is for the terminally ill patients.

Withdrawing and withholding treatment can be "voluntary," where the conscious patient authorizes it, or if unconscious, the patient had communicated to his next of kin that he would prefer not to be kept alive on life support. It can also be "nonvoluntary," where the decision to withdraw life support is made by the family of the patient, [16] or by the treating physicians.

At the end of life, the chronic heart patient, for example, often becomes increasingly symptomatic, and may have other life-limiting comorbidities as well. A clear mortality benefit with the use of implantable cardioverter defibrillators (ICDs) has been shown in patients with poor left ventricle and ventricular arrhythmia. However, patients who have an ICD may be denied the chance of a sudden cardiac death, and instead are committed to a slower terminal decline, with frequent electrical shocks that can be painful and decrease the quality of life, greatly contributing to their distress and that of their families during this period.

Deactivating an ICD or not performing a generator change is both legal and ethical, and is supported by guidelines from both sides of the Atlantic. Patient autonomy is paramount, and no patient is committed to any therapy that they no longer wish to receive [17].

Terminally ill Muslim patients are permitted to have life-sustaining treatments withheld or withdrawn when the physicians are certain about the inevitability of death and the treatment is futile, does not improve the patient's condition or quality of life, involves great complications, delays the dying process, or involves suffering. However, it should be a collective decision acquired on the basis of informed consent after consultation with the patient's family and all individuals involved in providing care. In these situations, death is allowed to take its natural course [18, 19].

The definition of **futility** is elusive and has been widely debated. The American Thoracic Society states that a treatment should be considered futile if it is highly unlikely that it will result in "meaningful survival" for the patient.

Resource utilization and outcomes in gravely ill patients must be observed. Futile treatments and medical interventions must be considered in light of outcomes.

If the treating physicians find a certain modality of treatment useless or going to increase the suffering of the patient, that modality of treatment should not be enforced from the start. The Prophet Muhammad (PBUH) says "above all do no harm" and this rule of non-maleficence is the cornerstone of all medical ethics. The intention must never be to hasten death, only to abstain from overzealous treatment [20].

Issues arising from withdrawal and withholding treatment have not reached total consensus among Muslim jurists. However, Article 63 of the Islamic code of medical ethics can be regarded as a clarion call on Muslim medical personnel. The article states that, "the treatment of a patient can be terminated if a team of medical experts or a medical committee involved in the management of such patient are satisfied that the continuation of treatment would be futile or useless." It further states that "treatment of patients whose condition has been confirmed to be useless by the medical committee should not be commenced" [21].

The following Fatwa is a landmark in regulating resuscitative measures, stopping of machines in cases thought to be not suitable for resuscitative measures. The decision should be based on medical criteria and decided by at least three competent physicians. The family should be approached and the facts discussed fully with them [22].

The Permanent Committee for Research and Fatwa, Fatwa No. 12086 on 28/3/1409 (1989). Question from Military Hospital (N.W. region) on using resuscitative measure on the following cases:

Q. 1. If a person who arrives to the hospital is already dead?
A. 1. There is no need to use any resuscitative measures in such a case.
Q. 2. If the medical file of the patient is already stamped: "Do not resuscitate," according to the patient's or his proxy's will and the patient is unsuitable for resuscitation.
A. 2. If three competent specialized physicians agree that he is unsuitable for resuscitation, then there is no need to do any resuscitative measures.
Q. 3. If three physicians have decided that it is inappropriate to resuscitate a patient who is suffering from a serious irremediable disease and that his death is almost certain.
A. 3. If the disease is irremediable and his death is almost certain, as witnessed by three competent physicians, there is no need to use resuscitative measures.
Q. 4. If the patient is mentally or physically incapacitated and is also suffering from stroke or late stage cancer or having severe cardiopulmonary disease or already had several cardiac arrests.
A. 4. If the condition of the patient is as described and the decision not to resuscitate has been reached by three competent specialist physicians, then it is permissible not to resuscitate.
Q. 5. If the patient had irremediable brain damage after a cardiac arrest?
A. 5. If the condition is authenticated by three competent specialist physicians, then there is no need for resuscitative measures as they will be useless.

Q. 6. If the treating physicians decided that resuscitation will be useless in a certain patient, is it permissible not to resuscitate even though the patient or his relatives asked for resuscitative measures to be carried on.

A. 6. If resuscitative measures are deemed useless and inappropriate for a certain patient in the opinion of three competent specialist physicians, then there is no need for resuscitative measures to be carried out. The opinion of the patient or his relatives should not be considered, both in withholding or withdrawing resuscitative measures and machines, as it is a medical decision and it is not in their capacity to reach such a decision" [23].

Islamic law permits withdrawal of futile and disproportionate treatment on the basis of the consent of the immediate family members who act on the professional advice of the physician in charge of the case or, as the Saudi Fatwa implies, it should be a clear medical decision by the treating physicians (at least 3).

Muslim jurists recognize, as a legal competent, the patient's informed refusal of treatment or a living will, which allows a person to die under circumstances in which there are no medical reasons to continue treatment [24]. The Prophet (PBUH) himself lauded those who refused treatment and many of the Sahaba (companions) refused to be treated in their final illness.

The basic human rights of the patient, which include being provided with food, drink, nursing, and painkillers, must still be provided and this can be done at home or hospice. The patient should be allowed to die peacefully and comfortably [25]. Thus, the removal of such basic necessities of life such as food and water will amount to actively killing the patient.

Social workers and religious affairs personnel will be needed for both the social and religious and spiritual needs of the patient and his family.

Supportive care is compassionate, humane, integrated, and responsive to the patient and family's physical, psychological, and spiritual needs at the end of life.

Do Not Resuscitate

Resuscitation is a medical procedure which seeks to restore cardiac and/or respiratory function to individuals who have sustained a cardiac and/or respiratory arrest. Cardiopulmonary resuscitation (CPR) is now routinely performed on any hospitalized patient who suffers cardiac or respiratory arrest. The frequent performance of CPR on patients who are terminally ill or who have little chance of surviving has prompted concern that resuscitation efforts may be employed too broadly. Advanced invasive procedures and treatments that may promote and sustain life may not confer any foreseeable benefit, and in fact may cause further suffering to the patient and the family [26].

Therefore, CPR may be withheld if, in the judgment of the treating team, an attempt to resuscitate the patient would be futile.

Do Not Resuscitate ("DNR") is a medical order to provide no resuscitation to individuals for whom resuscitation is not warranted.

The Islamic Medical Association of North America (IMANA) believes that when death becomes inevitable, as determined by physicians taking care of terminally ill patients, the patient should be allowed to die without unnecessary procedures. While the patient is still alive, all ongoing medical treatments can be continued. IMANA does not believe in prolonging misery on mechanical life support in a vegetative state. All of the procedures of mechanical life support are temporary measures. When a team of physicians, including critical care specialists, have determined, no further or new attempt should be made to sustain artificial support. Even in this state, the patient should be treated with full respect, comfort measures, and pain control. The patient should be allowed to die peacefully and comfortably. No attempt should be made to enhance the dying process in patients on life support [27]. Hydration and feeding should continue and no attempt should be made to withhold nutrition and hydration. Otherwise, it will be considered by Islamic Law (Shari'ah) as a murder case. If hydration and feeding is stopped the patient does not die peacefully and comfortably. He suffers dehydration and hunger for 10–14 days. It would be more humane to inject him and let him die in seconds or a few minutes rather than torturing him for 2 weeks, but this is considered as Euthanasia which is emphatically prohibited by Islamic jurists.

If the patient is competent enough; it should be discussed with him. He should be ensured of being given all necessary care and medication to alleviate pain and distressing symptoms.

If the patient is not competent enough, DNR should be discussed with the family members, especially the most appreciative and comprehending person.

The Fatwa of the high council of ulama of Saudi Arabica should be explained and given to the family. If the family still insists on doing everything possible, then they should be offered the possibility of transferring their patient to whichever hospital they wish.

A clear policy from the ministry of health regarding DNR, brain death, and end-of-life issues is urgently needed for all hospitals and health providers in most (if not all) Muslim and Arab countries.

A DNR is acceptable in Islamic law in certain situations [28]. In Saudi Arabia, for example, DNR policies that are practiced are mainly used in the hospital arena and are not valid outside the hospitals.

According to the fatwa, families and guardians cannot decide on the application or removal of resuscitation measures or procedures, as they are not considered qualified under the Fatwa. This is an important difference from the practice in the United States. The DNR Form in Saudi Arabia, for example, is valid only on the condition that it is signed by three qualified physicians (mainly 2 consultants, and 1 staff physician), and only acceptable within the hospital during the patient's admission. When signed, the form is kept in the patient's record, and it has to be reviewed by the physicians according to the institution's policies.

Do not resuscitate in pediatric practice

The ethical issues that attend the implementation of DNR orders to elderly patients are obviously different from those that are relevant to the neonatal or pediatric patient, who has just begun their life [29].

Children with irreversible or progressive terminal illness may benefit temporarily from CPR, only to deteriorate later. Painful and invasive procedures may be performed unnecessarily, and the child could be left in a poorer condition. A DNR order indicates that the treating team has decided not to have CPR attempted in the event of cardiac or pulmonary arrest.

Optimal ethical decision making requires open and timely communication between members of the pediatric team and the family, respecting their values, beliefs, and the fundamental principles of ethics [30].

It is never permissible to withdraw procedures designed to alleviate pain or promote comfort. For example, withholding hydration or antibiotics to treat transient infections is not justifiable. These infections may cause distress and pain, and treating them represents an important element of good palliative care.

Discussion of end-of-life issues in Neonatal Intensive Care Unit (NICU)

The subject of withholding or withdrawing treatment thus needs to be broached with considerable sensitivity and awareness, as not only is this an emotionally challenging time for parents, but there may also be important ethico-religious imperatives that parents will need to consider and sometimes seek advice on. Generally, parents and relatives are reluctant to make life-and-death decisions themselves, but are willing to transfer authority for such decisions to professionals who they trust will work in the interests of their baby while at the same time respecting the principles of their faith [31].

The decision of DNR is always a medical decision taken by the treating physicians (at least 3) and should be fully discussed with the family.

Breaking news of babies death

Telling parents that their baby has died using the words (your baby is now in the loving care of the Lord) or the Qur'anic expression "To Allah we belong and to Allah is our return" [32] can provide comfort. We also remind parents of Prophet Muhammad's (PBUH) reassurances that those who bear this loss with patience their babies, who are pure, will be their forerunners into Paradise [33].

Palliative Care at End-of-Life

The World Health Organization (WHO) defines palliative care as an approach that improves the quality of life of patients and their families facing the problems associated with life-threatening illness, through prevention and relief of suffering by means of physical, psychosocial, and spiritual means. The WHO has gone so far as to assert: "A palliative care program cannot exist unless it is based on a rational drug policy including…ready access of suffering patients to opioids."

Palliative care involves much more than the alleviation of physical pain but rather encompasses "total pain" including emotional, psychological, social, and spiritual pain [34].

Based either on assessment of available palliative care services or on the consumption of opioid analgesics, it is clear that palliative care is severely lacking in Muslim-majority countries (MMCs). This is true not only in the low- and middle-income MMCs (e.g., Pakistan, Bangladesh, and the MMCs of Africa) but also in the higher income countries of the Arab Gulf [35].

Ideally, these services would encompass consultative services within each hospital, dedicated beds for a palliative care unit, stand-alone hospices, and home-care palliative care and hospice services.

Issues regarding spirituality, religious beliefs, and practices can come to the forefront in patients' advanced illnesses [36]. Many patients may wish to discuss their beliefs with their healthcare providers [37] and it would appear obvious that for these discussions to be optimally useful, healthcare providers should possess cultural and religious knowledge and sensitivity relevant to the patients being treated. Healthcare providers should involve religious or spiritual persons in dealing with such patients and their families.

Historically, care for the dying has been seen as a family responsibility and death has been generally managed at home [38]. However, the lack of home-care services in most MMCs can lead to return trips to the hospital and/or extended stays and death in a hospital.

The core principles for end-of-life care are: (a) Respect the dignity of both the patient and the care giver. (b) Be sensitive to the patient's and family wishes (as far as possible). (c) Management of pain or other symptom. (d) Offer any therapy or measure that can improve quality of life. (e) Assess and manage psychological, social, spiritual needs of the patient and his family (as far as possible). (f) Respect the physicians' decisions to limit their intervention or forgo any specific treatment which they think to be of no use and probably harmful. (g) Hospice and home-care services should be the benchmark and bedrock of end-of-life care. (h) There is ample evidence that hospice and homecare provide better end-of-life care, with dignity. It is remarkably inexpensive compared to hospital care.

Relieving pain and suffering

True, there is pain and suffering at the terminal end of an illness, but Muslims believe there is immeasurable reward from God for those who patiently persevere in suffering. "Those who patiently persevere will truly receive a reward without measure" [39].

The Qur'an states that "Allah does not tax any soul beyond that which he can bear" and pain and suffering is not a punishment, but rather a "kaffarah" (expiation) for one's sins. But relieving pain or providing a sedative drug with the aim of pain relief is still allowed even if death is hastened (double effect), provided death was definitely not the intention of the physician [40].

The major disadvantage of controlling pain with morphine and its derivatives, especially. in patients where their respiratory centers are depressed or they are suffering from chronic obstructive lung disease, is further depression of the respiratory center and hence shortening the end of life.

Recently, cannabis and its derivatives have been introduced with good results in AIDS patients and other near-end-of-life cases. It reduces the sense of pain, gives some euphoria, and does not affect the respiratory center. The objection is by law and religion. Muslims prefer to be around until almost the very end, to make shahada and remember Allah. Opioids, cannabis, and other drugs may obscure consciousness. Alleviation of pain can also be done with nerve injection or other minor surgical procedures.

In the Islamic perspective, medication-related sedation could be looked at from two different angles. On the one hand, alleviation of the suffering of a human being is considered righteous. On the other hand, maintaining a level of consciousness as close to normal as possible is of great importance to allow for observance of the worship rites for the longest period possible before death. In terminally ill patients, it may be difficult to maintain a state of equilibrium allowing for optimal symptom control and a normal level of consciousness. In these situations, the pros and cons should be clarified to the patient and family, who may prefer to endure a slightly higher degree of symptoms in order to maintain a better level of consciousness [41].

End-of-Life Practices

Terminally ill patients should be entitled to the respect and dignity of a good death according to Islamic tradition. Tayeb et al. described three important domains in the end-of-life care of dying Muslim patients. The first domain of religious preferences at the time of dying includes: the presence of someone to prompt the dying person to say the "Shahadah (bearing witness that there is no true God but Allah and Muhammad is verily His Servant and His Messenger) as a final statement of faith"; the presence of someone at the bedside to recite chapters from the Holy Qur'an during the dying process; and positioning the dying patient to face the Kaaba at the Holy Mosque in Mecca. The second domain on self-esteem and image is preserving the bodily dignity in death, maintaining cleanliness of the body and clothing from bodily fluids (e.g., urine, stool, vomit), the eyes and mouth of the deceased should be closed, and ensuring normal appearance of the body after death (e.g., removing external medical devices, catheters, and indwelling tubes) and the limbs straightened.

When Muslims are sick, their friends and relatives tend to visit and sometimes in rather large numbers for rather extended visits. Western trained healthcare workers may find this somewhat unusual, but consideration should be given to the point where the visitors are not in some way impeding the delivery of care [42].

When death of the patient occurs, it is important to assist the family in preparation for burial which is to be performed as quickly as possible. Autopsy is not generally done except for legal or possible public health reasons.

The third domain is the wellbeing of surviving relatives, whereby the dying person feels secure that surviving family members will not be burdened with psychosocial and/or financial difficulties after one's death [43].

The Muslim person is required to make A "Wasyiah," will, testament especially if he has financial deals, debts, or commitments to others. The physician, the social worker, or the religious adviser should remind the competent patient of this religious and social duty. The treating physician should offer the family home care if they wish and arrange for home visits if needed.

He should recognize the special needs of the patient, e.g.: A family member can stay with the patient all the time. Food and comfort measures should be allowed to be brought from home. Support to the patient and family psychologically, socially, and spiritually is extremely important. Spiritual care and pastoral service for non-Muslims should be arranged, if requested through their embassies/consulates.

Disclosure

Some families may not wish their dying relative to be fully informed regarding his/her illness. While this is certainly not unique to Islam, it is perhaps somewhat more common in Muslim families than in Western families today. In some instances, the patients and relatives may be engaging in what has been termed "mutual pretense" i.e., both the patient and his/her family know that the patient is dying but the topic is avoided with each pretending that the other does not know the real situation [44].

The physician can withhold information from the patient if he has good reason that divulging the information to the patient is going to cause harm or impair management or cause distress. The physician should document this fact in the patient's file and should get the consent of the substitute decision maker (legal representative).

Nutrition at end of life

Prophet Muhammad (PBUH) discouraged forcing the sick to take food or drink. However, Muslim families tend to express great concern when the nutritional intake of a patient is jeopardized. Some Muslim families may demand for medical intervention to compensate for this decreased nutritional intake. Reference to the teachings of the Prophet (PBUH) on this matter helps to address the concerns of families and to facilitate their understanding of the anorexia/cachexia syndrome associated with malignancy. However, in patients who are slowly deteriorating, one should maintain the minimal amount of nutrition and hydration until the last moments of life. The reason for this approach is to prevent the potential feelings of guilt and sorrow that could be experienced by the family if nutritional or hydration support was withdrawn or withheld completely.

Basic nutrition should not be discontinued because such an action would starve a patient to death—a crime in the Islamic faith [45].

Advance Directives

Death is an inevitable phenomenon which strikes at any time during a person's infancy, youth, or old age. But, one cannot overlook the fact that before the inevitable (i.e., death) does take place a person may become a victim of a terminal illness, or may lapse into irreversible coma, or (PVS) [46]. The contemporary sophisticated medical care of terminally ill patients increasingly utilizes life support technologies and procedures that many individuals prefer to avoid when they reach that stage [47].

The Living Will (Advance Medical Directive) is a document in which a healthy person explains in writing which medical treatment he/she would accept or refuse at that critical juncture when he/she may not be in a position to express his/her wishes in case of emergencies, terminal illnesses, and situations where they may be incapable of making decisions. In other words, this document assists the attending physician to withhold or withdraw certain medical procedures and allow the patient to die naturally.

There are two types of advance directives: a living will and a durable or medical power of attorney.

Living wills and advance directives, which are legal documents in the United States, are used to make decisions regarding the person's type of care to receive in situations in which they cannot speak for themselves.

A durable power of attorney of health care is acceptable for Muslim patients. Patients not capable of making healthcare decisions can call upon an authorized representative to express his or her wishes and make treatment decisions on behalf of their best interests [48].

The question that arises here is whether it is permissible for a Muslim to include an advance medical directive in his his/her wasiyyah? Attention should be drawn here to the fact that the Living Will cannot form part of the wasiyyah, since what is incorporated in the wasiyyah will be executed only after one's demise.

Prophet Muhammad (PBUH) asked his wives, when he was ill, not to pour medicament in the side of his mouth (Ladood), if he would become unconscious, but his wives did. When he came around, he scorned them and asked them to do the same for themselves.

The following may be incorporated into the living will:

- Request to discontinue treatment
  A terminally ill Muslim patient can request that treatment be discontinued if the treatment would not in any way improve his/her condition or quality of life based on the Islamic juridical principle of *la darar wa la dirar* (no harm and no harassment). The intention here is not to hasten death, but the refusal of "overzealous" treatment. However, "palliative" care in the sense of maintaining personal hygiene and basic nutrition should not be discontinued.

- Instruction to switch off the life-support equipment

  A healthy Muslim may instruct that should he/she, as a result of a terminal illness or massive head injury, be diagnosed as brain dead, then the life-support equipment should be switched off. In this regard the International Islamic Fiqh Academy of the Organization of the Islamic Conference, during its third session held in Amman–Jordan from 8 to 13 Safar 1407 Hijri/11–16 October 1986, resolved that a person whose brain activity has ceased and the physicians confirm that such a cessation is irreversible and that the brain has entered the state of decomposition, under such circumstances the ventilator could be stopped even though some organs of his body, like the heart, continue to function artificially with the help of life-support equipment [49]. Other Fatwas on this issue allowed stopping the ventilators whenever brain death was diagnosed. They have been discussed in the Chap. 14.

- Inclusion of organ donation (Please refer to chapter on Organ transplantation).

- Power of attorney (wakalah)

  In the alternative Living Will it would be prudent on the part of a Muslim to entrust someone with the power of attorney and mention that person by name in his/her Living Will. This would safeguard that should he/she become non-competent, then his/her wishes as stated in the Living Will would be expressed by his/her wakil [50] (authorized representative) to family members and the attending physicians. The document should be dated and signed by the person giving the advanced medical directive, his/her wakil, and that of two witnesses. Muslims may draw up an alternative Living Will and include in it instructions pertaining to the cessation of treatment, switching off the life-support equipment, and organ donation. The wakil (authorized representative) would be morally bound to express and convey the wishes of the person concerned to members of the family and the attending physicians. If none of the clauses of the Living Will contradicts the broad teachings of the Qur'an and Sunnah of Prophet Muhammad (PBUH) there would be no justification to ignore the directives given therein [51].

  A prototype of an Islamic Living Will has been developed by the Ethics Committee of the Islamic Medical Association of North America (IMANA). It was published in The Journal of the Islamic Medical Association of North America, Volume 37, Number 1, July 2005. p. 37.

Euthanasia

Euthanasia is a Greek word composed of two syllables: EU means Good or Easy, Thanatos means Death [52]. Thus, the meaning becomes good death or easy death, and nowadays proponents like to call it "mercy killing."

Types of euthanasia:

Voluntary euthanasia is defined as: "The intentional administration of lethal drugs in order to painlessly terminate the life of a patient suffering from an incurable condition deemed unbearable by the patient, at this patient's request," while Assisted suicide is defined as: "intentionally assisting a person, at this person's request, to terminate his or her life."

Nonvoluntary euthanasia is defined as: "The intentional administration of lethal drugs in order to painlessly terminate the life of a patient suffering from an incurable condition deemed unbearable, not at this patient's request" [53].

Islam and Euthanasia

A subject of great importance is the subject of life. Life is given by God and cannot be taken away except by Him or with His permission. Preservation of life is one of the five basic purposes of the sacred law [54].

Human beings are considered to be responsible stewards of their bodies, which are viewed as gifts from God. The sanctity of human life is affirmed in the Qur'an. One cannot take the life of another: "Do not take life which God has made sacred except in the course of Justice" [55].

Thus, the person who intentionally ends his life will be punished because of his disobedience to Allah, and for denying His mercy, on judgment day. The Sunnah, a teaching of Prophet Muhammad (Hadith) describes one such instance. He (PBUH) said in one of the Hadith: "Whoever kills himself with an iron instrument will be carrying it forever in hell. Whoever takes poison and kills himself will forever keep sipping that poison in hell. Whoever jumps off a mountain and kills himself will forever keep falling down in the depths of hell" [12].

Life saving is a duty and the unjustifiable taking of life is considered a grave sin.

Islam and the Islamic law clearly prohibit euthanasia in all circumstances. However, the wishes of patient not to have his dying prolonged artificially in the presence of hopeless prognosis are well preserved. Such wishes may be declared in accepted standing Do Not Resuscitate (DNR) orders in certain hopeless medical conditions [56].

The Holy Qur'an says: "...One who has killed a person except in lieu of murder or mischief on earth; it would be as he slew the whole mankind and whoever saves the life of a human being, it is as if he has saved the life of all mankind ... ." [39].

One cannot also take one's own life: "Do not kill yourselves, for verily God has been to you most merciful." [57].

God says in the Qur'an: "It is He who created death and life, that He may try which of you is best in deed ... ." [58].

He also says: "... Nor can they control death nor life nor resurrection." [59].

The physician therefore has no right to terminate any human life under his care. This also applies to the unborn baby since clear evidence indicates that human life starts at the time of ensoulment (120 days from fertilization).

Taking away life should be the domain of the One Who gives life. The Qur'an emphasizes that "it is the sole prerogative of Allah to bestow life and to cause death," and therefore euthanasia is never allowed [24].

These sources from the Qur'an and hadith illustrate the sanctity of human life, prohibition of killing a human being with no justification, and prohibition of killing oneself. Thus, killing a person to ease his suffering even though it is at the request of the person will be inconsistent with Islamic law, regardless of the different names given to the procedure, such as, active voluntary euthanasia, assisted suicide, or mercy killing. A person in such situation is expected to persevere patiently with the available medical treatment as reward for such patience in the Hereafter is tremendous as promised in Qur'an, in which Allah (swt) stated to the effect: "And those who patiently persevere will timely receive a reward without measure" [60].

The Islamic World League held in Jeddah [61] in May 1992 declared a strong rejection against so-called euthanasia under all circumstances. And those terminally ill patients should receive the appropriate palliative medication, utilizing all measures provided by God in this universe, and that in no way should one despair from Allah's mercy, and that doctors should do their best to support their patients morally and physically, irrespective of whether these measures are curative or not [62].

The Islamic Medical Association of North America (IMANA) is absolutely opposed to euthanasia and assisted suicide in terminally ill patients by healthcare providers or patients' relatives [27].

All the Fatwas refuse euthanasia and considered it a crime punishable both in this world and the Hereafter. The Laws in Islamic and Arab Countries criminalize euthanasia and the physician participating in it is punished. The consent of the deceased or the action on his repeated plea to end his life reduces the punishment from capital punishment to imprisonment and abrogation of the license of Practice of Medicine [63].

In summary, no one is authorized deliberately to end life, whether one's own or that of another human being. Saving life is encouraged, and reducing suffering with analgesia is however acceptable, even if, in the process, death is hastened. This rule is based on the central teaching that "actions are to be judged by their intentions." Withdrawal of food and drink to hasten death is therefore not allowed and is considered as a murder crime [64, 65].

References

1. The Holy Qur'an 40:68
2. The Holy Qur'an 2:20–21
3. The Holy Qur'an 29:57
4. The Holy Qur'an 4:78
5. The Holy Qur'an 16:61

6. Baddarni K (2010) Ethical dilemmas and the dying Muslim patient. Asian Pac J Cancer Prev 11(1):107–112
7. AlBukhari M, Sahih AlBukhari (1958) Cairo: Matabi Asshab (1378H) 1958(6351)
8. Albar M (1995) Organ transplantation: an Islamic perspective. In: An Albar M. Contemporary Topics in Islamic Medicine, pp 3–11. Saudi Publishing House, Jeddah
9. The Holy Qur'an 7:34
10. Ebrahim AM. End of life issues: making use of extraordinary means to sustain life. FIMA Year Book, 2005–2006, Jordan Society for Islamic Medical Sciences in Collaboration with Federation of Islamic Medical Associations (FIMA)
11. Ibid
12. AlBukhari M, Sahih AlBukhari (1958) Cairo: Matabi Asshab (1378H)
13. Asadi-Lari M, Madjd Z, Goushegir S (2008) Gaps in the provision of spiritual care for terminally ill patients in Islamic societies—a systematic review. Adv Palliat Med 7:73–80
14. Bernat JL (2002) Ethical issues in the persistent vegetative state patient. Neurology, 2nd edn, pp 283–305. Butterworth-Heinemann, Boston
15. Kassim PN, Adeniyi OB (2010) Withdrawing and withholding medical treatment: a comparative study between the Malaysian. English and Islamic law Med Law 29(3):443–461
16. Sachedina A (2005) End-of-life: the Islamic view. Lancet 366:774–779
17. Chamsi-Pasha H, Chamsi-Pasha MA, Albar MA (2014) Ethical challenges of deactivation of cardiac devices in advanced heart failure. Curr Heart Fail Rep 11(2):119–125
18. Daar AS, Khitamt AB (2001) Bioethics for clinicians: 21. Islamic Bioeth CMAJ 164(1):60–63
19. Sachedina. op.cit
20. Bülow HH1, Sprung CL, Reinhart K, Prayag S, Du B, Armaganidis A, Abroug F, Levy MM (2008) The world's major religions' points of view on end-of-life decisions in the intensive care unit. Intensive Care Med 34(3):423–30
21. Code of Conduct drawn at the International Conference on Islamic Medicine held in Kuwait, 1981, known as "The Islamic Code of Medical Ethics," p 67
22. Albar MA (2007) Seeking Remedy, abstaining from therapy and resuscitation: an islamic perspective. Saudi J Kidney Dis Transpl 18(4):629–637
23. Fatwas regarding medicine and patients. Department of Religious Sciences, Research and Fatwa, Riyadh. Supervised by Saleh Al Fowzan 1424H/ 2004 AD Fatwa No 12086 on 28/3/ 1409 H (1989) pp 322–324
24. Sachedina A. op. cit
25. Islamic Medical Ethics by IMANA Ethics Committee, www.imana.org
26. Jan MM (2011) The decision of do not resuscitate in pediatric practice. Saudi Med J 32:115–122
27. IMANA Ethics Committee (2005) Islamic medical ethics: the IMANA perspective. J Islamic Med Assoc 37:33–42
28. Ur Rahman M, Arabi Y, Adhami NA, Paker B, Al-shimemeri A (2004) The practice of do-not-resuscitate orders in the Kingdom of Saudi Arabia: the experience of a tertiary care center. Saudi Med J 25:1278–1279
29. Goldberg DS (2007) The ethics of DNR orders as to neonatal and pediatric patients: the ethical dimension of communication. Houston J Health Law Policy 1:57–83
30. Jan MM. op. cit
31. Gatrad AR, Muhammad BJ, Sheikh A (2008) Reorientation of care in the NICU: a Muslim perspective. Semin Fetal Neonatal Med 13(5):312–314
32. The Holy Qur'an 2:156
33. Gatrad AR. op. cit
34. Mehta A, Chan LS (2008) Understanding the concept of total pain: a prerequisite for pain control. J Hospice Palliat Nurs 10:26–32
35. Aljawi DM, Harford JB (2012) Palliative care in the Muslim-majority countries: the need for more and better care. In: Contemporary and innovative practice in palliative care. www.intechopen.com

36. Williams AL (2006) Perspectives on spirituality at the end of life: a meta-summary. Palliat Support Care 4:407–417
37. Ehman JW, Ott BB, Short TH, Ciampa RC, Hansen-Flaschen J (1999) Do patients want their physicians to inquire about their spiritual or religious beliefs if they become gravely ill? Arch Intern Med 159:1803–1806
38. Gatrad AR, Sheikh A (2002) Palliative care for Muslims and issues before death. Int J Palliat Nurs 8:526–531
39. The Holy Qur'an 5:32
40. Sachedina A. op. cit., da Costa DE, Ghazal H, Khusaiby SA, Gatrad AR (2002) Do not resuscitate orders in a neonatal ICU in a Muslim community. Arch Dis Child Fetal Neonatal Ed 86:F115–F119
41. Al-Shahri MZ, Al-Khenaizan AM (2005) Palliative care for Muslim patients. J Support Oncol 3(6):432–436
42. Baddarni K. op. cit
43. Tayeb MA, Al-Zamel E, Fareed MM, Abouellail HA (2010) A "good death": perspectives of Muslim patients and health care providers. Ann Saudi Med 30(3):215–221
44. Aljawi DM. op. cit
45. Jericho BG, Morgenweck CJ (2009) End of life issues: withdrawal of life-sustaining therapy. Am Soc Anesthesiologists Newslett 73(9):24–25
46. Ebrahim AF (2000) The living will (Wasiyat Al-Hayy): a study of its legality in the light of Islamic jurisprudence. Med Law 19(1):147–60
47. Ebrahim AF. The living will (Wasiyat Al-Hayy): a study of its legality in the light of Islamic jurisprudence FIMA Year Book 2005–2006. Jordan Society for Islamic Medical Sciences in Collaboration with Federation of Islamic Medical Associations (FIMA)
48. Babgi A (2009) Legal issues in end-of-life care: perspectives from Saudi Arabia and United States. Am J Hosp Palliat Care 26(2):119–27
49. Resolution No. (5) of the third session of the council of the Islamic Fiqh Academy in Organisation of the Islamic Conference's Islamic Fiqh Academy—Resolutions and Recommendations. Jeddah. Matabi` Shirkat Dar al-`Ilm li al-Tiba`ah wa al-Nashr. 1406–1409H/1985-1989, p 30
50. For an account as to who can be appointed as the wakil see Kitab al-Fiqh `ala al-Madhahib al-Arba`ah, vol 3, pp 170–171
51. Ebrahim AF (2005–2006). op.cit
52. Emanuel EJ (1994) The history of euthanasia debates in the United States and Britain. An Intern Med 121(10):793–802
53. Van den Branden S, Broeckaert B (2011) Living in the hands of God. English Sunni e-fatwas on (non-) voluntary euthanasia and assisted suicide. Med Health Care Philos 14(1):29–41
54. Al-Shatibi I (1997) Al-Muwafaqat, 2. Dar Ibn Affan, Khobar, p 20
55. The Holy Qur'an 6:151
56. Takrouri MS, Halwani TM (2008) An Islamic medical and legal prospective of do not resuscitate order in critical care medicine. Internet J Health 7 [Electronic Version]
57. The Holy Qur'an 4:29
58. The Holy Qur'an 39:10
59. The Holy Qur'an 25:3
60. The Holy Qur'an 39:10
61. Islamic Fiqh council of Islamic World League. Jeddah, Saudi Arabia. May 1992
62. Dayeh AJ. Euthanasia. FIMA Year Book 2005–2006. op.cit
63. Abulgawad M. Islamic medicine 4th conference, held in Pakistan (1407 H). Islamic Organization for Medical Sciences Kuwait, vol 4, pp 762–777
64. Gatrad AR. op.cit
65. Misha'l AA. Commentary. End of life medical interventions. FIMA Book 2005–2006. op.cit

Glossary

Aql reason; an authoritative source of law for Shiite Islam (after Qur'an and Sunna)

Aqd contract

Arsh compensation for a wound

Advance directive (AD) a legally binding statement of preferences for treatment at the end of life

Akhlaq virtue ethics; ethics in general

Al-Akhlāqiyāt Ethics as related to human behavior or conduct

Alim singular of ulama; a religious authority; literally, one who knows

ART assisted reproductive technology; methods of assisting infertile couples to have children

Ash'ari a school of Islamic theology, very influential in Sunni Islam; founded by Abu hasan al-Ash'ari (d.circa 941)

Asnad (singular, Sanad) statement of chain of authorities in a tradition of the Prophet

Batil void

Bayyina proof positive

Cadaveric donations organs removed from donors after death

Ḍarūrah Dire necessity; external mitigating factors; an essential rule which renders a forbidden act permissible under certain critical conditions

Diyya blood money payable in respect of unintentional homicide

DNR a do-not-resuscitate order in the case of heart or lung failure, extensive disease, multiple organ failure, widespread cancer etc., where Cardio Pulmonary Resuscitation (CPR) is considered unsuitable and will only increase the suffering of the patient

© The Author(s) 2015

M.A. Al-Bar and H. Chamsi-Pasha, *Contemporary Bioethics*,
DOI 10.1007/978-3-319-18428-9

Fatwā (pl. fatāwā) A non-binding, context specific Islamic ethico-legal assessment or ruling issued by a trained Islamic jurist. The Fatwa of the highest authority in the country is binding to that country

Fiqh Jurisprudential understanding or an ethico-legal ruling; legal discourse

Fuqaha jurists; those trained in the discipline of fiqh

Fitra a Qur'anic doctrine that signifies "innate nature" or "disposition" with which humans have been created

Furu' al-fiqh (branches of jurisprudence) an elaboration of rules which govern ritual and social activities

Ghayb Unseen realm

Hadd a prescribed penalty for certain specific offenses

Hadith record of the traditions or sayings of the Prophet Muhammad, revered and received as a major source of religious law and moral guidance, second only to the authority of the Qur'an, the holy book of Islam

Hanafi the most widespread of the four Sunni schools of law, dominant in Turkey, the Eastern Mediterranean, and South Asia. Hanafī legal thought (madhhab) developed from the teachings of the theologian Imām Abū Ḥanīfah (c. 700–767) by such disciples as Abū Yūsuf (d. 798) and Muhammad ash-Shaybānī (749/750–805) and became the official system of Islāmic legal interpretation of the 'Abbāsids, Seljuqs, and Ottomans

Hanbali the least widespread of the four Sunni schools of law, dominant in the Arabian Peninsula. It is based on the teachings of Aḥmad ibn Ḥanbal (780–855). the Ḥanbalī legal school (madhhab) emphasized virtually complete dependence on the divine in the establishment of legal theory and rejected personal opinion (ra'y), analogy (qiyās)

Haram forbidden by law; taboo; one of the five values of legal action

Hurma sanctity of the human body, Places of worship e.g. mosques and the inviolability of freedom of religion, human life

Ḥukm (pl. aḥkām) Ruling; Judgment; decree

IFC of Islamic World League Islamic Fiqh council of Islamic World League, Makkah Al Mukaramah (Majma al-fiqhi al-islami of the Muslim World League, Makkah)

Ifta the giving of legal opinions (fatwas) by muftis

Idda the period during which a divorced or widowed woman may not re-marry

Ijhad (isqat) abortion whether spontaneous or induced

Ijmā' Consensus agreement, usually of the scholars; an authoritative source for Islamic law; after Qur'an and Sunna

Ijtihad Juristic effort or methodology used to construct a fatwa in a novel or unprecedented case

Ijtihad jama'i The process of group decision making based on uṣūl al-fiqh within a council of Islamic juris consults

Illa effective cause (on which ta'lil is based)

Imam Sunnism: the leader of prayer or of a congregation; a political leader

Imam Shiism: one of the twelve descendants of the Prophet who led the community; the twelfth Imam remains hidden and will return

IOMS Islamic Organization of Medical Sciences (Kuwait)

IUD intrauterine device, a form of contraceptive

IVF in vitro fertilization, fertilization of the egg outside of the womb

Istihsan in Jurisprudence the method of prioritization of two or more equally valid judgments through juristic practice; also known as "juristic preference" usually used by Hanafi Jurists

Istislah one of the major principles in promoting and securing benefits and preventing and removing harms in the public sphere. Maslaha has been linked to the term istislah that is, "to seek to promote and secure common good". It was first introduced by Iman Malik but accepted by all others with difference details

Ittibā' Following the example of (an individual)

Ja'fari the dominant Shiite school of law, found among the Imami (Twelver) Shiites

La darar wa la dirar fi al-islam various meanings are taken into consideration. Among these are: "In islam there shall be no harm inflicted or reciprocated"

Madarra in the context of public good, an obligation to prevent and remove evil. It comes close to the principle of "non-maleficence" in secular bioethics

Madhhab (pl. madhāhīb) doctrine, The 'schools' of Islamic law which have tradition-based legal theories; group of scholars sharing a common outlook on sources and their interpretation

Maliki one of the four Sunni schools of law, dominant in North and West Africa

Mālikiyyah also called Madhhab Mālik, English Malikites, one of the four Sunnī schools of law. Founded in the eighth century and based on the teachings of the imam Mālik ibn Anas, the Mālikiyyah stressed local Medinese community practice (sunnah), preferring traditional opinions (ra'y) and analogical reasoning (qiyās) to a strict and reliance on Ḥadīth (traditions concerning the Prophet's life and utterances) as a basis for legal judgment

Manfa'a in the context of public good, an obligation to seek and promote good. It comes close to the principle of "beneficence" in secular bioethics

Makruh disapproved, reprehensible; one of the five legal categories; but not prohibited by Islamic Law. However, the Hanafi school use the word Makruh in two different meanings (i) Prohibited things not officially mentioned in the Qur'an or Hadith as Prohibited; (ii); Preferable to avoid but if committed not considered as sin (Haram)

Maqasid al-shari'a the aims of the shari'a; principles perceived as underlying Islamic law

Maslaha general principle of "public good". A variably interpreted source of Islamic law. This principle is evoked in providing solutions to majority of novel issues in biomedical ethics. Maslaha can refer to actions that customarily agree with what reasonable people do

Masalih al-mursala al the phrase signifies public good that is established by reason. Technically, al-mursala means "extra-revelatory" that is not requiring scriptural proof. When used with maslaha, the phrase signifies seeking the good of the people without any reference to a particular text in the revelation

Mubah allowable, indifferent; one of the five legal categories

Muftī/faqīh Islamic ethicist; Juris consult, authoritative person who renders a legal opinion (fatwa) in response to a query

Mu'tazali a school of Islamic theology, very influential in Zaidi Shiite Islam, and to some extent in other Shiite groups and Ibadiya group found in Oman, Algeirs some part of Libya

Mu'tazilah (Arabic: Those Who Withdraw, or Stand Apart) English Mutazilites, in Islām, political or religious neutralists; by the tenth century the term came to refer specifically to an Islāmic school of speculative theology that flourished in Basra and Baghdad (eighth–tenth centuries ad).
The name first appears in early Islāmic history in the dispute over 'Alī's leadership of the Muslim community after the murder of the third caliph, 'Uthmān (656). Those who would neither condemn nor sanction 'Alī or his opponents but took a middle position were termed the Mu'tazilah

Nafs Self, sometimes used interchangeably with rūḥ (Soul)

Nasab blood relationship

Naskh abrogation, repeal, supersession

Naṣṣ Textual sources of the Islamic ethico-legal tradition, such as the Qu'ran and the Sunnah

Niyya intention

"No harm, no harassment" functions both as a principle and a source for the rule that states "hardship necessitates relief"

OIC Organization of the Islamic Conference (Jeddah), an intergovernmental organization representing fifty-seven Muslim states

OIC-IFA The International Islamic Fiqh Academy of Organization of Islamic Conferences (Majma al-fiqhi al-islami of the Organization of the Islamic Conference, Jeddah)

Oocytes human egg cells

"Preventing harm has a priority over promoting good" this principle is the main source for careful analysis of harm and benefit when for example, a medical procedure prolongs the life of a terminally ill patient without advancing long term cure

Qāḍī A judge who is given legal authority by an Islamic government

Qawa'id fiqhi primary rules in juridical methodology for deducing rulings. See also: qawa'id usul

Qawa'id usul primary principles in Islamic juristic ethics that are stated as obligations and their derivatives are stated as qawa'id fiqhi

Qiyas reasoning and deduction of rules of law by analogy with Qur'an, Sunna and Ijma; a formal source (uṣūl) of Islamic law

Qur'an God's revelation to the Prophet Muhammad; the most authoritative document in Islam

Ra'y, al "Sound opinion" formulated by a jurist in order to promote the good of the people. Accepted, mainly by Hanafi jurists

Rūḥ Soul

Ruwat (Singular Rawi) narrators

Shafi'i one of the four Sunni schools of law, dominant in Egypt and Southeast Asia, South Yemen. Somalia etc.

Shāfi'īyah also called Madhhab Shāfi'ī, English Shafiites, one of the four Sunnī schools of religious law, derived from the teachings of Abū 'Abd Allāh ash-Shāfi'ī (767–820). This legal school (madhhab) stabilized the bases of Islāmic legal theory, admitting the validity of both divine will and human speculation. Imam Shāfi'ī introduced Qiyas (Analogy) as a source of reaching Hokum (plural Ahkam) after the Qur'an, Sunna and Ijma. It was agreed also by others

Shari'a, Sharī'ah Islamic law; the correct path of action as determined by God

Shiites Shi'a, a Muslim sect that differs from Sunnis in several ways, especially their veneration of the Prophet's family; Imami Shiites are dominant in Iran and Iraq; Isma'i'li s are found in South Asia and East Africa; Zaydis dominate in Yemen

Shura juristic rule of consultation, a feature of Islamic communitarian ethics, against the dominant principle of autonomy that is based on liberal individualism. Muslims are exhorted to conduct their affairs "by mutual consultation"

Sufi one concerned with the esoteric side of religious belief; a mystic

Sunna "Tradition" a hadith report, collected and compiled to form the basis for legal ethical rulings, the second authoritative source for Muslims; the correct way of doing things; the Prophet Muhammad exemplary action as recorded in hadith

Sunnah (Arabic: "habitual practice") also spelled Sunna, the body of traditional social and legal custom and practice of the Islamic community. Along with the Qur'ān (the holy book of Islam) and Hadith (recorded sayings of the Prophet Muhammad), it is a major source of Sharī'ah, or Islamic law

Sunni the majority sect of Muslims, as opposed to Shiite

Sura one of the 114 chapters of the Qur'an

Tafsir interpretation, usually of the Qur'an

Talaq dissolution of marriage by the husband; Repudiation or divorce;

Tazir a doctrine of punishment; (literally) disgracing

Ulama religious scholars, literally, the people of knowledge. The term refers to scholars of the Islamic tradition trained in Islamic seminaries. A near-equivalent term or synonym is Fuqahā' (singular Faqīh), meaning, "scholars of fiqh," which specifically refers to Islamic scholars of law and ethics

U'rf (also ada) usage; custom; refers to the social practice and norms of a community. It is regarded as one of the important sources in deriving judicial rulings based on conventions and customs of the region, but it should not contradict a rule of Qur'an, Sunna, Ijma or Qiyas

Umma Muslim community; supercedes all other loyalties

Uṣūl al-fiqh Islamic legal theory or moral theology; the science identifies the sources of ethicolegal knowledge and lays down the discursive rules for moral-ethical reasoning; literally, roots of jurisprudence

Wahy inspiration

Walī Guardian and protector; one who is responsible for someone else

Wilāyah Authority and governance

Yaqīn Absolute certainty

Zahiri a historically important school of law, emphasizing literal interpretation of the sources Ẓāhirīyah, (Arabic: "Literalists") followers of an Islamic legal and theological school that insisted on strict adherence to the literal text (ẓāhir) of the Qur'ān and Ḥadīth (sayings and actions of the Prophet Muḥammad) as the only source of Muslim law. It rejected practices in law (fiqh) such as analogical reasoning (qiyas) and pure reason (ra'y) as sources of jurisprudence and looked askance at consensus (ijmā). Theologically, the school formed the extreme rejection of anthropomorphism (tashbih), attributing to God only those essential elements and qualities set forth clearly in the Qur'ān. **Ẓannī** refers to a judgment (or proof text interpretation) that is probability based

Zaydi a subgroup of Shiites, found in Yemen

Zina illicit sexual intercourse

Printed in the United States
By Bookmasters